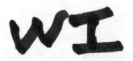
W9-BSM-676

WI

Living a Healthy Life with Chronic Pain

Sandra LeFort, MN, PhD • **Lisa Webster**, RN
Kate Lorig, RN, DrPH • **Halsted Holman**, MD
David Sobel, MD, MPH • **Diana Laurent**, MPH
Virginia González, MPH • **Marian Minor**, PT, PhD

Bull Publishing Company
Boulder, Colorado

Published by Bull Publishing Company
P.O. Box 1377
Boulder, CO, USA 80306
www.bullpub.com

Library of Congress Cataloging-in-Publication Data

LeFort, Sandra M.

  Living a healthy life with chronic pain / Sandra M. LeFort, MN, PhD, Lisa Webster, RN, Kate Lorig, DrPH,
Halsted Holman, MD, David Sobel, MD, MPH, Diana Laurent, MPH, Virginia Gonzalez, MPH, Marian Minor,
RPT, PhD.

    pages cm

  Summary: "Nobody wants chronic pain in their lives. Unfortunately, about 30 percent of people
worldwide live with chronic pain conditions, many of which have no identifiable cause. We wrote this
book to help these people explore healthy ways to manage and live with their chronic pain condition
so they can enjoy more fulfilling, satisfying lives"-- Provided by publisher.

  Includes bibliographical references and index.

  ISBN 978-1-936693-77-1 (paperback)

1. Chronic pain--Popular works. 2. Chronic diseases--Popular works. 3. Self-care, Health.
I. Webster, Lisa. II. Lorig, Kate. III. Holman, Halsted, 1925- IV. Sobel, David. V. Laurent, Diana.
VI. Gonzalez, Virginia. VII. Minor, Marian A. (Marian Adams)

RB127.L384 2015
616'.0472--dc23

                                                                                       2015002233

Printed in U.S.A.
19 18 17 16 15   10 9 8 7 6 5 4 3 2 1

Interior design and project management: Dovetail Publishing Services
Cover design and production: Shannon Bodie, Lightbourne, Inc.

This book is dedicated to the memory of Howard Montrose Genge for his love, courage, and wisdom in the face of pain; Mary Ellen Jeans, PhD, for believing in education for people in pain; and people of all ages and their families who struggle with pain in their lives.

Acknowledgments

Many people helped us write this book. Among the most important are the first 110 participants of the Chronic Pain Self-Management Program study funded by the National Health Research and Development Program of Health Canada. That study paved the way for thousands of workshop participants in Canada, the United States, Denmark, and other countries. All of these people, along with our wonderful workshop leaders, told us what information they needed and helped us make adjustments along the way. All of you have informed this new North American edition of our book.

Many professionals also assisted us, including Lynn Beatie, PT, MPT, MHA, Bonnie Bruce, RD, DrPH, Norman Buckley, MD, FRCPC, Beth Darnall, PhD, John W. Doyle, BA, Steven Feinberg, MD, Chaplain Bruce Feldman, MD, Shelley Gershman, RN, Peg Harrison, MSW, Noorin Jamal, RN, MN-NP, Mary Ellen Jeans, PhD, Roman Jovey, MD, Michael McGillion, PhD, RN, Patrick McGowan, PhD, Ronald Melzack, PhD, Yvonne Mullin, MSc, RD, Sheila O'Keefe-McCarthy, PhD, RN, Catherine Regan, PhD, Ned Pratt, BFA, Kathleen Rowat, PhD, Richard Seidel, PhD, and Judith Watt-Watson, PhD, RN. A special thanks to Nicolaj Holm Faber, Chief Consultant, Danish Committee on Health Education, whose support has been invaluable. To all of you, your help has been gratefully received.

A special thanks to Jon Peck, Jon Ford, and Erin Mulligan, who helped us every step of the way. Editors are unsung heroes of good books. We wish to acknowledge their fine contributions to making this a more readable, understandable book. We would also like to thank our T-Trainers, Master Trainers, and Leaders. There are now hundreds of you, and you all have made important suggestions that helped us craft this book.

We would like to thank DRx, publisher of *The Healthy Mind, Healthy Body Handbook* (also published as *Mind & Body Health Handbook*) by David Sobel, MD, and Robert Ornstein, PhD, for permission to adapt sections of their book.

Finally, many thanks to Jim Bull, Claire Cameron, and the team at Bull Publishing. Bull Publishing has been a strong supporter of health-related books for more than 40 years. Jim's support and encouragement have been essential to the development of this book. We couldn't have done it without you!

If you would like to learn more about our continuing research, online programs, trainings, and materials, please visit our website:

www.patienteducation.stanford.edu

We are continually revising and improving this book. If you have any suggestions or comments, please send them to

self-management@stanford.edu.

Contents

CHAPTER 1

Overview of Self-Management and Pain

NOBODY WANTS CHRONIC PAIN in their lives. Unfortunately, about 30 percent of people worldwide live with chronic pain conditions, many of which have no identifiable cause. We wrote this book to help people explore healthy ways to manage and live with their chronic pain condition so they can enjoy more fulfilling, satisfying lives.

This may seem like a strange concept. How can you live a healthier, happier life when you are hurting? To answer this, we need to explore what happens with most chronic health problems. Whether it's heart disease, diabetes, depression, or any of a host of others, the conditions that cause chronic pain also cause fatigue, loss of physical strength and endurance, emotional distress, and a sense of helplessness or even hopelessness. A healthy way to live with chronic pain is to work at managing the physical, mental, and emotional problems caused by the condition. The challenge is to learn how to function at your best even with the difficulties pain can present. The goal is to achieve the things you want to do, to get pleasure from life, and to be as healthy

1

as possible. That is what this book is all about. Before we go any further, let's talk about how to use this book. It is not a textbook; in fact you might want to think of it as a workbook rather than as a traditional book. You do not need to read every word in every chapter. Instead, we suggest you read the first two chapters and then scan the table of contents to find the specific information you need. Read the sections that feel most relevant to your situation. Feel free to skip around and to make notes right in the book.

You will not find any miracles or instant cures in these pages. What you will find is hundreds of tips and ideas to make your life easier. This advice is from physicians, psychologists, physical therapists, registered nurses, and other health professionals who specialize in working with people in chronic pain. It also is from people like you who have learned to positively manage their own chronic pain.

Please note that we said "positively manage." If you have chronic pain, there is no way to avoid managing it, but there are different ways to approach it. If you choose to do nothing but sit and watch TV all day, that is one way of managing. If you rely on medication alone

to manage your pain, that is another management style. But the management style we advocate in this book is different from these two approaches. This book teaches you to be a positive self-manager by being proactive about your pain and working with your health care professionals. We believe that if you adopt this positive management style, you will live a healthier life.

In this chapter we begin by discussing the importance of being your own self-manager and the self-management skills that will help you successfully live with your chronic pain condition every day. These skills are useful not just for chronic pain management but for the management of any chronic disease condition. This is good news because people often have more than one chronic condition. Learning these key self-management skills will allow you to successfully manage not just a single condition but your entire life. After introducing the basics of self-management, we then go on to define pain and discuss the difference between acute and chronic pain. We also cite the most common problems experienced by people with chronic pain and provide a list of resources so you can learn more about pain.

Understanding Your Role as a Self-Manager

The first responsibility of any chronic pain self-manager is understanding your condition. This means more than learning about pain and what you can do about it. It also means carefully observing how chronic pain and its treatment affect your physical and mental health and how

it affects those around you. With experience, you and your family will become experts at this.

Your second responsibility as a self-manager is communicating your unique situation, experiences, and preferences to your doctor and others on the health care team. They need to know how you are feeling and how the pain is impacting all aspects of your life. In other words, to effectively manage your condition you must be an observant person who communicates openly with his or her health care providers.

When you develop a painful condition, you become more aware of your body. Minor symptoms that you ignored may now cause concerns. For example, you may wonder is this pain in your arm a signal of a heart attack? Is this pain in your leg a sign that you should stop exercising? Is your pain spreading to other parts of your body? Does the pain in your back signify something more serious? There are no simple, reassuring answers to questions like these. Nor is there always a fail-safe way of sorting out serious signals from minor, temporary symptoms that can be ignored.

Even though chronic pain can be unpredictable, it is helpful to be aware of the natural rhythms of your particular condition. Chronic illnesses usually wax and wane in intensity. Symptoms do not follow a steady path. Most times, chronic pain is like that too—although sometimes you may feel as if it's all a downward path and the outlook is bleak. In general, you should check with your doctor if symptoms are unusual or severe. You also should contact your doctor if symptoms occur after you start a new medication or treatment plan.

Throughout this book we give specific examples of what actions to take if you experience certain symptoms. However, you should not rely solely on the information in this book. Partnership with your health care provider is critical. Self-management does not mean going it alone.

Get help or advice whenever you are concerned or uncertain.

Think of self-management like this: Both at home and in the business world, managers direct the show. But they don't do everything themselves. Managers work with others, including consultants, to get the job done. What makes them managers is that they are responsible for making decisions and making sure those decisions are carried out.

As the manager of your chronic pain condition, your job is much the same as any other manager. You gather information and work with a consultant or team of consultants consisting of your physician and other health professionals. Once they have given you their best advice, it is up to you to follow through.

In this book, we describe many self-management skills and tools to help you address the problems of living with your condition. We do not expect you to use all of them. Pick and choose. Experiment. Set your own goals. *What you do may not be as important as the sense of confidence and control that comes from successfully doing something proactive to deal with your situation.*

Whenever we try a new skill, our first attempts may be clumsy, slow, and show few results. When this occurs, it is often easier to return to old ways than to continue trying to master new and sometimes difficult tasks. The best way to master new skills is through practice, perseverance, and thoughtful evaluation of the results. Always keep this in mind as you develop effective self-management skills for your chronic pain condition.

Self-Management Skills

Throughout this book we examine ways of breaking the cycle of chronic pain illustrated in Figure 1.2 on page 13 and overcoming feelings of physical and emotional helplessness. A first step in the right direction is becoming aware of the essential management skills you need to learn in order to live a healthier, more satisfying life with your chronic pain condition. Table 1.1 lists these important skills.

Table 1.1   Self-Management Skills

- Problem solving and responding to your chronic pain condition day to day
- Maintaining a healthy lifestyle that features stress management, regular exercise, healthy eating, and sound sleep habits
- Managing common symptoms
- Making decisions about when to seek professional help and what treatments to try
- Working effectively with your health care team
- Using medications safely and effectively while minimizing side effects
- Finding and using community resources
- Talking about your condition with family and friends
- Participating in work, volunteer, and social activities

Perhaps the most important skill of all is learning to respond to your chronic pain on an ongoing basis in order to solve the daily problems associated with your condition. After all, you live with your condition 24 hours a day; your health care provider sees you only a tiny fraction of that time. This means that *you* are primarily responsible for managing your chronic pain. (See Chapters 4 and 5.)

Some of the most successful self-managers are people who think of their chronic pain as a journey or a path along life's way. Sometimes this path is flat and smooth and you can travel along with few problems. At other times the way is rough, and you must slow down to think about your next move or to take a rest.

To negotiate this path one has to use many strategies. Good self-managers are people who have learned three types of skills:

- **Skills to deal with chronic pain.** Chronic pain, like any health condition, requires that you adapt and do new things to deal with it. These may include practicing relaxation and stress reduction techniques regularly, monitoring your pain levels in order to balance activity with rest, and learning specific exercises and developing a physical activity program. Your condition may mean you may have more frequent interactions with your health care providers. You may need to take medications or treatments on a daily basis. All chronic pain conditions benefit from day-to-day self-management skills.

- **Skills to continue a normal life.** Chronic pain does not mean that life stops. There are still household tasks that need to get done, friendships to maintain, work to perform (whether you have a job or do volunteer work), and important family relationships to nurture. You just may need to learn new skills or adapt the way you do things in order to maintain the things you need and want to do in your life.

- **Skills to deal with emotions.** When you are diagnosed as having a chronic pain condition, your future changes. With these changes come changes in plans and changes in emotions. Many of the new emotions are negative. They may include anger ("Why me? It's not fair"), fear ("I am afraid to move my body in case I hurt myself"), depression ("I can't do anything anymore, so what's the use?"), frustration ("No matter what I do, it doesn't make any difference. I can't do what I want to do"), or isolation ("No one understands. No one wants to be around someone who is in pain all the time"). Negotiating the path of chronic pain means learning skills to work with these negative emotions.

Self-management involves using skills to manage the work of living with your pain condition, continuing to take part in normal daily activities, and successfully dealing with your emotions so you can start enjoying a healthier, happier life.

What Is Pain?

Pain is a part of being alive. It is nearly universal, something we all share as human beings. At the same time, it is a most personal, individual, and subjective experience. One person's experience of pain is not the same as another person's. Throughout human history, pain has been regarded as mysterious and unknowable. Because we can't see another person's pain, it seems invisible. But when we feel pain ourselves, it is all too real.

Humans have always tried to understand pain. The ancient Greeks described pain as a "passion of the soul," an emotion like sadness or grief. This idea of pain as an emotion is called the *affect theory of pain* and this view of pain was prevalent until the seventeenth century.

In 1664, a famous French philosopher and scientist, René Descartes, developed a new concept of pain. He believed that there were special places in the body called pain receptors that sent pain impulses along a pain pathway that went directly to a single pain center in the brain. He also believed that the mind and body were completely separate and that one did not affect the other. According to Descartes, pain was purely physical, and it was a straightforward, simple process. This was called the *specificity theory of pain*, and it persisted for 300 years.

But it wasn't until the late 1800s that scientists started to use observation and experiments to study pain. Descartes' idea that pain was purely physical just didn't fit the facts. But progress was slow. Then, in 1959, two scientists—Dr. Ronald Melzack from McGill University and Dr. Patrick Wall from Oxford University—set out to unravel the puzzle of pain. They met while working at the Massachusetts Institute of Technology (MIT) in Cambridge, Massachusetts. Together they developed new ideas about pain that they called the *gate control theory*. Their ideas revolutionized pain research.

New Ideas about Pain

Nerve endings all over our body are sensitive to types of stimuli that can cause us harm and signal danger. Exposure to things like heat, cold, pressure, or chemicals cause particular patterns of nerve or electrical impulses. If the stimuli are strong enough, these nerve impulses travel along the nerves to the spinal cord and up to the brain.

Let's say you just stubbed your toe. Within nanoseconds, the nerve endings in your toe that respond to pressure send a pattern of nerve impulses along the 'nerve highway'—the nerves in your toe, foot, leg, buttock and up to the spinal cord in your back. The spinal cord is like a super highway of nerves that connect to your brain. It's your brain that asks: *"How dangerous is this really?"* It's only when the brain thinks the pattern of nerve impulses are dangerous that pain is felt. In other words, pain is not in your toe, although it sure feels like that. *Pain is produced by your brain to tell you and your body to take action.* Because this is so important, it bears repeating: *All pain is 100 % in the brain.*

Melzack and Wall said that there is a transmission station in the spinal cord that influences the flow of nerve impulses to the brain. They called this transmission station a 'gate'. Think of it just like a gate you can open or close to get to your backyard. Two things can happen when nerve impulses from your toe reach the gate:

- If the gate is open, the impulses pass through and continue up the spinal cord to the brain. If the brain senses 'danger', you experience pain.

- If the gate is closed or partially closed, then only some or none of the nerve impulses travel to the brain. The brain might then interpret the signals as a little danger—not enough to worry about—or no danger. So you experience minimal or no pain.

The gate can be opened or closed in a number of ways, including by the brain itself. The brain can send electrical messages down nerve pathways to close the gate and shut out or reduce the flow of nerve impulses to the brain, or send messages that do just the opposite. Many factors can open or close the gate.

Some of these factors arise from our mind. They include our past experience, what we have learned about pain from our culture and social environment, our expectation about what might happen, our beliefs about pain, how much attention we direct towards the pain, and our emotions. For example, positive mood, distraction, and deep relaxed breathing can act to close or partially close the gate while strong emotions like fear, anxiety, and expecting the worst can open the gate.

So research on the *gate control theory* has explained a lot. It tells us that pain results from many interactions and information exchanges at different levels of our nervous system—in billions of nerve cells, the spinal cord and the brain. Our physical bodies, our feelings and emotions, our thoughts and beliefs and other factors are all involved in the experience of pain. And all pain is produced in the brain. The mind and body are completely connected. They influence each other all the time.

But the story does not stop here. The *gate control theory* mostly explained what is happening when nerve impulses travel to the spinal cord. But what is going on within the brain itself? Answers are coming from several sources: advanced brain imaging studies, studies of the link between pain and genetics, research into the immune system and our response to stress, and Dr. Melzack's latest *neuromatrix theory of pain.*

It turns out that at least seven (and probably more) areas of the brain are active when we experience pain. Some of these brain regions control our emotions, our thinking (or cognitive function), and the processing of body

sensations. These body sensations include stimuli that might cause us to feel pain as well as things like light touch, vision, hearing, and other body sensations. These areas of the brain are connected to each other through a complex widespread network of nerve cells and neurochemicals. Dr. Melzack called this network a 'neuromatrix'. The purpose of the neuromatrix is to organize the huge amount of information coming into the brain so that we experience our body as a single unified whole. How this network gets developed in the first place is mostly due to our genetics. But after that, many things affect how the network changes to influence how we experience our body.

Look at Figure 1.1. You can see that information from at least three different sources goes to this network in the brain. Our thoughts and emotions, whether positive or negative, influence network activity. Nerve impulses from all over our body—our skin, muscles, tissues, our eyes, ears, etc.—impact the network. All this information is processed by the network to produce a pattern of nerve impulses. If the brain thinks this pattern means that our body is in "danger", then a number of things happen.

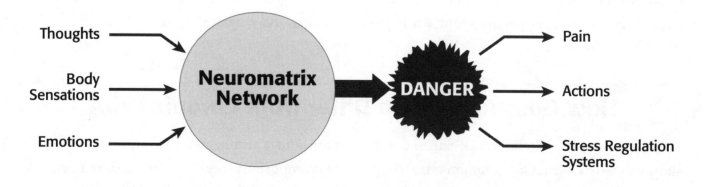

Figure 1.1 **Pain and the Brain**

- We experience pain—its location, strength, and how it feels (sharp, dull, burning, miserable, etc).

- We take action to protect the body. Think of your stubbed toe. You start hopping around, raise your foot, and rub your toe. You might sit down and decide not to walk on your foot until the pain is better. Often, actions are unconscious like tensing muscles or holding our breath. Movements can even occur during sleep.

- Our body releases neurochemicals throughout the nervous system and brain that attempt to regulate the stress caused by pain. These include stress hormones that ready our body for action, hormones from our immune system that fight inflammation, sex-related hormones like estrogen, morphine-like substances such as endorphins that decrease pain, and others.

Probably the most difficult thing to understand is that pain is not injury. It's our brain's assessment of danger. That's why there is no exact relationship between how strong a stimulus is, the amount of injury it causes if any, and the amount of pain we feel. So two people can be in the same potentially pain-producing situation but have very different experiences. One person can be in excruciating pain while the other feels little pain or discomfort. Or the same person may experience extreme pain in one situation but not in another even when the amount of damage to body tissues is exactly the same or there is no damage at all. That's because our central nervous system and brain actively process information and assess the meaning it has for each of us as individuals at this particular time and place—is there 'danger' or 'no danger'?

So, pain is really complex. There is still a lot more research that needs to be done before we have all the answers. But we don't have to wait until then to take action to manage our pain. Science supports the important role of thoughts, emotions and physical sensations in the experience of pain at all levels of the nervous system and the brain. That's why this book emphasizes ways to use your mind and your breathing to regulate your thoughts and emotions. These techniques can help close the gate in the spinal cord and influence the complex network of nerve cells in the brain. This book also emphasizes how participating in normal physical activity and exercise does not pose a danger to you. In fact, increasing your activity can change the way your brain processes information about movement and physical sensation. The good news is that you can learn to calm your nervous system, reduce your stress, and re-train your brain so you can live a healthier, happier life.

How Does Acute Pain Differ from Chronic Pain?

A truly satisfactory definition of chronic pain simply does not exist. One common misconception is that chronic pain is just like acute pain, except that chronic pain persists. But acute pain and chronic pain are different in some very important ways. Understanding these differences, which are listed in Table 1.2 on page 9, is essential for you to better cope with and

Table 1.2 **Differences Between Acute and Chronic Pain**

	Acute Pain	Chronic Pain
Duration	Short or time-limited.	Long term. Lasts beyond the usual time for healing and recovery.
Intensity	Often intense, depending on the cause.	Varies in intensity, from mild to very severe.
Location	Most often felt in one body area.	Felt in one or many body areas.
Purpose	Has survival value. It warns of danger and harm and causes us to take action.	Has no survival value. It no longer warns of immediate danger.
Cause	Biological mechanisms of acute pain are well understood. Usually due to tissue damage.	Biological mechanisms of pain are amplified and exaggerated. The brain is mis-interpreting nerve impulses as "danger". But body tissues have healed.
Emotional response	Associated with anxiety and fear, but these feelings go away.	Associated with ongoing irritability, fatigue, isolation, helplessness, etc. Chronic pain is like a form of chronic stress.
Diagnosis	Commonly accurate.	Often difficult.
Treatment	Treatments usually effective, and cure is common.	Many treatments used. The goal is to calm the nervous system and retrain the brain.
Role of activity and exercise	Rest is often best. Rest allows healing to begin.	Activity and exercise, balanced with rest, are essential. Healing of damaged tissues has already occurred.
Role of professionals	Diagnose and treat.	Serve as teacher and partner.
Role of person with pain	Follow treatment advice.	Become a pain self-manager and partner with health care professionals.

manage your chronic pain condition. It is also important for your family to understand these differences, because an informed support system is an important part of successful self-management of pain.

Acute Pain

All of us have experienced acute pain. Whether it is the stubbed toe we talked about on page 6, a sore throat, a toothache, or the aftereffects of surgery, these are pains that have an identifiable cause and usually go away once healing has taken place. Pain in these situations is a very important part of the body's defense mechanism because it warns us of danger and harm. It has survival value. We pay attention to the pain. We take action and do what we can to alleviate it.

The biological mechanisms of acute pain have been studied extensively and are well understood. An injury or illness opens the gate in the spinal cord (see page 6) to allow nerve signals to go to the brain. At the same time, the brain and spinal cord release substances that start the healing process and help us cope with the pain (See Figure 1.1 and page 7).

It is important to understand that, because acute pain has a survival function, our approach to its management is very different from our approach to chronic pain. In the early stages, acute pain can be linked to anxiety and fear. We wonder: *What is the cause of the pain? How bad will the pain get? Will it go away?* But once we understand the cause and seek treatment, and we start to feel better, our emotional response usually subsides.

The brain also instructs the body to protect the injured area. Muscles can go into spasm. We can unconsciously hold our muscles in tension. If it hurts enough, we stop, rest, and conserve our energy so healing can take place. If, for example, we have had surgery or are feeling the aches and pains of influenza, being too active can slow healing. Rest is best. As the pain subsides and the healing improves, the protective mechanisms diminish. We gradually increase our activity and get back to normal.

When dealing with acute pain, our role and the role of our health care providers are clear: we go to the doctor for a diagnosis and to get advice on how to treat our condition. For the most part, we follow that advice. We don't usually argue about whether we need surgery for a burst appendix or whether we should take antibiotics for a severe chest infection. As a result, healing occurs and the pain usually goes away.

But what if the pain does not go away? What if the brain network continues to interpret nerve impulses as "dangerous," even when they are not?

Chronic Pain

There are many ways to classify chronic pain. In this book, we talk about two main kinds of chronic pain. One is pain associated with a chronic disease. Examples include pain from arthritis or angina. In these cases, pain is a symptom of a generally well-understood disease process, and medical pain management is often specific to the disease that's causing the pain.

The other kind of chronic pain is idiopathic pain. Idiopathic means that there is no known cause for the pain. Examples of idiopathic chronic pain include musculoskeletal pain (such as chronic neck, shoulder, and lower back pain), whiplash injuries, fibromyalgia, chronic regional pain syndromes, repetitive strain injuries, postsurgical pain, phantom limb pain, chronic pelvic pain, neuropathic or neuralgia pain, and central pain that persists after a stroke. Persistent headache and pain from poorly understood chronic conditions such as irritable bowel syndrome, Crohn's disease, and interstitial cystitis are other examples. Initially, these pains may have been triggered by an event like a workplace injury, a minor fall, a surgical procedure, or a virus. Sometimes the pain may stem from nothing in particular. In either case, these conditions started as acute pain and should have gone away but did not. As such, chronic pain is defined as pain lasting longer than three to six months, which is beyond the normal time for healing and recovery.

Things to Know about Pain

- Pain is 100% in the brain. Your brain thinks you are in danger and wants you to act.

- There is no one "pain center" in the brain. Billions of nerve cells in the spinal cord and in many areas of the brain are involved in pain.

- There is no single pathway for nerve impulses to travel to the brain to be interpreted as pain. There are several pathways. Some go up to the brain from the spinal cord and others travel down from the brain to the spinal cord.

- The central nervous system and the brain are "plastic." (This is termed "neuroplasticity.") This means that our central nervous system and brain are changing and adapting to new information all the time. *We can influence our nervous system and our brain.*

- At least 350 genes and probably more are thought to be involved in the regulation of pain.

- Our immune system and stress response system are very involved in pain regulation.

- When our brain thinks 'danger', our bodies want to protect us. This works in acute pain because we stop, rest and let healing begin. In chronic pain, protective mechanisms like tensing muscles and limiting movement work against us. Healing has already occurred.

Unlike acute pain, chronic pain can vary considerably in intensity, and it is often unpredictable. Some days the pain is mild and other days it is very intense. It can affect just one area of the body or be felt in multiple areas. Once pain has persisted beyond the normal time for healing, it no longer warns us of danger or harm. But the brain network misinterprets the pattern of nerve impulses and keeps signaling that the body is in danger. However, injured tissues have already healed entirely or as much as they are going to. In these circumstances, the pain has no survival value any more. But it still must be managed.

The mechanisms that result in acute pain (see pages 6–7 and Figure 1.1) become amplified and exaggerated in chronic pain. Healing should calm down the nervous system. Instead, nerve cells continue to fire even though there is no new tissue damage. And our brain continues to interpret these signals as 'danger'. Pain, action responses, and stress responses just get stronger. Imagine that you set the thermostat to 68 degrees but your furnace keeps turning on so that the house is 85 degrees and rising. Something is wrong. It could be the thermostat, the wiring, or the furnace that's broken . . . or maybe it's a combination of all three. Chronic pain is like that—it's a disturbance of a complex interactive system that includes billions of nerve cells, the spinal cord, and the brain, as well as the immune system, our stress response system, and our individual genetic makeups.

When the body is bombarded with persistent intense nerve signals that are interpreted as pain, our nervous system eventually loses its ability to respond effectively. As a result, areas of the spinal cord and brain fundamentally change over time. These changes cause some people to become more sensitive to weaker body signals. They develop a hypersensitivity to even mild stimuli that would normally not cause pain. For others, pain that was once located in only one body part seems to spread to other areas, causing widespread pain. That's why people don't get "used to" having chronic pain, because it changes.

Another finding is that people with chronic pain may have an increase in some neurochemicals and a decrease in others. For example, some people have excess release of cortisol that can itself produce destruction of tissues and more chronic pain. Others have reduced amounts of endorphins, serotonin (important for sleep and mood regulation), and others that help regulate stress and immune responses. It's as though the body can't keep up with the demand for neurochemicals. The good news is that there are things you can do to increase the levels of these helpful neurochemicals, including exercise, relaxation and meditation, positive thinking, and even just laughing. Exercise can play an important role in chronic pain management. Note that unlike acute pain that initially requires rest, you need to be active when you have chronic pain. Exercise can help your brain reinterpret body movements as safe and not dangerous.

Understandably, the emotional response to chronic pain is different from the response to acute pain. In a very real sense, chronic pain is a form of chronic stress and can be associated with ongoing tension, anxiety, fatigue, and a host of difficult emotions such as frustration and anger. This can lead to feelings of helplessness, hopelessness, and depression. Nagging questions inevitably arise: *Why me? Why is the pain persisting? What do I really have? How can I explain this to other people when I can't understand it myself? What does the future hold?* All these questions and concerns are very real. But the way forward is to look for solutions about how to manage your pain, not what caused it, because you may never know what caused it. Learn as much as you can about your condition and how to manage it. Instead of obsessing about your pain, be kind to yourself, and make a decision to enjoy your life even with chronic pain.

This brings us to the appropriate relationship between you, as the person with pain, and your health care providers. Collaboration and partnership are the cornerstones of effective care. Health care professionals may well be experts in disease, but you are the expert in your own life, and you are the expert in your daily experience with chronic pain. Because you are responsible for managing your condition day-to-day, the advice and lifestyle changes proposed by health professionals must be based on your needs.

If you are interested in exploring concepts about pain beyond this brief introduction, review the multiple resources provided for you at the end of this chapter and other chapters in this book. The sources listed in the Suggested Further Reading section of the chapter are great places to go to find out more about this important topic. You will also find more information on strategies to "close the gate" and retrain the brain in Chapters 4 and 5.

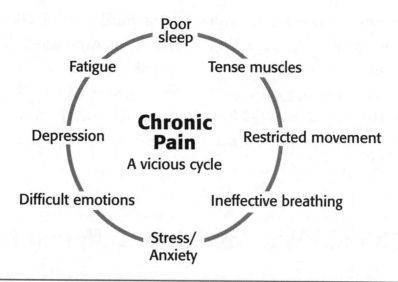

Figure 1.2 **The Vicious Cycle: Chronic Pain and Symptoms**

Chronic Pain Symptoms

Unlike acute pain, where full recovery is expected, chronic pain usually leads to additional symptoms and sometimes loss of functioning. With chronic pain, many people assume that the symptoms they are experiencing are due to the pain itself. While chronic pain can certainly cause fatigue, restricted movement, depression, and the like, it is not the sole cause. What's more, each of these symptoms can feed off each other. For example, depression causes fatigue and tight, tense muscles cause physical limitations, both of which can lead back to poor sleep and more fatigue. The interactions of these symptoms make the pain condition worse. It becomes a vicious cycle, illustrated in Figure 1.2, that doesn't stop unless we find a way to break the cycle.

Whether your chronic pain is caused by a known disease process like arthritis or is idiopathic like lower back pain or whiplash, the problems it causes are similar (see Figure 1.2). For example, most people with chronic pain suffer fatigue and loss of energy. Sleeping problems are also common. Furthermore, when part of the body hurts, our natural response is to tense the muscles in that area in an effort to protect or "guard" the area from further harm. Usually people are not aware they are doing this. Muscle tension causes us to restrict our movement and ultimately results in muscles becoming weak from not being used. This can lead to physical disability for some. Muscle tension can also cause shallow, ineffective breathing so that our bodies do not receive the oxygen needed to function efficiently. This can make fatigue even worse.

Other significant components of chronic pain are stress, anxiety, and fear. Fear of movement is common. So is fear for the future. Concerns and worries can wear us down and lead to such difficult emotions as anger, frustration, and feelings of helplessness. These emotions in turn can feed symptoms of "feeling blue," which can lead to depression. Feelings of sadness or discouragement are normal when dealing with a problem like chronic pain. It can be hard to maintain a cheerful disposition when your condition is constantly annoying and unlikely to go away completely. However, if these sad feelings last for more than a few weeks, there may be an imbalance in brain chemicals often associated with depression. Depression is linked to fatigue, and the more depressed and tired you feel, the more pain you feel. More pain leads to more stress, which leads to more depression and fatigue. And so the cycle continues.

Same Chronic Pain Condition—Different Response

Fred suffers from chronic lower back pain. He is in pain most of the time and has difficulty sleeping because of it. He took early retirement because of his pain and now, at age 55, he spends his days sitting at home watching TV or lying down resting. He avoids most physical activity because of his pain, weakness, and fatigue. Fred doesn't pay much attention to his diet. He has become very irritable. It even seems too much trouble when the grandchildren he adores come to visit. Most people, including his family, no longer enjoy his company.

Joyce, age 66, also suffers from chronic lower back pain. Every day she manages to walk several blocks to the local library or the park. When the pain is severe, she practices relaxation techniques and tries to distract herself. She has learned to plan her activities around her condition so she can still do things she enjoys, like meeting her friends for coffee and visiting her grandchildren. She even manages to take care of the grandkids sometimes when her daughter has to run errands. Her husband is amazed at how much zest she has for life.

Fred and Joyce both live with the same condition and similar physical problems. Yet their abilities to function and enjoy life are very different. Why? In part, the difference lies in their respective attitudes toward their chronic pain. Fred has allowed his physical and emotional capacities to wither. Joyce has learned to take an active role in managing her pain. Even though she has limitations, *she* controls her life instead of letting the pain control it.

A good attitude cannot cure your chronic pain. But a positive attitude and certain self-management skills can make it much easier to live with. Much research now shows that the experience of pain, discomfort, and disability can be modified by circumstances, beliefs, thoughts, mood, and the attention we pay to symptoms. For example, excessive negative thinking and focusing attention on pain has been found to be a strong contributor to increased levels of pain and disability in people with neck, shoulder, and back pain, arthritis, different types of neuropathic pain, and phantom pain. What goes on in a person's mind is as important as what is going on in the person's body.

Important Points to Keep in Mind As You Deal with Chronic Pain

- **You are not to blame.** You are not responsible for causing your pain or failing to cure it. Chronic pain is caused by a complex combination of genetic, biological, environmental, and psychological factors. But although it is not your fault, you *are* the one who is responsible for taking action to manage your pain condition.

- **Don't do it alone.** One of the side effects of chronic pain is a feeling of isolation. As supportive as friends and family members may be, they often cannot understand your struggle to cope every day. However, there are others who know firsthand what it is like to live with a chronic condition just like yours. And many are coping successfully. Connecting with these people can reduce your sense of isolation. They can help you understand what to expect and introduce you to practical tips on how to manage symptoms and feelings. Reaching out can even give you the opportunity to help others cope with their condition, help you appreciate your strengths, and inspire you to take a more active role in managing your pain. Support can come from reading a book, article, or newsletter about how someone lives with chronic pain. Or it can come from talking with others on the telephone, attending support groups, or even by linking with them online through websites devoted to your particular condition.

- **You are more than your pain.** When you have chronic pain, too often the focus of attention becomes your pain. But you are more than pain—you are a person. It is essential to cultivate areas of your life that you enjoy. Small daily pleasures can help balance your efforts to manage uncomfortable symptoms or emotions. Find ways to enjoy nature by growing a plant or watching a sunset. Indulge in the pleasure of human touch or a tasty meal. Seek out companionship with family or friends. Focus on your abilities and strengths rather than disabilities and problems. Celebrate small improvements. If chronic pain teaches anything, it is to live each moment more fully. Your pain condition presents legitimate limits to what you can do, but there are many ways to enhance your function, sense of control, and enjoyment of life.

- **Illness can be an opportunity.** As strange as it may sound, challenges like chronic pain can provide opportunities for personal growth. Pain can make you reevaluate what is really important, shift priorities, and move in new directions that you may never have considered before.

David developed chronic hip and leg pain after a car accident. He has had four surgeries but still is in pain 15 years later. During his journey, he became involved in a support group as a way to cope. Now he is the director of a national

Resources on the Web

Understanding Pain and what to do about it in less than five minutes. Hunter Integrated Pain Service (HIPS). Australia. YouTube, 5:00

Why Things Hurt. Dr. Lorimer Moseley. TED talk. YouTube 14:33

chronic pain association. He feels that before the accident he would never have thought he had the skills to be a leader. Chronic pain, he says, taught him to be persistent and work toward a goal. For him, "knowing that I'm involved and helping others" is the key.

Chronic pain often necessitates a change in lifestyle. To do some of the things they like to do, people with chronic pain have to be smarter and wiser in choosing the activities they want to pursue. They may decide to spend more time deepening relationships with family and friends,

or they may pick up an old hobby they used to enjoy. For example, Melanie has had fibromyalgia for three years. She loves music and learned to play the guitar when she was younger, but she hadn't played for years because she was too busy. After her diagnosis, she started playing again and discovered a whole new network of friends in the city where she lives as well as online. She feels her life is richer because of music and her new friends. So although chronic pain is a difficult condition to have and may close some doors, you can, like Melanie, choose to open new ones.

Suggested Further Reading

To learn more about the topics discussed in this chapter, we suggest that you explore the following resources:

Butler, David and G. Lorimer Moseley. *Explain Pain*. NOI Group Publishing, Australia, 2013.

Caudill, Margaret A. *Managing Pain Before It Manages You*. New York: Guilford Press, 2009.

Corey, David. Pain: *Learning to Live Without It*. Toronto: MacMillan Canada, 1993, 2004. Available as a free download at www.healthrecoverygroup.com/pmp/pain_handbooks.htm Part 1: Why We Hurt: The Human Body and Pain.

Cousins, Norman. *Anatomy of an Illness as Perceived by the Patient*. New York: W. W. Norton, 2005.

Foreman, Judy. *A Nation in Pain: Healing Our Biggest Health Problem*. New York: Oxford University Press, 2014.

Gruman, Jessie. *AfterShock: What to Do When the Doctor Gives You—or Someone You Love—a Devastating Diagnosis*. New York: Walker, 2010. See also Gruman's website, which offers a selection of further resources: www.aftershockbook.com.

Kabat-Zinn, Jon. *Full Catastrophe Living: Using the Wisdom of Your Body and Mind to Face Stress, Pain, and Illness.* New York: Bantam, 2013.

Melzack, Ronald, and Patrick Wall. *The Challenge of Pain.* London: Penguin, 2008.

Moseley, G. Lorimer. *Painful Yarns, Metaphors and Stories to Help Understand the Biology of Pain.* Dancing Giraffe Press, Australia. 2007

Selak, Joy H., and Steven S. Overman. *You Don't Look Sick: Living Well with Invisible Chronic Illness.* Binghamton, N.Y.: Haworth Medical Press, 2005.

Sobel, David, and Robert Ornstein. *The Healthy Mind, Healthy Body Handbook.* Los Altos, Calif.: DRx, 1996.

Sobel, David, and Robert Ornstein. *Healthy Pleasures*, Reading, Mass.: Addison-Wesley, 1989.

Sobel, David, and Robert Ornstein. *Mind and Body Health Handbook: How to Use Your Mind and Body to Relieve Stress, Overcome Illness, and Enjoy Healthy Pleasures,* 2nd ed. Los Altos, Calif.: DRx, 1998.

Turk, Dennis C., and Frits Winter. *The Pain Survival Guide: How to Reclaim Your Life.* Washington, D.C.: American Psychological Association, 2006.

Weil, Andrew. *Healthy Aging: A Lifelong Guide to Your Physical and Spiritual Well-Being.* New York: Anchor Books, 2005.

CHAPTER 2

Becoming an Active Self-Manager

SOME PEOPLE MANAGE THEIR CHRONIC PAIN by withdrawing from life. They rest almost all the time, socialize less, and even withdraw from their family. The pain becomes the center of their existence. Other people with the same condition and symptoms somehow manage to get on with life. They may change some of the things they do or the way certain things get done. Sometimes, they may say no to things they used to do. Nevertheless, life for them continues to be full and active.

The difference between these two extremes is not the pain itself but rather how the person with chronic pain decides to manage his or her condition. Please note the use of the word *decides* in the previous sentence. Self-management is always a decision: a decision to be active or a decision to do nothing; a decision to seek help or a decision to suffer in silence. This book will help you with these decisions.

Remember: *you* are the manager when it comes to your health. And, like the manager of an organization or household, you are responsible for the following tasks:

1. Determine what your problem is and think about how you can solve it.

2. Make a decision about what you want to accomplish.

3. Take action by setting your goal and evaluating your options.

4. Make a short-term action plan.

5. Carry out your action plan.

6. Check the results.

7. Make mid-course corrections to your action plan as needed.

8. Reward yourself for your success.

The material in this chapter will help get you started on accomplishing the responsibilities outlined in this list. Like any skill, active self-management must be learned and practiced. This chapter starts you on your way by presenting the three most important self-management tools: problem solving, making decisions, and taking action.

We begin by discussing the importance of problem solving.

Problem Solving

Problems sometimes make themselves known with a feeling of general uneasiness. Let's say you are unhappy but not sure why. Your first goal is to identify the problem. Upon closer examination, you find that you miss having contact with some relatives who live far away. With the problem identified, you consider different ways to address it and ultimately decide to take a trip to visit the relatives you miss.

In the past you have always driven, but you now find it tiring to drive. You consider leaving at noon instead of early in the morning, making the trip in two days instead of one, or asking a friend along to share the driving. You decide none of these are viable options, so you seek other ways of travel. There is a train that stops close to your destination, or you could fly. After comparing the price of air and rail tickets, you decide to take the train.

The trip still seems overwhelming, so you decide to write down all the steps necessary to make it a reality. These include finding a good time to go, buying a train ticket, figuring out how to handle luggage, seeing if you can make it up and down the stairs on the train, determining if you can walk on a moving train to get food or visit the restroom, and figuring out how you will get to the station. Each of these steps can be addressed as part of an action plan.

To start your action planning, you promise yourself that this week you will call and find out how much the railroad can help. You also decide to start taking a short walk each day, including walking up and down a few steps, so you will be steadier on your feet. You then carry out your action plans by calling the railroad and starting your walking program.

A week later you check the results. Right away, you see that a single call answered many questions. The railroad offers help to people who have mobility problems and has ways of dealing with many of your concerns. However, even though you are walking better, you still feel unsteady on your feet. You make a change in your action plan by asking a physical therapist about this, and he suggests using a cane or walking stick. Although you don't like using one, you realize that a cane will give you the extra security needed on a moving train.

You have just engaged in problem solving to achieve your goal to take a trip. This example illustrates some of the steps of problem solving. In the material that follows we discuss in more detail the specific steps in problem solving.

The following steps for solving problems are summarized in Table 2.1:

1. **Identify the problem.** This is the first and most important step in problem solving— and usually the most difficult step as well. You may anticipate, for example, that the stairs on the train might pose a problem, but it may take a little more exploration to determine that the real problem you need to address is your fear of falling.

2. **List ideas to solve the problem.** You may be able to come up with a good list of ideas yourself. And you can also call on friends, family, members of your health care team, or community resources. But remember: these folks cannot help you if you do not clearly identify and describe the problem. For example, there is a big difference between saying that you can't walk because your feet

Table 2.1 **Problem-Solving Steps**
1. Identify the problem.
2. List ideas to solve the problem.
3. Pick an idea to try.
4. Check the results.
5. Pick another idea if the first doesn't work.
6. Seek additional resources.
7. Accept that the problem may not be solvable now.

hurt and saying that your feet hurt because you cannot find walking shoes that fit properly. The first is a vague complaint; the second is an identifiable problem that can be rectified.

3. **Pick an idea to try.** Start with the idea that you feel has the most promise to solve your problem. As you try it, remember that new activities can be difficult sometimes. Be sure to give your potential solution a fair chance before deciding it doesn't work.

4. **Check the results.** After you've given your idea a fair trial, evaluate the results. If all went well, your problem has been solved.

5. **Pick another idea if the first doesn't work.** If you still have the problem, pick another idea from your list and try again.

6. **Seek additional resources.** Turn to your family, friends, and health care providers for more ideas if you still do not have a solution to the problem.

7. **Accept that the problem may not be solvable now.** If you have exhausted all your ideas and the problem is still unsolved, your problem may not be solvable right now. You

may have to accept that fact. This is sometimes hard to do. But just because a problem can't be solved right now doesn't mean that it won't be solvable later. It also doesn't mean that other problems cannot be solved. Even if your path is blocked, there are probably alternative paths waiting to be discovered. Don't give up. Keep going.

Making Decisions

Like solving problems, making decisions is an important tool in your self-management toolbox. The steps for making decisions resemble the steps for problem solving. They are as follows:

1. **Identify your options.** Sometimes your options can be a simple choice between changing a behavior or not changing at all. For example, you may have to make a decision about getting help with housework or continuing to do it all yourself.

2. **Identify what you want.** It may be important for you to continue your life as normally as possible or to have more time with your family. Perhaps you no longer want to be responsible for certain chores, such as shoveling the walkways or mowing the lawn. Sometimes identifying your core values (such as spending time with family and friends) will help you set your priorities. Identifying your values and what you want can even increase your motivation to change.

3. **Write down pros and cons for each of your options.** List as many items as you can for each side.

4. **Rate each pro and con on your list.** Rate each pro or con on a scale from 0 to 5, with 0 indicating "not at all important" and 5 indicating "extremely important."

5. **Add up your ratings for each column and compare them.** The option in the column with the highest total should be the option you choose. If the totals are close or you are still not sure, skip to the next step.

Living with Uncertainty

Living with uncertainty can be difficult. The diagnosis of a chronic pain condition takes away some of our sense of security and control, which can be frightening. Even as we work with health professionals to pursue and begin new treatments, this uncertainty continues.

When we have a chronic condition, this feeling becomes an important part of our lives. We are uncertain about our future health, and perhaps about our ability to continue to do the things we want, need, and like to do. Many people find it very challenging to make decisions while accepting uncertainty. It is one of the hardest self-management tasks. If you feel uncertain in the face of chronic pain conditions, know that it is a normal reaction and it is something you can learn to address.

Figure 2.1 **Decision-Making Example**

Should I get help in the house?

Pro	Rating	Con	Rating
I'll have more time	4	It's expensive	3
I'll be less tired	4	It's hard to find good help	1
I'll have a clean house	3	They won't do things my way	2
		I don't want a stranger in the house	1
Total	11		7

6. **Apply the "gut test."** For example, does going back to work part-time feel "right" to you? If so, you have probably reached a decision. If not, the way you feel should probably win out over the math.

You can see a decision-making example and a blank decision-making chart in Figures 2.1 and 2.2.

In the example shown in Figure 2.1, the clear decision is to get help because the pro score (11) is significantly higher than the con score (7). If a decision made in this way feels right in your gut, you have the answer.

Now it's your turn! Try making a decision using the chart in Figure 2.2. It's okay to write in your book.

Figure 2.2 **Decision to be Made**

Decision to be made:

Pro	Rating	Con	Rating
Total			

Taking Action

We have just discussed how to identify problems and make difficult decisions. These are important first steps but often knowing what to do is not enough. Now, it is time to do something, to take action. We suggest you start by doing one thing at a time. In the material that follows we outline the steps to taking action. First, set a goal and evaluate your options for achieving that goal, then begin by making a short-term action plan.

Setting Your Goals

Before you can take action, you first must know what you want to do. Be realistic and specific when stating your goal. One self-manager wanted to climb 20 steps to her daughter's home so she could join her family for a holiday meal. Another wanted to overcome his fatigue and attend an evening class once a week. Still another wanted to continue to ride his motorcycle regularly even though he could no longer handle his 1,000-pound bike like he used to.

Take a few minutes and write your goals in the chart in Figure 2.3. Feel free to add more lines if necessary.

Figure 2.3 **Goals**

_____

_____

_____

_____

Put a star (★) next to the goal you would like to work on first.

Evaluating Your Options

There are many ways to reach any specific goal. For example, our self-manager who wanted to climb 20 steps could climb a few steps each day at first, begin a slow walking program, or look into holding the family gathering at a different place. The man who wanted to attend evening classes could plan rest periods throughout the day, go on very short outings, ask a friend to go along for assistance, or talk to the health care team about his fatigue concerns. Our motorcycle rider could buy a lighter motorcycle or a three-wheeled model, use a sidecar, or put "training wheels" on his bike.

As you can see, there are many options for reaching each goal. Your job is to list the options and then choose one or two to try out.

Sometimes it is hard to think of all the options yourself. If that's true for you, share your goal with family, friends, and health professionals. You can call community and national organizations such as the American Chronic Pain Association or the Canadian Pain Coalition for advice. Or you can research potential options on the Internet. Don't, however, ask others what you *should* do; rather, ask for *suggestions* about what to do. It is a subtle but important distinction. It is always good to have a full list of options, but in the end *you* must prioritize them and pursue the ones that you feel are the most promising.

A note of caution: you may not seriously consider some options because you assume they are unworkable. Never make this assumption until you have thoroughly investigated the option. One woman we know had lived in the same town all her life and felt that she knew all about the community resources. When she was having problems with her health insurance, a friend from another city suggested contacting an insurance counselor. The woman dismissed this suggestion because she was certain this service did not exist in her town. It was only when the friend came to visit and called the Area Agency on Aging (which exists in most counties in the United States) that the woman learned there were three insurance counseling services nearby. Then there's our motorcycle rider who thought that training wheels on a Harley was a crazy idea, but he overcame his skepticism and investigated the possibility. He added 15 years to his riding life using training wheels. In short, never assume anything. Assumptions are major self-management enemies.

Write a list of options for your main goal in Figure 2.4. Place a star (★) next to the two or three options you would most like to pursue.

Figure 2.4 **Options**

_____

_____

_____

_____

One last note about goals: not all goals are achievable. Chronic pain may mean having to give up some options. If this is true for you, don't dwell on what you can't do. Rather, start working on another goal you would like to accomplish. One self-manager we know who uses a wheelchair talks about the 90 percent of things he *can* do—not the 10 percent he has had to quit

doing. He devotes his life to developing this 90 percent to the fullest.

Making a Short-Term Action Plan

Once you've identified a goal and narrowed down your list of options, you should have a pretty good idea of where you are going. However, the path ahead may be overwhelming. *How will I ever move? How will I ever be able to garden again? How will I ever* _____*?* (You fill in the blank.) One of the problems with goals is that they often seem like dreams. They are so far off, big, or difficult that we are overwhelmed, so we don't even try to accomplish them.

The secret is to not try to do everything at once. Instead, look at what you can realistically expect to accomplish within the next week. We call this an action plan. An action plan is short-term, is doable, and sets you on the road toward your goal.

Action plans are probably your most important self-management tool. They help you do the things you know you should do in order to achieve your ultimate goals. For example, most people with chronic pain can walk. Some can make it just across the room, others can walk for half a block. Many can walk several blocks, and some can walk a mile or more. However, few people have a systematic exercise program to improve their ability to walk even with chronic pain. In the material that follows, we discuss the steps for making a realistic action plan.

First, decide what you will do this week. For the person who wants to climb 20 steps, the goal for the first week might be climbing just three steps on each of four consecutive days. The man who wants to continue riding his motorcycle might spend half an hour on two days researching lighter motorcycles and motorcycle training wheels.

Make very sure your plan is action-specific. For example, instead of just planning to "lose weight" (which is not an action but the result of an action), plan to "drink tea instead of soda with meals."

You can get specific about your plan by answering the following questions:

- **Exactly WHAT are you going to do?** If you want to lose weight, are you going to walk? Eat less? Practice distraction techniques? Again, be specific. "Losing a pound this week" is not an action plan because it does not involve a specific action; "not eating after dinner for four days this week," by contrast, is a fine action plan.

- **HOW MUCH will you do?** Answers to this question often involve time, distance, repetitions, or quantities. Will you practice relaxation exercises for 15 minutes? Will you walk one block, or make two trips up the stairs each afternoon? Will you eat half portions at lunch and dinner?

- **WHEN will you do it?** Again, this must be specific: before lunch, in the shower, upon coming home from work. Connecting an action plan with an old habit is a good way to trigger the new behavior and make sure it gets done. For example, make brushing your teeth your reminder to take your new medication. Make a plan to do your new activity before an old favorite activity such as reading the paper or watching a favorite TV program.

- **HOW OFTEN will you do it?** This is a bit tricky. We would all like to do things every day, but that is not always possible. We recommend initially aiming for three or four times a week. If you do more, so much the better. However, if you are like most people, you will feel less pressure if you can do your activity a few times a week and still feel successful. (Note that taking medications is an exception. This must be done exactly as directed by your health care provider.)

There are some other general guidelines for developing your action plan that may help. First, the action plan should be about something *you* want to do or accomplish. Do not make action plans to please your friends, family, or doctor.

Second, "start where you are," or start slowly. If you can walk for only one minute, start your walking program by walking one minute once every hour or two, not by trying to walk a block. If you have never done any exercise, start with a few minutes of light stretching. If your goal is to lose weight, base your plan on your existing eating behaviors, such as having half portions of some of your usual foods.

Third, give yourself some time off. All people have days when they don't feel like accomplishing much. That is a good reason for planning to do something three times a week instead of every day.

Fourth, once you've made your action plan, ask yourself the following question: "On a scale of 0 to 10, with 0 being totally unsure and 10 being totally certain, how sure am I that I can complete this entire plan?"

If your answer is 7 or above, you probably have a realistic action plan. If your answer is below 7, look at your plan again. Ask yourself why you are unsure. What problems do you foresee? Then see if you can either solve the

Table 2.2 **Basics of a Successful Action Plan**

- It is something *you* want to do.
- It is achievable (something you can expect to be able to accomplish that week).
- It is action-specific.
- It answers the questions *What? How much? When?* and *How often?*
- On a scale from 0 (not at all sure) to 10 (absolutely sure), you are confident you will complete your entire plan at a level of 7 or higher.

problems or change your plan to make yourself more confident of success. Table 2.2 summarizes the features of a successful action plan.

Once you have come up with a plan you are happy with, write it down and post it where you will see it every day. Thinking through an action plan is one thing. Writing it down makes it more likely you will take action. Keep track of how you are doing and the problems you encounter. (A blank action plan form is provided at the end of this chapter. You can find more at the end of the book.)

Carrying Out Your Action Plan

If your action plan is well written and realistically achievable, completing it is generally pretty straightforward. Ask family or friends to check to see how you are doing. Having to report your progress is good motivation.

Successful managers typically keep lists of what they want to accomplish. Do the same, and check things off your to-do list as you complete them. If you are not checking off many things, perhaps your plan was not realistic. Along with your to-do list, make daily notes about your actions, successes, and failures. Later these notes may be useful in determining a pattern to use for problem solving.

For example, our stair-climbing friend never did her climbing. Each day she had a different problem. One day, she didn't have enough time. Another she was too tired. On a third day, the weather was too cold, and so on. When she looked back at her notes, she realized she was

Success Improves Health

The benefits of change go beyond the payoffs of adopting healthier habits. Obviously, you feel better when you exercise, eat well, keep regular sleeping hours, stop smoking, and take time to relax. But there's also evidence that your health improves when you simply experience the feelings of self-confidence and control that come from making any successful change over your life. By changing and improving even one area of your life, such as boosting your physical fitness or learning a new skill, you regain a sense of optimism and vitality. By focusing on what you can do rather than what you can't do, you're more likely to lead a more positive and happier life.

coming up with excuses every day. She began to realize that the real problem was her fear of falling with no one around to help her. So she altered her action plan. She decided to use a cane while climbing stairs, and to climb when a friend or neighbor was around.

Checking Your Results

At the end of each week, check in to see if you are closer to accomplishing your goal. Are you able to walk farther? Have you lost weight? Do you have more energy? Taking stock is important. You may not see progress each day, but you should see a little progress each week. If you are not accomplishing what you want to by the end of each week, it may be time to revisit your plan and use your problem-solving skills.

Making Midcourse Corrections (Back to Problem Solving)

When you are trying to overcome obstacles, your first plan may not turn out to be the most effective one. If something doesn't work, don't give up; try something else. Modify your short-term action plan so that the steps are easier. Give yourself more time to accomplish difficult tasks. Choose a new action plan, or check with your consultants for advice and assistance. If you are not sure how to go about this, go back and read pages 24–27.

Rewarding Yourself

The best part of being a good self-manager of your pain condition is the reward that comes from accomplishing your goals and living a fuller and more satisfying life. However, don't wait until this ultimate goal is reached to celebrate your progress. Reward yourself frequently for your short-term successes. In fact, build these rewards into your action plan. For example, decide not to read the paper or your favorite magazine until after you exercise. Thus reading becomes your reward. One self-manager we know buys only a few pieces of her favorite fruit at a time. She has to walk the half mile to the supermarket every day or two to get more. In this way, the fruit becomes the immediate reward for her exercise. Another self-manager who stopped smoking used the money he would have spent on cigarettes to have his house professionally cleaned. There was even enough left over to go to a baseball game with a friend. Rewards don't have to be fancy, expensive, or calorie-laden. Focus on healthy pleasures that add both enjoyment and benefit to your life.

Now that you understand the meaning of self-management, you are ready to begin learning to use the tools that will make you successful at it. The rest of the book is devoted to teaching you about these tools. Your toolbox will include practical

How People Change

Thousands of studies have been done to learn how and why people change—or don't change. Here's what we know about people and change:

- Most people change on their own, and only when they are ready. Although physicians, counselors, spouses, and self-help groups may coax, persuade, nag, and otherwise try to assist people to change their lifestyle and habits, most people make changes without much help from others.

- Change is not a smooth, steady process. It happens in stages. Most of us think of change as occurring one step at a time, each step an improvement over the one before it. Although a few people do make changes this way, it is rare. More than 95 percent of people who successfully quit smoking, for example, do so only after a series of setbacks and relapses.

- Relapses are not failures; they are merely setbacks. Relapsing can actually be a helpful way to maintain change, because it provides feedback about what you are doing that isn't working.

- Efficient self-change depends on doing the right things at the right time. For example, making an elaborate written plan of action when you really haven't psychologically committed yourself to change is a prescription for failure. You're likely to get bored, discouraged, or frustrated before you even start.

- Confidence in your ability to change is the key ingredient for success. Your belief in your own ability to succeed predicts whether you will attempt change in the first place, whether you will persist if you relapse, and whether you will ultimately be successful.

strategies to help you succeed with exercise and movement, nutrition and healthy weight management, pain management techniques, good communication skills, family and intimacy issues, decision making about the future, and finding resources and information. We talk about medications and their uses in Chapters 15 and 16. Chapter 18 contains information on some of the more common chronic pain problems and Chapter 19 is about chronic angina pain. If your specific pain problem is not covered, we are sure that this book can still be helpful for you. Fortunately, most self-management skills are applicable to many types of chronic pain.

My Action Plan

In writing your action plan, be sure it includes all of the following:

1. What you are going to do (a specific action)

2. How much you are going to do (time, distance, portions, repetitions, etc.)

3. When you are going to do it (time of the day, day of the week)

4. How often or how many days a week you are going to do it

Example: This week, I will walk (what) around the block (how much) before lunch (when) three times (how many).

This week I will _____ (what)

_____ (how much)

_____ (when)

_____ (how often)

How sure are you? (0 = not at all sure; 10 = absolutely sure) _____

Comments

Monday _____

Tuesday _____

Wednesday _____

Thursday _____

Friday _____

Saturday _____

Sunday _____

CHAPTER 3

Finding Resources

A N IMPORTANT ASPECT OF BECOMING A SELF-MANAGER is knowing how to find help when you need it. When you seek help, you are no longer a victim of your condition; you are a good self-manager. Start by evaluating your condition. As you do so, you may discover that there is a gap between what you can do and what you want to do. If so, it may be time to get help so you can do the things that are most important to you.

Locating the Resources You Need

As we begin to look for help, most of us start by asking family or friends. Sometimes this can be difficult. We are afraid that others will see us as weak, and our pride gets in the way. The truth is that most people want to be helpful but do not know how. Your job is to tell the people around you what you need. Finding the right words to ask for help is discussed in Chapter 10.

Unfortunately, some people either do not have family or close friends or find it difficult to ask them for help if they do. Sometimes family or friends cannot offer all the help that is needed. Thankfully, we have another wonderful resource to turn to: our community.

Finding resources can be a little like a treasure hunt. As in a treasure hunt, creative thinking wins the game. Finding what you need may be as simple as visiting a website or looking in the telephone book and making a couple of phone calls. Other times it may take sleuthing. The community resource detective must find clues and follow them. Being a good detective even involves starting over when a clue leads to a dead end.

The first step is to define the problem and then decide what you want. For example, suppose you find it difficult to prepare meals because standing for a long time is painful. After some thought, you decide that you want to continue cooking for yourself. You could do this if you could cook while sitting. Your treasure hunt involves figuring out how to do this.

You look at kitchen stools and soon determine they will not work, so you decide that you need to redesign the kitchen. Now the hunt begins in earnest. Where can you find an architect or contractor who has experience in kitchen alterations for people with physical limitations? You start with the phone book, which has pages of ads and listings for architects and contractors. Some advertisers say they specialize in kitchens, but none mention designing to accommodate physical limitations. So you must call and ask. After calling a few contractors, you come to realize that none are experienced in kitchens for the physically limited. Next you turn to the Internet. You find a company that seems to be just what you need, but it is located more than 200 miles away.

Now what? You could contact the rest of the contractors listed in the phone book, but this would be time-consuming. And even if you found someone suitable, you would still have to check references.

Who else might have the information you need? Maybe someone who works with people with physical disabilities would know. This opens a long list of possibilities: occupational and physical therapists, medical supply stores, the local Center for Independent Living, and nonprofit organizations that understand pain problems, such as the Arthritis Foundation or Arthritis Society. You decide to ask a friend who is a physical therapist. Unfortunately your friend does not have any ideas about local contractors who do this sort of work. So now what?

In addition to formal organizational resources, there are people in every community who are natural resources. These "naturals" or "connectors" seem to know everyone and everything about their community. They tend to be folks who have lived a long time in the community and have been closely involved in it. They are also natural problem solvers and enjoy being helpful, so people often turn to them for advice. It could be a friend, a business associate, the mail carrier, your physician, your pet's veterinarian, your hairdresser or barber, the checker at the corner grocery, the pharmacist, a bus or taxi driver, the school secretary, a real estate agent, the chamber of commerce receptionist, or the librarian. Sometimes the natural will taste the thrill of the hunt and, like a modern-day Sherlock Holmes, announce that "the game is afoot!" and promptly join you in your search. You are about to start researching local organizations when you start to think about all the people you regularly come in contact with and realize that some of them are naturals.

Say the person in your community who fills this role is a friend who runs a local business. You tell him about your problem the next time he comes to your house and he tells you about a contractor whose wife uses a wheelchair. He knows this because the guy just did a great job on the kitchen of one of his co-workers. You call the contractor and find he is perfect for your situation. Problem solved!

Let's review the lessons from this example. The most important steps in finding the resources you need are:

1. Identify the problem.

2. Identify what you want or need to solve the problem.

3. Look for resources in the phone book and on the Internet.

4. Ask friends, family, and neighbors for ideas.

5. Contact organizations that might deal with similar issues.

6. Identify and ask naturals in your community.

One last note: the best sleuth follows several clues at the same time. This will save you lots of time and shorten the hunt. Watch out, though—once you get good at thinking about community resources creatively, you may become a natural in your own right!

Resources for Resources

When we need to find goods or services, there are certain resources we can call on. One resource often leads to another. The natural is one of those resources, but our "detective's kit" needs a variety of other useful tools.

The phone book and Internet search engines are the most frequently used tools, and for most searches that is where to start. These tools are particularly helpful if you are looking for someone to hire, but they can also lead you to a number of other resources.

Information and Referral Services

Almost all communities have one or more information and referral service. Sometimes these are related to a geographic area such as a city, county, or region, or they are specific to a demographic group, such as the Area Agencies on Aging. Other times they are specific to a condition, like fibromyalgia or migraine headaches.

There are several types of agencies that operate these services. Online, search under "United Way Information and Referral," "Senior Information and Referral" (or "Area Agency on Aging," "Council on Aging," or "Seniors Resource Center"), "Community Services Council" or just "information and referral" and the area in which you live, such as your state or province. If you are using a phone book, be sure to check your city, county, or regional government listings. These services maintain huge files of contact information. Just about any help you might need is available. Even if they don't have the answer you seek, they will almost always be able to refer you to another agency that might.

Nonprofit, Community, and Other Organizations

Nonprofit agencies such as the American Pain Society, the American Chronic Pain Association, the Chronic Pain Association of Canada, and the Canadian Pain Coalition are great sources of information. Other organizations such as the American Heart Association and the Canadian Heart and Stroke Foundation are also excellent resources. There are similar organizations in most other countries. Many of them have wonderful websites, and in our new world of cyberspace, you can live in rural North Dakota or the Canadian Arctic and still access the help provided by Chronic Pain Australia.

These organizations provide up-to-date information about pain problems. They also provide support and direct services to people with chronic pain. Often, they may fund research to improve our understanding of pain and its treatment and to help people live better with their condition. In some instances you can become a member of one of these organizations. Membership may entitle you to receive regular bulletins by mail or e-mail. You do not, however, have to be a member to qualify for their services; they are there to serve you.

There are also local resources in your community that offer information and direct services. These include the local chapter of AARP (formerly known as the American Association of Retired Persons) or CARP (the Canadian equivalent of AARP), senior centers, community centers, and fitness and recreation facilities. Besides information and referrals, these places offer classes, recreational opportunities, nutrition programs, legal and tax help, and social programs. There is probably a senior center or community center close to you. Your city or regional government office or local librarian can tell you where to find these resources. The calendar section of your newspaper will usually have information about their programs as well.

Most religious groups provide information and social services to persons who need it, either directly through the place of worship or through organizations such as the National Council of Churches or Jewish Family Services. To get help from religious organizations, start with a local place of worship. You usually need not be a member of the congregation or even of the religion to receive help.

The medical community is another resource for you. Call your local hospital, clinic, or health insurance plan and ask for the social service department. Your primary care provider will also be aware of the physical and mental health services available through his or her practice, as well as other services available in your area.

Libraries

Your public library is a particularly good resource when you are looking for information about your chronic condition. Even if you know your way around a library, it's a good idea to ask the reference librarian for assistance. These people are familiar with volumes of material that you may overlook, and they usually are knowledgeable about the community. (They're probably among the ranks of the local naturals.) Even if you cannot make a visit to your library, you can always call or e-mail with your questions.

In addition to city or county libraries, there are other, more specialized health libraries. Ask your information and referral service if there is a health library in your community that specializes in health-related resources. These places usually have a searchable computer database along with the usual print, audiotape, and videotape materials. These libraries are often maintained by nonprofit organizations and hospitals, so they sometimes charge a small fee for use.

Universities and colleges also have libraries with helpful staff. By law, the regional "government documents" sections of these libraries must be open to the public at no charge. There are government publications on just about any subject, and health-related publications are particularly extensive. You can find information on everything from your chronic pain condition to organic gardening to detailed nutritional recipes. These publications represent "your tax dollars at work."

If you are fortunate enough to have a medical school in your community, you may be able to use its medical library. It will only be a resource for information, however, not for help with tasks. Naturally, you can expect to find a great deal of information about disease and treatment at a medical library. Unless you have special knowledge about medicine, however, the detailed information you find in a medical library can be confusing and even frightening. Use medical libraries with care.

Books

Books can be useful—indeed, you are reading a book now! Many books on chronic pain and other conditions contain reading and resource lists, either at the ends of chapters or at the back of the book. These lists can be very helpful. We identify useful books at the ends of a number of the chapters in this book.

Newspapers and Magazines

Your local newspaper can be an excellent resource, especially if you live in a smaller community. Be sure to look in the calendar of events. Even if you are not interested in a particular featured event, you might find what you are looking for by calling the contact number or visiting the website. Look in other logical places for news stories that might be of interest. If, for example, you are looking for an exercise program for people with your health problem, check the sports and fitness section. The pages around the calendar section sometimes feature articles about local health-related events.

Sometimes you can find clues in the classified section. Review the index of classified headings (it is usually printed at the front of the section near the rate information). Look under "announcements," "health," or any other heading that seems promising.

The Internet

Today most people have access to the Internet. Even if you are not an Internet user, you almost certainly know someone who is. Even if you do not have a computer, you can use one in your local library or ask a friend for help.

The Internet is the fastest-growing source of information today. New information is being added to it every second of every day. The Internet not only offers information about health (or anything else you can imagine), it also provides several ways to interact with people all over the world. For example, someone who has interstitial cystitis, a painful and sometimes embarrassing condition, might find it difficult to find others with the same problem where she or he lives. The Internet can put that person in touch with a whole group of such people; it doesn't matter whether they are across the street or on the other side of the world.

The good thing about the Internet is that anyone can maintain a website, a Facebook or other social network page, a blog, or a discussion group. That is also the bad thing about the Internet. There are virtually no controls over who is posting information or the accuracy or even safety of what is posted. So although there is a lot of very useful information out there, you may also encounter incorrect or even dangerous information. Therefore, never assume that information found on the Internet is automatically trustworthy. Rather, approach it with skepticism and caution. Ask yourself: Is the author or sponsor of the website clearly identified? Is the author or source reputable? Are credentials listed, and are they verifiable? Is the information contrary to what everyone else seems to be saying about the subject? Does common sense support the information? What is the purpose of the website? Is someone trying to sell you something or win you over to a particular point of view?

One way to analyze the purpose of the website is to examine its URL. The URL is the website's address on the Internet. You will find it in a bar in the upper-left corner of the computer screen. It will start with the letters http or www. The URL will usually look something like this:

www.patienteducation.stanford.edu

or

www.stanford.edu

At the end of the main part of a U.S.–based website's URL, you will most commonly see another group of letters preceded by a period: .edu, .org, .gov, or .com. This will give you a clue about the nature of the organization that owns the site. A college or university's website URL ends in .edu, a nonprofit organization in .org, a governmental agency in .gov, and a commercial organization in .com. The URLs for some of our

Some Pain Resources on the Web

In the search box on any of the following websites, enter such phrases as "chronic pain," "pain management," or your specific condition:

American Chronic Pain Association: theacpa.org

American Pain Society: www.americanpainsociety.org

Arthritis Foundation: www.arthritis.org

Arthritis Society: www.arthritis.ca

Canadian Pain Coalition: www.canadianpaincoalition.ca

Canadian Pain Society: www.canadianpainsociety.ca

Chronic Pain Association of Canada: chronicpaincanada.com

eMedicineHealth: http://www.emedicinehealth.com

Mount Sinai Beth Israel Hospital: www.stoppain.org

National Center for Complementary and Alternative Medicine: nccam.nih.gov

WebMD: www.webmd.com

Women's College Hospital: www.womenshealthmatters.ca

favorite reliable websites are listed above and at the end of this chapter.

As a general rule of thumb, American sites with URLs ending in .edu, .org, and .gov are fairly trustworthy (although a nonprofit organization can be formed to promote just about anything). Many Canadian-based websites end in .ca, so you will have to investigate whether a site is affiliated with a school, nonprofit organization, government agency, or commercial enterprise. A website with .com in the address may be trying to sell you a product or service. This doesn't mean that a commercial website can't be a good source of information or assistance. On the contrary, there are many outstanding commercial sites dedicated to providing high-quality, trustworthy information.

Social Networking Sites

Social networking sites and blogs are exploding on the Internet. These are websites where people with similar interests connect to socialize, discuss issues, or share information. Sites such as Facebook, Blogger, and PatientsLikeMe are currently very popular, but new ones may have emerged by the time this book is published.

These sites enable the average person to communicate easily with others who want to listen to or read what she or he has to say. Some sites, such as Facebook, require users to control who is allowed to read their posts. Others, such as sites hosted through Blogger, are more like personal journals that are open to anyone.

Many such websites have been started by people living with particular health conditions.

These authors are eager to share their experiences. The information and support offered can be valuable, but again, be cautious: some sites can be proposing unproven and dangerous ideas. If you are unsure about something you find on the Internet related to chronic pain, ask your health care provider for his or her opinion.

Discussion Groups

Yahoo, Google, and other websites offer discussion groups where people can post about just about anything you can imagine. Anyone can start a discussion group about any subject. The groups are run by the people who start them. Given any one health problem, there are probably dozens of discussion groups. You can join groups and partake in the discussions if you wish, or you can just "lurk" (read without interacting). For the person with interstitial cystitis, for example, a discussion group may allow her to connect with people who share her experiences. This may be her only opportunity to talk with someone else with her rare condition. Similarly, for someone with depression associated with chronic lower back pain who finds it difficult to talk with someone face-to-face about his problems, the Internet offers an alternative.

To find discussion groups, go to the Google or Yahoo (or any other) home page and search for a link to "groups." You may have to create an account with the sponsoring company before you can view or participate in the discussions, but this is quick and free to do. Despite the fact that it is an "account," you do not have to provide financial information to sign up, nor are you under any obligation to purchase something. An account simply provides you access to the community of online groups hosted there.

Keep in mind that the Internet changes constantly. Our guidelines reflect conditions at the time this book was written. Things may have changed by the time you read this. Becoming an effective resource detective is one of the jobs of a good self-manager. We hope this chapter has given you some ideas about the process of finding resources in your community and beyond. If you find resources that you think we should add to future editions, kindly e-mail them to us at:

self-management@stanford.edu.

Further Resources

To learn more about the topics discussed in this chapter, we suggest that you explore the following resources:

- ☐ Association of Cancer Online Resources (ACOR): www.acor.org
- ☐ Canadian Institutes of Health Research (CIHR): www.cihr.ca
- ☐ CarePages: www.carepages.com
- ☐ CaringBridge: www.caringbridge.org
- ☐ Center for Advancing Health: www.cfah.org

☐ Centers for Disease Control and Prevention (CDC): www.cdc.gov

☐ HealthCentral: www.healthcentral.com

☐ Mayo Clinic: www.mayoclinic.org

☐ MedlinePlus: www.nlm.nih.gov/medlineplus

☐ Memorial Sloan Kettering Cancer Center: www.mskcc.org

☐ National Cancer Institute: www.cancer.gov

☐ National Institutes of Health (NIH): www.nih.gov

☐ National Institutes of Health Office of Rare Diseases Research: www.rarediseases.info.nih.gov

☐ National Library of Medicine tutorial for evaluating Internet health information: www.nlm.nih.gov/medlineplus/evaluatinghealthinformation.html

☐ PatientsLikeMe: www.patientslikeme.com

☐ Psych Central: psychcentral.com

☐ QuackWatch: Your Guide to Quackery, Health Fraud, and Intelligent Decisions: www.quackwatch.org

☐ U.S. Department of Health and Human Services (HHS): www.healthfinder.gov

CHAPTER 4

Understanding and Managing Common Symptoms and Problems

C HRONIC PAIN CONDITIONS ARE ACCOMPANIED by symptoms. These symptoms are signals from your body that something unusual is happening. In addition to pain itself, symptoms may include fatigue, poor sleep, depression, anger, stress, and memory problems. Usually symptoms cannot be seen by others, can be difficult to describe, and can occur at unexpected times. Although some symptoms are common, the ways in which they affect us are very personal. What's more, these symptoms can interact with each other. This interaction may worsen existing symptoms and pain and even lead to new symptoms or problems.

Regardless of the causes of symptoms, you can deal with them in similar ways. Again, our self-management tools are the key to success. In this chapter we discuss several common symptoms, their causes, and some of the tools you can use to manage them. There is also a section on how to cope with unemployment. Additional cognitive tools—ways you can use your mind to calm your nervous system and help deal with many of these symptoms—are discussed in Chapter 5.

41

Dealing with Common Symptoms

Learning to manage symptoms is very similar to problem solving, discussed in Chapter 2. First, identify the symptom you are experiencing. Next, determine why you might be having the symptom at this time. This may sound like a simple process, but it is not always easy.

You may experience many different symptoms, and each symptom may have various causes. The ways in which these symptoms affect your life also differ. All these factors can become very tangled, like the frayed threads of a cloth. To successfully manage symptoms, you need to figure out how to untangle the threads.

One way to approach this is a daily diary or journal. Keeping a journal can be as simple as writing your symptoms on a calendar along with some notes about what you were doing before the symptom started or worsened, as shown in the example in Figure 4.1. After a week or two, you may see a pattern. For example, you may notice that on nights when you

go out to dinner, you have trouble sleeping. Once you realize that, you become aware that when you go out, you tend to overeat and drink a couple cups of coffee after the meal (something you don't do at home). Now you know to adjust your behavior in the future to avoid experiencing sleep problems after a night out on the town. Or you may notice that after every time you babysit the grandchildren you experience more pain than usual. This may cause you to consider what kinds of activities you are doing with the grandkids. Can you modify those activities to include a nap for the kids and a rest break for you? Or is it one particular activity that is causing your pain flare-up? Recognizing patterns is the first step in symptom self-management for many people.

As you read this chapter, note that many of the symptoms we discuss have the same causes. Also, note how one symptom can lead to other symptoms. For example, pain may cause you to

---

Figure 4.1 **Sample Calendar Journal**

Mon.	Tue.	Wed.	Thur.	Fri.	Sat.	Sun.
Grocery shop	Babysit grandkids Pain P.M.	Tired	Water exercise Feel great	Little stiff Clean house	Dinner out Poor sleep	Tired
Mon.	**Tue.**	**Wed.**	**Thur.**	**Fri.**	**Sat.**	**Sun.**
Grocery shop	Babysit grandkids Pain P.M.	Tired	Water exercise Feel great	Clean house	Feel great	Feel great Dinner out Poor sleep

Using Symptom-Management Tools

■ Choose a tool to try, and be sure to give it a fair trial. We recommend that you practice using any new tool for at least two weeks before deciding whether or not it is going to be helpful.

■ Try a variety of tools, giving each a similar trial period. It is important to try more than one tool because some may be more useful for certain symptoms, or you may find that you simply prefer some symptom-management techniques over others.

■ Think about how and when you will use each tool. For example, some of these tools may require more lifestyle modification than others. The best symptom managers learn to use a variety of techniques depending on their conditions and what they want and need to do each day.

■ Place some cues in your environment to remind you to practice these techniques. When mastering new skills, consistency is important. For example, place stickers or notes where you'll see them, such as on your mirror, near the phone, in your office, on your computer, or on your car's dashboard. Change the notes from time to time so you'll continue to notice them.

■ Try linking each new tool with one of your established daily behaviors or activities. For example, practice relaxation before you go to bed or as part of your cool-down after exercise.

■ Ask a friend or family member to remind you to practice each day. He or she may even wish to participate.

unconsciously tense your muscles in the area where you are hurting. As a result, you change your posture, and then you are not standing straight and tall. Instead you are stooping a little. This change in posture may change the way you walk. This new way of walking may change your balance, generate a new pain, or cause you to fall. As you gain a better understanding of this cycle of symptoms, you will be able to identify better ways to address them. You may also find ways to prevent or lessen certain symptoms.

Read on to learn what you can do to lessen some of the more common symptoms experienced by people with chronic pain conditions.

Common Symptoms

The following common symptoms are discussed in this chapter:

Pain

Pain or physical discomfort is *the* universal problem shared by all people with chronic pain conditions. As with most symptoms, pain can have many causes. We discussed reasons why chronic pain develops in Chapter 1, pages 5–16. You might want to revisit that material before reading the next section. What follows is a brief description of some of the most common causes of pain:

- **The pain condition or disease itself.** Pain can come from inflammation, damage in or around joints and tissues, insufficient blood supply to muscles or organs, and an irritated nervous system, to name just a few sources. In some cases, there is no known cause for the pain. Whatever the initial cause, the ultimate result is a malfunctioning or disturbance of a complex interactive network of nerve cells in the spinal cord and the brain—in other words, chronic pain.

- **Tense muscles.** When something hurts, the muscles in that area become tense. This is your body's natural reaction to pain—to try to protect the area that hurts. Stress can also cause you to tense your muscles. Chronic muscle tension can lead to increased soreness or pain.

- **Muscle deconditioning.** With chronic pain, it is common to become less active. This leads to a weakening of the muscles, or muscle deconditioning. When a muscle is weak, it tends to complain anytime it is used. This is not because it is damaged but because it has not been used in a while.

- **Lack of sleep or poor-quality sleep.** Pain often interferes with your ability to get either enough sleep or good-quality sleep. Poor sleep can also make pain worse, and it can lessen your ability to cope with it.

- **Stress, anxiety, and emotions such as anger, fear, frustration, and depression.** These feelings are all normal responses to living with a condition like chronic pain, and they can amplify the experience of pain. This does not mean that the pain is not real. It is all too real. It just means that emotions such as stress and fear and other symptoms such as depression can make a painful situation worse.

- **Medications.** The medicines you are taking can sometimes cause pain, weakness, changes in your thinking, or abdominal or other physical or emotional discomfort. Ask your doctor or pharmacist about the potential side effects of all your medication.

Controlling Pain

We are not helpless in the face of pain. The brain can regulate the flow of pain messages by sending signals that open and close "pain gates" along nerve pathways in the spinal cord and in the brain itself (see the material on the Gate Control Theory Chapter 1, pages 6–7).

For example, the brain can release powerful opiate-like chemicals such as endorphins that effectively block or reduce the pain we feel. For example, when people are seriously injured, they sometimes experience little pain while they are focused on survival. How you focus your attention, your mood, and the way you view your situation—your thoughts and feelings—can open or close the gates.

Your day-to-day pain level is based on how your mind and body respond to pain. Here are four ways in which the mind and body interact when you are experiencing pain.

■ **Inactivity.** Because of pain, you tend to avoid physical activity. This avoidance in turn causes you to lose strength and flexibility. The weaker and more out of condition you become, the more frustrated and depressed you feel. These negative emotions can open the gates and cause pain levels to rise.

■ **Overdoing.** You may be determined to prove that you can still be active, so you overexert and push yourself to finish a task. At the same time, you ignore the signals your body sends about its need for rest. Pushing yourself only leads to more pain, which leads to more inactivity, more depression, and more pain.

■ **Misunderstanding.** Your friends, family, boss, and coworkers may not understand that you are suffering and may dismiss your pain as "not real." This can evoke anger or depression.

■ **Overprotection.** On the other hand, friends, family, and coworkers might coddle you and make excuses for you. This can lead you to feel and act more dependent and disabled.

Fortunately, you can interrupt this downward spiral of negative mind-body interaction. If you've been told you have to live with pain, it doesn't mean you cannot have a happy, fulfilling life. Learning to live with pain means learning to accept it and manage it. It can be a new beginning. You can learn techniques such that retrain the brain and calm your nervous system such as:

■ Redirecting your attention to control pain

■ Challenging negative thoughts that support pain

■ Cultivating more positive emotions

■ Developing relaxation techniques

■ Slowly increasing your activity and reconditioning yourself

■ Learning pacing techniques to balance activity and rest

Here's an example of how one of these techniques might work. If you find yourself waking up in pain and thinking, "I'm going to be miserable all day; I won't get anything done," challenge this negative thinking or self-talk with more positive thoughts. Tell yourself instead, "I've got some pain this morning, so I'll start with some relaxation and stretching exercises. Then I'll do some of the less demanding things I want to get done today." Use your mind to counteract the negative thinking. You will find more about positive thinking, relaxation, imagery, visualization, distraction, meditation, and other ways to use your mind in Chapter 5.

Tools for Managing Localized Pain

For localized pain in an area such as the neck, back, or knee, the application of heat, cold, and massage have all been found to be helpful. These three tools work by stimulating the skin and other tissues surrounding the painful area. Heat and massage increase the blood flow to these areas, while cold makes the area feel numb. All

Keep a Pain Diary

To clearly understand how your moods, activities, and conditions affect your pain, keep a pain diary. This is an expanded version of the calendar journal in Figure 4.1 on page 42. Begin by recording your activities and pain levels three times a day, at regular intervals. For each entry, do the following:

1. Record the date and time.

2. Describe the situation or your activity (watching TV, doing housework, arguing, and so on).

3. Describe the pain (for example, "deep aching pain in left lower back").

4. Rate the physical sensation of the pain on a scale from 0 (no pain) to 10 (worst pain).

5. Describe any emotional distress (for example, "felt very angry" or "wanted to cry").

6. Rate the emotional distress on a scale from 0 (no distress) to 10 (terribly distressed).

7. Describe what you did, if anything, to alleviate the discomfort (quit cleaning, took medication, massaged the area, did a relaxation exercise, took a walk, and so on) and its effect.

Look for patterns in your entries. For example, is your pain worse after sitting for a long time? Is it less when you are engaged in a favorite hobby? Such factors as your mood, fatigue, and muscle tension may affect how much you notice pain.

It's important to distinguish between physical pain sensations (physical stabbing, burning, and aching sensations) and emotional pain distress (the accompanying anger, anxiety, frustration, or sadness). This is useful because even if your pain sensations cannot be changed, you can work on changing how you feel about the pain. By doing so, you can experience less distress, anxiety, helplessness, and despair and live a healthier, happier life.

---

three methods can close the gate and change the way the brain interprets body sensations.

Apply heat with a heating pad or a warm bath or shower (with the water flow directed at the painful area). You can improvise a heating pad by placing uncooked rice or dry beans in a sock, knotting the top of the sock, and heating it in a microwave oven for three to four minutes. Before use, be sure to test the heat so you don't burn yourself. Do not use popcorn!

Some people prefer cold for soothing pain, especially if the pain is accompanied by inflammation. A bag of frozen peas or corn makes an inexpensive, reusable cold pack. Whether using heat or cold, place a towel between the source and your skin. Also, limit the application to 15 or 20 minutes at a time (longer can burn or freeze the skin).

Massage is one of the oldest forms of pain management. Hippocrates (c. 460–380 B.C.E.) said, "Physicians must be experienced in many things, but assuredly also in the rubbing that can bind a joint that is loose and loosen a joint that is too hard." Self-massage is a simple procedure that you can perform with little practice or preparation. Simply rubbing or stretching the painful area with a little applied pressure stimulates the skin, underlying tissues, and muscles. Always use a nonirritating skin cream or oil to provide lubrication. If you prefer a cooling effect, use a mentholated cream.

There are three basic approaches to self-massage:

■ **Stroking.** Place your hand on the muscle you want to massage. When you slightly cup the hand, the palm and fingers will glide over the muscle as you massage. A slow, rhythmic movement repeated over the tense or sore area works best. Experiment with different pressures. If you have an affliction such as complex regional pain syndrome, try putting your hand in a bath of warm water and then firmly stroking the painful area with your warmed hand.

■ **Kneading.** If you ever reached up and squeezed your tense neck or shoulder muscles, you were kneading. Grasp the muscle between the palm and fingers or between the thumb and fingers as if you were kneading dough. Then slightly lift and squeeze it. Don't pinch the skin; work more deeply into the muscle. A slow, rhythmic squeeze and release works best. Don't knead one spot for more than 15 or 20 seconds.

■ **Deep circular movement.** To create soothing heat (friction) that penetrates into muscle, make small circular movements with the tips of the fingers, the thumb, or the heel of the hand, depending on how large an area you are massaging. Keeping the fingers,

thumb, or palm in one place, begin lightly making small circles and slowly increase the pressure. Don't overdo it. After 10 seconds, move to another spot and repeat.

Massage is not appropriate for all cases of pain. Do not use self-massage for a "hot" joint (one that is red, swollen, and hot to the touch) or an infected area. Avoid massage if you are suffering from phlebitis (inflammation of a vein), thrombophlebitis (a blood clot in a vein), or any kind of skin bite or eruption.

Medications and other treatments can also be useful to manage localized pain. These are discussed in Chapter 16.

Tools for Managing Chronic Pain

Managing chronic pain is a complex task. Like mastering all new tasks, it requires knowledge, practice, and patience. Sometimes you can't manage pain directly unless you use medications or other treatments your doctor might recommend. (These topics are discussed in detail in Chapter 16.) But often, without medication or medical intervention, you can self-manage other symptoms that are related to chronic pain, such as stress, poor sleep, and depression. If you can address even a couple of these symptoms, you will feel more in control of your pain. The rest of this chapter and Chapter 5 are about how to self-manage common symptoms.

In addition to managing common symptoms, you can make important lifestyle choices that will positively influence your pain, your health, and your life. These include making physical activity and exercise a regular part of your week, eating healthy, managing your stress, improving your family and partner relationships, working with your health care providers, and planning for the future. That's what the rest of this book is about. Taken together, these are all tools for you to use to manage chronic pain. Just as you cannot build a house with one tool, you often need many tools to manage chronic pain.

Ineffective Breathing

Shallow or labored breathing prevents your body from getting the oxygen it needs. Like other symptoms, it can have several causes.

Causes of Breathing Problems

Pain from weak, tense muscles can lead to ineffective breathing. When an area of the body hurts, the natural response is to tense the muscles in that area. This is so automatic you are often unaware of how much tension you are carrying. Muscle tension can change how you move. You may move more slowly, or your posture may change so that your chest is not as open, leaving less room for your lungs to expand effectively.

Shallow breathing may ultimately result in muscles becoming weak and deconditioned. And this doesn't only affect your breathing muscles; the core muscles of your abdomen and the small muscles of your back can also be affected. When muscles become deconditioned, they are less efficient at doing what they are supposed to do. They require more energy (and oxygen) to perform activities.

Excess weight can also cause shortness of breath. Additional weight increases the amount of energy you use and therefore the amount of oxygen you need. Weight also increases the workload for the heart. If excess weight is coupled with restricted movement and poor posture, your body struggles to get the oxygen it needs.

Certain chronic pain conditions can directly impact posture and thereby reduce lung capacity. The list includes scoliosis, osteoporosis, and some severe forms of arthritis that attack the bones in the neck and back. Other causes of breathing problems include chronic lung diseases such as emphysema, chronic bronchitis, and asthma. These conditions usually require special medications and sometimes supplemental oxygen in addition to self-management techniques.

Shortness of breath can be frightening, and this fear can cause two additional problems. First, when you are afraid, you release hormones such as epinephrine. This causes more muscle tension and more shortness of breath. Second, you may stop activity altogether for fear it will hurt you. If this happens, you cannot build up the endurance necessary to help manage your chronic pain and breathing issues.

Breathing Self-Management Tools

Just as there are many causes of ineffective breathing, there are many things you can do to manage this problem. When you feel short of breath, don't stop what you are doing or hurry to finish up. Instead, slow down. If shortness of breath continues, stop for a few minutes. If your doctor has prescribed medication for this problem, then take it.

The basic rule is to take things slowly and gradually. Increase your activity, by not more than 25 percent each week. For example, if you are currently able to garden comfortably for 20 minutes, next week increase your time in the garden by a maximum of 5 minutes. Once you can garden comfortably for 25 minutes, you can again add a few more minutes. Chapters 6 through 9 discuss ways to increase your physical activity safely.

Finally, it is very important that you don't smoke. It might seem strange to think that smoking affects chronic pain, but it does. Recent studies have found a 20 percent increased risk of chronic musculoskeletal pain (such as back pain) in smokers.

Since we know that being exposed to secondhand smoke is also a health risk, you may want to avoid smokers as well. This can be difficult because smoking friends may not realize how they may be impacting your health. Your job is to tell them. Explain that you would appreciate it if they would not smoke when you are around. Also, make your house and especially your car "no smoking" zones. At home, ask people to smoke outside. In the car, tell them they can smoke before they get in or after you reach your destination.

There are several tools that can help with better, more effective breathing. Here we describe two effective techniques:

Diaphragmatic Breathing

Ineffective breathing can be caused by a deconditioned diaphragm (a large muscle at the bottom of your rib cage) and breathing muscles in the chest, as well as by poor posture. In either case, the lungs are not able to function properly—that is, they do not fill well, nor do they get rid of old air effectively. Most of us mainly use our upper lungs and chest for breathing. But we can breathe more deeply if we use diaphragmatic breathing, called "belly breathing." When you do this breathing technique properly, the diaphragm moves down into the abdomen and allows your lungs to expand fully with air. Diaphragmatic breathing strengthens the breathing muscles and makes them more efficient, so breathing is easier and more oxygen is available to the body.

Interestingly, babies belly breathe instinctively with little effort. For adults, though, deep breathing requires a little practice to learn to fully expand the lungs. These are the steps to practice diaphragmatic breathing:

1. Lie on your back with pillows under your head and knees.

2. Place one hand on your stomach (at the base of your breastbone) and the other hand on your upper chest.

3. Breathe in slowly through your nose, allowing your stomach to expand outward. Imagine your lungs filling with fresh air. The hand on your stomach should move upward, and the hand on your chest should not move or should move only slightly.

4. Breathe out slowly, through pursed lips. At the same time, use the hand that is on your stomach to gently push inward and upward on your abdomen.

5. Practice this technique for 10 minutes, three or four times a day, until it becomes

automatic. If you begin to feel a little dizzy, rest or breathe out more slowly.

You can also practice diaphragmatic breathing while sitting in a chair.

1. Relax your shoulders, arms, hands, and chest. Do not grip the arms of the chair or your knees.

2. Think about your posture. Sit straight, gently slide your chin back, and feel your neck lengthen. Imagine the top of your head being gently tugged upward toward the ceiling. You may notice your abdominal muscles tightening just a little.

3. Put one hand on your stomach and the other on your chest.

4. Breathe in through your nose, filling the area around your waist with air. The hand on your chest should remain still and the hand on your stomach should move.

5. Breathe out without force or effort.

Once you are comfortable with this technique, you can practice it almost anytime, while lying down, sitting, standing, or walking. Diaphragmatic breathing and paying attention to your posture can help strengthen and improve the coordination and efficiency of the breathing muscles. It also decreases the amount of energy needed to breathe and reduces overall muscle tension in your body. It can be incorporated with any of the relaxation techniques that use the power of your mind to manage your symptoms (see Chapter 5).

Pursed-lip Breathing

A second technique, pursed-lip breathing, usually happens naturally for people who have problems emptying their lungs. It can also be used if you are short of breath or breathless.

1. Breathe in, and then purse your lips as if to blow across a flute or into a whistle.

2. Using diaphragmatic breathing, breathe out through pursed lips without any force.

3. Relax the upper chest, shoulders, arms, and hands while breathing out. Check for tension. Breathing out should take longer than breathing in.

By mastering this technique while doing other activities, you will be better able to manage your shortness of breath.

Fatigue

Chronic pain can drain your energy, making fatigue a very real problem for people who experience chronic pain. Fatigue, not just pain, can keep you from doing things you'd like to do. Unfortunately, fatigue is often misunderstood by people who do not live with chronic pain. After all, others cannot usually see your fatigue.

Spouses, family members, and friends sometimes do not understand the unpredictable way in which the fatigue associated with your condition can affect you. They may think that you are just not interested in certain activities or that you just want to be alone. Sometimes you may not even know why you feel so tired.

To manage fatigue, it is important to understand that your fatigue may be related to several factors, including the following:

■ **Chronic pain itself.** When a chronic pain condition or other illness is present, the body uses energy less efficiently. This is because the energy that could be consumed by everyday activities is instead being redirected to the parts of your body affected by your condition. Therefore, your brain may release chemical signals to conserve energy and make you rest more. Also some chronic conditions are associated with anemia (low blood hemoglobin), which can contribute to fatigue.

■ **Inactivity.** Muscles that are not used regularly become deconditioned, lose strength, and are less efficient at doing what they are supposed to do. This can happen to all the muscles in our body, including the heart, which is made of muscle tissue. When the heart becomes deconditioned, its ability to pump blood is decreased. Your blood carries necessary nutrients and oxygen to other parts of the body. When muscles do not receive these nutrients and oxygen, they cannot function properly. Deconditioned muscles tire more easily than muscles in good condition.

■ **Poor nutrition.** Food is our basic source of energy. If we eat poor-quality food, eat too much food, or improperly digest food, fatigue can result. Chronic pain can cause a change in appetite. Some people overeat and gain weight. Extra weight causes fatigue by increasing the energy we need to perform daily activities. Other people lose their appetites. Eating too little, being underweight, or eating the wrong kinds of food can cause muscle tissue to break down. Less muscle means less strength and less energy. This leads to fatigue.

■ **Not enough rest.** Some people with chronic pain overdo activity and do not balance activity with rest. Others suffer from lack of sleep or poor-quality sleep. Either situation can result in fatigue. We discuss how to manage sleep problems in more detail later in this chapter, and we review ways to balance activity and rest in Chapter 6.

■ **Emotions.** Anxiety, fear, boredom, and depression can all cause fatigue. It can be exhausting to deal with the ongoing stresses that can accompany chronic pain. Being bored and not having enough to occupy your mind can also lead to fatigue. Most people are aware of the connection between stress and feeling tired, but fewer are aware that fatigue is a major symptom of depression.

■ **Medications.** Some medications, including those you may be taking for your pain, can cause fatigue. If you think your fatigue is related to your medication, talk to your doctor. Sometimes medications or dosages can be changed.

If fatigue is a problem, start by trying to determine the cause. Again, a journal may be helpful. Consider the possible causes of fatigue that are within your control to improve. Are you eating healthy foods? Are you exercising? Are you pacing your activities with rest periods? Are you getting enough good-quality sleep? Are you effectively managing stress? If you answer no to any of these questions, you may have found one or more of the reasons for your fatigue.

The important thing to remember is that your fatigue may be caused by things *other than your pain*. Therefore, to combat and prevent fatigue, you must address all the possible causes. This may mean trying a variety of self-management tools.

If your fatigue is the result of not eating well, such as eating too much junk food or drinking too much alcohol, then the solution is to eat better-quality foods in the proper quantities or to drink less alcohol. For some, the problem may be a decreased interest in food, leading to decreased food consumption and weight loss. Chapter 13 discusses some of the problems associated with eating and provides tips for healthy eating.

People often say they can't exercise because they feel fatigued. This misconception creates a vicious cycle: they are fatigued because of a lack of exercise, and they don't exercise because of the fatigue. Believe it or not, motivating yourself to exercise and be more physically active might be the answer. You don't have to run a marathon; just get outdoors and take a short walk. If that is not possible, walk around your house or try some gentle exercises like the Moving Easy Program in Chapter 8. See Chapters 7 and 9 for more information about starting an exercise program.

If emotions are causing your fatigue, rest will probably not help. In fact, it may make you feel worse, especially if your fatigue results from depression. We talk about how to deal with depression later in this chapter on pages 57–63. If you feel that your fatigue may be related to stress, read the section on managing stress on pages 65–69.

Sleep Problems

Sleep problems are common for people with chronic pain. Two out of every three people with chronic pain, and almost everyone with fibromyalgia, report poor-quality sleep. They may have trouble falling asleep, wake too early and can't get back to sleep, wake up frequently in the night, or wake up feeling tired and achy. Sleep and pain experts think that the neurochemicals that are low in people with chronic pain are critical for regulating sleep and mood. That may be one of the reasons why chronic pain, poor sleep, and depression often go together. The problem of sleep and pain is even more complicated because some prescribed pain medicines, such as morphine or codeine, can also fragment sleep.

Sleep is a basic human need, like food and water. Good-quality sleep makes you feel refreshed, rested, and reenergized, ready to face the day. When you sleep, the body heals and repairs your muscles and tissues and provides energy to your vital organs, including the brain. Sleep may also play an important role in regulating appetite. When we do not get enough good-quality sleep, we may experience a variety of symptoms. These include fatigue, inability to concentrate, irritability, increased pain, and weight gain. Of course, this does not mean that all these symptoms are always caused by a lack of sleep. Remember, the symptoms associated with chronic pain can have many causes.

Nevertheless, improving the quality of your sleep can help you manage many of these symptoms, regardless of their cause. In fact, because sleep is so important, sleep and pain experts suggest that *improving sleep quality should be a major goal of all chronic pain treatment.*

How much sleep do you need? The amount varies from person to person. Most people do best with about 7½ hours. Some feel refreshed with just 6, while others need 8 to 10 hours to function well. If you are alert, feel rested, and function well during the day, chances are you're getting enough sleep. But if you get less good sleep than you require night after night, your mood and quality of life will suffer.

Getting a Good Night's Sleep

Improving your sleep habits is one of the key steps you can take to help manage your pain. The self-management techniques we offer here are clinically proven to improve sleep quality for most people. They are not quick fixes like sleep medications, but they'll give you more effective (and safer) results in the long run. Allow yourself at least two to four weeks to see some positive results and 10 to 12 weeks for long-term improvement.

Things to do before you get into bed

- **Get a comfortable bed.** Your bed should allow for ease of movement and provide good body support. This usually means a good-quality, firm mattress that supports the spine and does not allow the body to sink in the middle of the bed. A bed board made of 1/2- to 3/4-inch (1 to 2 cm) plywood can be placed between the mattress and the box spring to increase firmness. Heated waterbeds, air beds, or foam mattresses are helpful for some people with chronic pain because they support weight evenly by conforming to the body's shape. If you are interested in one of these options, try one out at a friend's home or a hotel for a few nights to decide if it is right for you. An electric blanket or mattress pad, set on low heat, or a wool mattress pad are also effective at providing heat while you sleep. If you decide to use electric bedding, be sure to follow the instructions carefully to prevent burns.

- **Keep your hands and feet *warm* with gloves or socks.** For painful knees, it may help to cut the toes off warm stockings and wear the cut sock as sleeves over your knees.

- **Find a comfortable sleeping position.** The best position depends on you and your condition. Sometimes small pillows placed in the right places can relieve pain and discomfort. Experiment with different positions and pillow placement. Also check with your health care provider for specific recommendations given your condition. One caution: do not prop your head up on a mountain of pillows. This will aggravate a neck or back problem.

- **Elevate the head of the bed 4 to 6 inches (10 to 15 cm).** Do this if you have a problem with breathing, heartburn, or gastric reflux. You can prop sturdy wooden blocks under the bed legs or purchase an adjustable bed to raise your head during sleep.

- **Keep the room at a comfortable temperature.** This may be warm or cool. Each of us requires different conditions to sleep better.

- **Use a vaporizer if you live where the air is dry.** Warm, moist air often makes breathing and sleeping easier. If you prefer cool air at night, use a humidifier.

- **Make your bedroom safe and comfortable.** Keep a lamp and telephone by your bed, within easy reach. Get rid of scatter rugs by your bed that may be a hazard and cause you to trip and fall. If you use a cane, keep it by the bed where you can reach it easily and use it when you get up during the night.

- **Keep eyeglasses by the bed.** This way if you need to get up in the middle of the night, you can easily put on your glasses and see where you are going!

Things to avoid

- **Do not eat before bedtime.** You may feel sleepy after eating a big meal, but overeating is not an appropriate route to falling asleep quickly and getting a good night's sleep. Sleep affords your body time to rest and recover. When it is busy digesting food, the body redirects valuable time and attention from the healing process. If you find that going to sleep feeling hungry keeps you awake, try drinking a glass of warm milk at bedtime.

- **Avoid alcohol.** You may think alcohol helps you sleep better because it makes you feel relaxed and sleepy, but in fact, alcohol disrupts the sleep cycle. Alcohol consumption in the evening can lead to shallow sleep and frequent awakenings throughout the night.

- **Avoid or limit caffeine.** Caffeine is a stimulant, and it can keep you awake. Coffee, tea, colas and other sodas, and chocolate all contain caffeine. If you drink caffeinated beverages, drink them early in the day. If you have significant sleep problems, eliminate caffeine altogether to see if this has a positive effect on your sleep. If you have been a regular caffeine user, don't stop caffeine suddenly. This can cause withdrawal symptoms such as headaches and the jitters. Instead, keep a log for a couple of days that tracks the number of caffeinated drinks you have each day. Gradually reduce the number of drinks you have each day by switching to noncaffeinated beverages as much as possible.

- **Stop smoking.** Aside from the fact that smoking can cause complications for your chronic pain, falling asleep with a lit cigarette can be a fire hazard. Furthermore, the nicotine contained in cigarettes is a stimulant. Like caffeine, it impacts sleep. Quitting smoking may not be easy, but doing so will be a huge step forward in managing your chronic pain condition. For help to stop smoking, talk to your doctor or contact your local public health department or lung association.

- **Do not take diet pills.** Diet pills often contain stimulants, which may interfere with falling asleep and staying asleep.

- **Do not take sleeping medication.** Although sleeping pills may seem like the perfect solution for sleep problems, they are not a viable long-term answer. For one thing, sleeping medications tend to become less effective over time. Also, many sleeping pills have a rebound effect—that is, if you stop taking them, it is even more difficult to get to sleep or stay asleep than it was before you began taking them. Sometimes your doctor may recommend a short course of sleeping pills (a few weeks at most) together with improving your sleep practices, such as limiting your time in bed and using your bedroom only for sleep and sex and nothing else. (See the *How to develop a routine* list below.) This combination of short-use medication and sleep-friendly practices may be helpful for people with chronic pain who have significant sleep problems. Sleep specialists agree that these sorts of approaches, instead of sleeping pills, offer the best long-term solution to poor sleep. Other types of medicines prescribed for your chronic pain may also improve sleep (see Chapter 16).

- **Do not use or watch any blue-light emitting devices such as computers, TVs, tablets, cellphones, or some e-readers for about an hour before you go to bed.** The light from these devices can disrupt your natural sleep rhythms.

- **Avoid diuretics (water pills) before bedtime.** If you are on diuretics, take them in the morning so your sleep is not interrupted by frequent trips to the bathroom. Unless your doctor has recommended otherwise, don't reduce the overall amount of fluids you drink, as fluids are important for your health. However, you may want to limit the amount you drink right before you go to bed.

How to develop a routine

- **Maintain a regular rest and sleep schedule.** Go to bed at the same time every night and get up at the same time every morning. Even though you may feel tired on some mornings, getting up at the same time each day helps your body maintain its natural sleep cycle. If you wish to take a brief nap, take one in the afternoon but only for 10 to 20 minutes, no more. Do not take a nap in the evening after dinner. Stay awake until you are ready to go to bed.

- **Reset your sleep clock when necessary.** If your sleep schedule gets off track (for example, you go to bed at 4:00 A.M. and sleep until noon one day), you need to reset your internal sleep clock. To do so, try going to bed an hour earlier (or later) each day until you reach the hour you want to go to sleep.

- **Exercise at regular times each day.** Not only does exercise help you sleep more soundly, it also helps establish a regular pattern for your day. However, avoid vigorous exercise in the evening before bedtime.

- **Get out in the sun every morning.** Exposure to sunlight is important, even if it is only for 15 or 20 minutes. A regular dose of morning sun helps regularize your body clock and rhythms.

- **Practice relaxation techniques at regular times each day.** This doesn't have to be complicated. Even 10 minutes of deep belly breathing can help. Just like regular exercise, this establishes a regular pattern to your day, and quiets your nervous system. To learn more about techniques that can help you relax as you prepare for sleep, see Chapter 5.

- **Do the same things every night before going to bed.** This can be anything from listening to calm music on the radio to reading a chapter of a book to taking a warm bath. By developing and sticking to a "get ready for bed" routine, you are letting your body know that it's time to start winding down and relax.

■ **Use your bedroom only for sleeping and sex.** If you have had pain for some time, you may have begun to use your bedroom for activities other than sleep. Awake activities such as watching TV or balancing your checkbook keep you alert. When you do these activities in your bed, being in bed becomes a signal for your body to be alert. So you cannot relax and fall asleep. If you carry out these activities in bed because you are in pain and need to recline, move to another room where you can relax comfortably and do all your awake activities there instead. Reserve your bedroom for sleep and sex only! If you find that you get into bed and you can't fall asleep, get out of bed and go into another room until you begin to feel sleepy again. Keep the lighting low when you are awake at night no matter what room you are in—bright lights signal to your body that it is time to be up and about.

What to do when you can't get back to sleep

Many people can get to sleep without a problem but then they wake up with the "early morning worries" and can't turn off their minds. This becomes a vicious circle, if they become even more worried because they cannot go back to sleep once they have awakened.

Keeping your mind occupied with pleasurable or interesting thoughts wards off the worries and helps you get back to sleep. For example, try a distraction technique to quiet your mind such as counting backward from 100 by threes or naming a flower or sports team for every letter of the alphabet. The relaxation techniques described in Chapter 5 may also be helpful. If you still can't fall sleep, get up, leave your bedroom, and do something—read a book, wash your hair, or play a game of solitaire (not on the computer). After 15 or 20 minutes, go back to your bedroom and go back to bed.

It can also help to set a "worry time." Does a racing mind regularly keep you awake? If it does, designate a regular time well before bedtime during which you write down your problems and concerns, and then make a to-do list. You can relax and sleep well at night, knowing that you have some ideas to address your concerns. You may not solve your worries right away, but there will always be tomorrow's worry time to come up with new ideas for your to-do list.

Sleep Apnea and Snoring

If you are tired when you wake up in the morning, even after a full night's sleep, you may have a sleep disorder. People who have the most common sleep disorder, obstructive sleep apnea, often do not know it. When they are asked about their sleep, they respond, "I sleep just fine." Sometimes the only clue is that others complain about their loud snoring. Sleep specialists believe that obstructive sleep apnea is very common and alarmingly under-diagnosed.

When people have sleep apnea, the soft tissue in the throat or nose relaxes during sleep and blocks the airway. This makes breathing an extreme effort. The person struggles against the blockage for up to a minute, wakes just long enough to gasp air, then falls back to sleep to start the cycle all over again. The person is rarely aware that he or she has awakened dozens of times during the night. This, in turn, leads to symptoms such as fatigue and pain, because the body does not get the deep sleep needed to restore energy and help with the healing process.

Sleep apnea can be a serious or even life-threatening medical problem. It has been linked to heart disease and stroke. Sleep experts suggest that people should be evaluated for sleep apnea or other disorders if they are tired all the time in spite of a full night's sleep or need more sleep now than when they were younger. It is especially urgent that you are checked if you (or your spouse) report snoring.

Getting Professional Help for Sleep Problems

You can self-manage many sleep problems with the techniques we have discussed, but there are times when you need professional assistance. When should you get help?

- If your pain causes sleep problems two to three times a night and you are unable to

fall asleep in a timely manner once you awaken

- If poor-quality sleep continues to seriously affect your daytime functioning (your job or your social relationships), after you have faithfully followed the self-help program described in this chapter

- If you have great difficulty staying awake during the day and your daytime sleepiness causes or comes close to causing an accident

- If your sleep is disturbed by breathing difficulties, including loud snoring with long pauses, chest pain, heartburn, leg twitching, or other related physical conditions

- If your sleep problems are accompanied by depression or problems with alcohol, sleeping medications, or addictive drugs

Don't put off asking for help. Most sleep problems can be addressed. Once sleep is improved, many people find that there is an improvement in their chronic pain and their mood.

Depression

Most people with chronic pain feel depressed sometimes. Scientists think that an imbalance of certain chemicals in your brain (such as the neurotransmitters serotonin and norepinephrine) is involved in chronic pain, depression, and sleep disorders. Just as there are different degrees of pain, there are different degrees of depression. These range from feeling occasionally sad or blue to serious clinical depression. Clinical depression, which is also referred to as

major depression, is characterized by a constant feeling of hopelessness and despair. About 27 percent of people with chronic pain who seek the care of a family doctor experience clinical depression. The rate of clinical depression is even higher for those who attend a pain clinic.

Sometimes a person may not realize he or she is depressed. And often people do not want to admit to being depressed. How you handle depression makes the difference.

What is Depression?

Feeling sad sometimes is natural. "Normal" sadness is a temporary feeling, often linked to a specific event or loss. We sometimes mistakenly use the word *depressed* to describe feeling sad or disappointed: "I'm really depressed about missing out on visiting with my friends." In these circumstances we feel sad, but we can still relate to others and find joy in other areas of our lives.

Sometimes sadness affects you more deeply or lasts longer, as when you lose a loved one or are diagnosed with a serious illness. If, however, those sad feelings are especially severe, long-lasting, and recurrent, you may be experiencing clinical depression. Clinical depression drains the pleasure out of life, leaving you feeling hopeless, helpless, and worthless. With clinical depression, you may become numb, and even crying brings no relief.

Depression affects everything: the way you think, the way you behave, the way you interact with others, and even the way your body functions.

What Contributes to Depression?

Depression is not caused by personal weakness, laziness, or lack of willpower. Heredity, chronic pain conditions, medications, even the weather may all play a role in depression. The way you think, especially negative thoughts, can also produce and sustain a depressed mood. Negative thoughts associated with depression can be automatic, recur endlessly, and often are not linked to any event or triggering cause.

Certain feelings and emotions also contribute to depression. They include:

- **Fear, anxiety, or uncertainty about the future.** Worries about finances, your family, or your pain condition or treatment can lead to depression. If you face these issues as soon as possible, both you and your family will spend less time worrying and have more time to enjoy life. This can have a healing effect. We talk more about these issues and how to deal with them in Chapter 20.

- **Frustration.** Frustration can have many causes. You may find yourself thinking, "I just can't do what I want," "I feel so helpless," "I used to be able to do this myself," or "Why doesn't anyone understand me?" The longer you accept these feelings, the more alone and isolated you are likely to feel.

- **Loss of control over your life.** When you are living with chronic pain, many things can make you feel like you are losing control. These include having to rely on medications, having to see a doctor on a regular basis, or having to count on others to help you do things you used to do yourself. Feeling like you have lost control can make you lose faith in yourself and your abilities. Even though you may not be able to do everything yourself, you can still be in charge. Remember: as a self-manager, you are the coach for your team.

A person may not even realize they have depression, or they may feel it but attempt to hide it. Sometimes unrealistic cheeriness masks what a person is really feeling, and only the wise and sensitive observer recognizes the brittleness or phoniness of the mood. Refusal to accept offers of help, even in the face of obvious need for it, is a frequent symptom of unrecognized depression.

Am I Depressed?

Here is a quick test for depression: Ask yourself what you do to have fun. If you do not have a quick answer, consider your mood over the past two weeks. Have you experienced any of the following symptoms?

- **Little interest or pleasure in doing things.** An inability to enjoy life or other people may be a sign of depression. Symptoms include not wanting to talk to anyone, go out, or answer the phone or doorbell.

- **Feeling down, depressed, or hopeless.** Feeling persistently blue can be a symptom of depression.

- **Trouble falling or staying asleep, or sleeping too much.** Awakening and being unable to return to sleep or sleeping too much and not wanting to get out of bed can signal a problem.

- **Feeling tired or having little energy.** Fatigue—feeling tired all the time—is often a symptom of depression.

- **Poor appetite or overeating.** This may range from a loss of interest in food to unusually erratic or excessive eating.

- **Feeling bad about yourself.** Have you felt that you are a failure or have let yourself or your family down? Do you doubt your self-worth or have a negative image of your body?

- **Trouble concentrating.** Have you found it hard to do such things as reading the newspaper or watching television?

- **Lethargy or restlessness.** Have you been moving or speaking so slowly that other people have noticed? Or the opposite—have you been much more fidgety or restless than usual? Either can be a sign of depression.

- **Wishing yourself harm or worse.** Thoughts that you would be better off dead or of hurting yourself in some way are often the hallmark of clinical depression.

Depressed people may also experience weight gain or loss, loss of interest in sex or intimacy, loss of interest in personal care and grooming, inability to make decisions, and more frequent accidents.

If several of these symptoms seem to apply to you, please seek help from someone you trust—your doctor, a member of the clergy, a psychologist, or a social worker. Do not wait for these feelings to pass. If you are thinking about harming yourself or others, get help now. Don't let a tragedy happen to you and your loved ones.

Fortunately, the treatments for depression including antidepressant medications, counseling, and self-help, are highly effective in decreasing its frequency, length, and severity. Depression, like other symptoms, can be managed.

Depression can lead to withdrawal, isolation, and cessation of physical activity. These behaviors can cycle back to create more depressed feelings. The paradox of depression-related behavior is that the more you engage in isolationist behavior, the more you drive away the people who can support and comfort you. Most of our friends and family want to help us feel better, but often they don't really know what to do. As their efforts to comfort and reassure us are frustrated, they may eventually throw up their hands and quit trying. Then the depressed person winds up saying, "See, nobody cares." This again reinforces the feelings of loss and loneliness.

All these factors, along with chronic pain itself, can contribute to an imbalance in the chemicals in your brain called neurotransmitters. This imbalance can result in changes in the way you think, feel, and act. Thinking and behaving in a more positive, proactive manner can be a powerful and effective way to change your brain chemistry, lighten depression, and even simply improve ordinary bad moods.

Treating Depression

The most effective treatments for depression are antidepressant medications, counseling, and self-help. We discuss each of these in the material that follows.

Medications

Antidepressant medications that help balance brain chemistry are highly effective. They can also help relieve pain directly, lessen anxiety, and improve sleep (see Chapter 16). It can take several days to several weeks for most antidepressant medications to begin to work. Then they usually bring significant relief. Don't be discouraged if you don't feel better immediately. Stick with it. To get the maximum benefit you may need to take some medications for six months or more.

Side effects of antidepressant medication are usually most noticeable in the first few weeks and then lessen or go away. If the side effects are not especially severe, continue to take your medication. As your body gets used to the medication, you will begin to feel better. It is important to remember to take your medication every day. If you stop because you're feeling better (or worse), you may relapse. Antidepressant medications are not addictive. If you have significant side effects or if the medications are not helping, talk with your doctor before stopping or changing the dose.

Counseling

Several types of psychotherapy, particularly cognitive-behavior therapy, can be highly effective in relieving symptoms of depression. As with medications, counseling rarely has an immediate effect. It may be weeks (or longer) before you see improvement. Therapy time can be brief, usually involving one to two sessions a week for several months. By teaching you new skills and ways to think and relate, psychotherapy may also help reduce the risk of recurrent depression.

Self-help

Self-help for depression can be surprisingly effective. You can learn many psychotherapy techniques on your own. For mild to moderate depression or just to lift your mood, the self-management strategies discussed here can be very productive. One study showed that reading and practicing self-help advice improved depression in nearly 70 percent of patients.

These skills and strategies can be used alone or to supplement medications and counseling.

- **Eliminate the negative.** Being alone and isolating yourself, crying a lot, getting angry and yelling, blaming your failure or bad mood on others, or using alcohol or other drugs usually leaves you feeling worse. Tranquilizers or narcotic painkillers such as Valium®, Librium®, Restoril®, Vicodin®, codeine, sleeping medications, or other "downers" intensify depression or may cause depression as a side effect. However, if you have been prescribed one of these medicines, do not stop taking it before first talking with your doctor. There may be important reasons for continuing its use, or you may experience withdrawal reactions.

Alcohol is also a downer. For most people, one or two drinks in the early evening is not a problem, but if your mind is not free of alcohol during most of the day, you are having trouble with this drug. Talk this over with your health care provider or seek help from Alcoholics Anonymous.

■ **Plan for pleasure.** When you are feeling blue or depressed, the tendency is to withdraw, isolate yourself, and restrict activities. That is, in fact, the wrong thing to do. Maintaining or increasing activities is one of the best antidotes for depression. Go for a walk, look at a sunset, watch a funny movie, get a massage, learn another language, take a cooking class, or join a social club. Activities like these can help keep your spirits up and prevent you from falling into a depression.

But sometimes having fun isn't such an easy prescription. You may have to make a deliberate effort to plan pleasurable activities. Don't leave good things to chance. Consider making a schedule of what you'd like to do with your free time during the week. Even if you don't feel like doing it, try to stick to your activity schedule. That nature walk, cup of tea, or half hour of listening to music may well improve your mood despite your initial misgivings.

If you are feeling hardly any emotion and the world seems devoid of color, make an effort to put some sensation back into your life. Go to a bookstore and look through your favorite section. Listen or dance to some upbeat music. Exercise or schedule a massage so you can reconnect with your body. Eat some spicy food. Treat yourself to a fragrant herbal bath, or try a cold shower. Go to a garden center and smell all the flowers.

Make plans and carry them out. Look to the future. Plant some young trees. Look forward to your grandchildren's graduation from college even if your own kids are in high school. If you know that one time of the year is especially difficult, such as Christmas or a birthday, make specific plans to be active during that period. Don't wait to see what happens. Be prepared.

■ **Take action.** Continue your daily activities. Get dressed every day and take pride in your appearance. Make your bed, get out of the house, go shopping, walk your dog. Plan and cook meals. Force yourself to do these things even if you don't feel like it.

Taking action to solve your most immediate problems provides the surest relief from negative feelings. More important than what you change or how much you change are the confidence-building feelings that come from successfully changing something—anything! Taking action is the important thing. You might decide to clean or reorganize a room, for instance, or a closet or even a desk drawer. Even a single simple action can boost your mood. Get a new magazine subscription, or call an old friend.

When you are feeling emotionally vulnerable, do not set difficult goals for yourself or take on a lot of responsibility. Break large tasks into small ones, set some priorities, and do what you can as best you can. Learn some of the proven steps for taking successful action (see Chapter 2). It may be wise not to make big life decisions when you are feeling depressed. For example, don't move without first visiting the new setting for a few weeks and learning about the resources available to you in this new community. Moving can be a sign of withdrawal, and depression often intensifies when you are in a location away from friends and acquaintances. Besides, many troubles may move with you. At the same time, the support you may need to deal with your troubles may have been left behind.

■ **Socialize.** Don't isolate yourself. Try to seek out positive, optimistic people who can lighten your heavy feelings. Make an effort to see family and friends you enjoy. Get involved in a church group, a book club, a community college class, a self-help class, or a nutrition program. If you can't get out, consider joining a group on the Internet. If you join an online group, be sure it is moderated—that is, that someone is in charge to enforce the rules of the group.

■ **Move your mood.** Physical activity lifts depression and negative moods. Depressed people often complain that they feel too tired to exercise. But the feelings of fatigue associated with depression are not due to physical exhaustion. Try to get at least 20 to 30 minutes of some type of exercise every day. It can be walking, yard work, chair dancing—anything. If you can get yourself moving, you may find that you have more energy (see Chapters 7 to 9).

■ **Think positive.** Many people tend to be excessively critical of themselves, especially when they're depressed. You may find yourself thinking groundless, untrue things about yourself.

Challenge your automatic negative thoughts by rescripting the negative stories you tell yourself (see Chapter 5). For example, one of your underlying beliefs may be, "Unless I do everything perfectly, I'm a failure." Perhaps this belief could be revised to, "Success is doing the best that I can in any situation." Also, when you are depressed, it's easy to forget that anything nice has happened at all. Make a list of some of the good or positive events in your life.

■ **Do something for someone else.** Lending a helping hand is one of the most effective ways to change a bad mood, but it is one of the least commonly used. Arrange to babysit for a friend, read a story to someone who is ill, or volunteer at a soup kitchen. When you're depressed, you may greet this advice with thoughts like, "I've got enough troubles of my own. I don't need anyone else's." But if you can bring yourself to help someone else, even in a small way, you'll feel better about yourself. Feeling useful is good for self-esteem, and you will be temporarily distracted from your own problems. Helping others who are needier than yourself can help you appreciate your own assets and capabilities. Your problems and difficulties may not appear as overwhelming. Sometimes helping others is the surest way to help yourself.

Don't be discouraged if it takes some time to feel better. If, however, these self-help strategies alone are not sufficient, seek help from your physician or a mental health professional. Often some "talk therapy" or the use of antidepressant medications (or both) can go a long way toward relieving depression. Seeking professional help and taking medications are not signs of weakness. They are signs of strength.

Anger

Anger and frustration are common reactions to chronic pain. The uncertainty and unpredictability of living with chronic pain may threaten your independence and control. You may find yourself asking, "Why me? It's so unfair." This is a normal response to a persistent pain problem that impacts all areas of your life.

You may be angry with yourself, family, friends, health care providers, God, or the world in general. For example, you may be angry at yourself for not taking better care of yourself. You may be angry at your family and friends because they don't do things the way you want. Or you might be angry at your doctor and other health care providers because they cannot fix your problems. Some people who are depressed or have anxiety disorders express their depression or anxiety through anger.

It is no wonder that people with chronic pain are upset at times. However, anger and frustration, especially when inappropriately expressed, are emotions that can block effective management of pain. Anger can result in lack of motivation, inactivity, hostility toward others, and "acting out" behavior (such as

blowing up, shouting, or other more aggressive actions). These behaviors can alienate those who can help you most. This can increase your sense of isolation and lead to more anger and frustration. The first step to self-managing your anger is recognizing and admitting that you are angry. The second step is identifying the reason for your anger. Managing your anger also involves finding constructive ways to express your emotions.

Managing your Anger

Research now suggests that people who vent their anger actually get angrier. But suppressing anger isn't the answer either. The angry feelings often smolder, only to flare up later. There are some strategies you can use to reduce hostile feelings including the following:

■ Raise your anger threshold—that is, allow fewer things to trigger your anger in the first place.

■ Choose how to react when you get angry— without either denying your feelings or giving in to the situation.

This sounds simple enough, but what gets in the way is our tendency to see anger as coming from outside ourselves—something over which we have little control. We see ourselves as helpless victims. We blame others and say, "You make me so angry!" We explode and then say, "I couldn't help it." We see spouses as selfish and insensitive, bosses as snobs or bullies, friends as unappreciative. So it seems that our only choice is an outburst of hostility. But with a little practice, even a seasoned hothead can master a new repertoire of healthy and more effective responses.

Strategies for Anger Management

There are several things you can do to help manage your anger.

Reason with yourself

How you interpret and explain a situation determines whether you feel angry about it. You can learn to defuse anger by pausing and questioning your anger-producing thoughts. If you change your thoughts, you can change your response. You can decide whether or not to get angry and then whether or not to act.

At the first sign of anger, count to three and ask yourself the following questions:

- **Is this really important enough to get angry about?** Maybe this incident isn't serious enough to merit the time and energy. Determine if the issue will really make a big difference in your life. If not, it doesn't warrant flying into a rage.

- **Am I justified in getting angry?** You may need to gather more information to really understand the situation. More information

may prevent you from jumping to conclusions or misinterpreting the intentions or actions of others.

- **Will getting angry make a difference?** More often than not, losing your cool does not work and may even be punishing. Exploding or venting increases your angry feelings, puts a strain on your relationships, and potentially damages your health.

Cool off

Any technique that relaxes or distracts you—such as meditating or taking a long walk—can help put out the fire within. Slow, deep breathing is one of the quickest and simplest ways to cool off (see page 49). When you notice anger building, take ten slow, relaxed breaths before responding. Sometimes withdrawing and spending some time alone can defuse the situation. Physical exercise also provides a good natural outlet for stress and anger.

Verbalize without blame

One important skill is to learn how to communicate your anger out loud, preferably without blaming or offending others. This can be done by learning to use "I" (rather than "you") messages to express your feelings. (Refer to Chapter 10 for a discussion of "I" messages.) However, if you choose to express your anger verbally, know that many people will not be able to help you address the cause of your anger. Most of us are not very good at dealing with angry people. This is true even if the anger is justified.

If you really feel the need to vent, you may find it useful to seek counseling or join a support group. Nonprofit organizations, such as the various chronic pain, heart, diabetes, arthritis, and other health-related associations, may be useful resources in this area.

Modify your expectations

You have modified your expectations throughout your life. For example, as a child you thought you could become anything—a fireman, a ballet dancer, a doctor, and so on. As you grew older, however, you reevaluated these expectations, along with your capabilities, talents, and interests. Based on this reevaluation, you modified your plans.

This same process can be used to deal with the frustration of having chronic pain in your life. For example, it may be unrealistic to expect that you will ever be "all better." However, it is realistic to expect that you can still do many pleasurable things. Changing your expectations can help you change your perspective. Instead of dwelling on the 10 percent of things you can no longer do, think about the 90 percent of things you can still do.

In short, anger is a normal response to having a condition like chronic pain. Part of learning to manage the condition involves acknowledging this anger and finding constructive ways to deal with it.

Stress

Stress is a common problem. But what is stress? In the 1950s, the physiologist Hans Selye described stress as "the nonspecific response of the body to any demand made upon it." Others describe stress as the body's way of adapting to demands, whether pleasant or unpleasant. You may feel stress after experiencing negative events, such as the death of a loved one, or even joyful events such as the marriage of a child.

How Does the Body Respond to Stress?

Your body is used to functioning at a certain level. When there is a need to change this level, your body adjusts to meet the demand. It reacts by preparing to take some action: your heart rate increases, your blood pressure rises, your neck and shoulder muscles tense, your breathing becomes more rapid, your digestion slows, your mouth becomes dry, and you may begin sweating. These are signals of what we call stress.

Why does this happen? To act, your muscles need to be supplied with oxygen and energy. Your breathing increases in an effort to inhale as much oxygen as possible and to get rid of as much carbon dioxide as possible. Your heart rate increases to deliver oxygen and nutrients to the muscles. At the same time, body functions that are not immediately necessary, such as the digestion of food and natural immune responses, slow down.

In general, these responses last only until the stressful event passes. Your body then returns to its normal level of functioning. Sometimes, though, your body does not return to its former comfortable level. If the stress is present for any length of time, your body begins adapting to it. This chronic stress can contribute to the onset of some chronic conditions and can make symptoms more difficult to manage.

Common Stressors

Regardless of the type of stressor, the changes in the body are the same. Stressors, however, are not completely independent of one another. In fact, one stressor can often lead to other stressors or magnify the effects of existing stressors. Several stressors can also occur at the same time. For instance, fatigue can cause anxiety, frustration, inactivity, and loss of endurance. Let's examine some of the most common sources of stress.

Physical stressors

Physical stressors include the physical symptoms of your chronic pain condition, but they also can be something as pleasant as picking up a new baby or going shopping. What do all these stressors have in common? They increase your body's demand for energy. If your body is not prepared to deal with this demand, the results may be anything from sore muscles to fatigue or a worsening of other symptoms.

Mental and emotional stressors

Mental and emotional stressors can also be either pleasant or uncomfortable. The joys you experience from seeing a child get married or meeting new friends may induce a similar stress response as your feelings of frustration about your illness. Although this fact may seem surprising, the similarity comes from the way your brain perceives the stress.

Environmental stressors

Environmental stressors, too, can be both good and bad. They may be as varied as a sunny day, a sandy beach, uneven sidewalks, loud noises, bad weather, a snoring spouse, or secondhand smoke. Each creates a pleasurable or apprehensive excitement that triggers the stress response.

Exercise is a Good Stressor

Some sources of stress can be good, such as a job promotion, a wedding, a vacation, a new friendship, or a new baby. These stressors make you feel happy but still cause the changes in your body that we have just discussed. Another example of a good stressor is exercise.

When you exercise or do any type of physical activity, a demand is placed on your body. The heart has to work to deliver blood to the muscles. The lungs are working harder, and you breathe more rapidly to keep up with your muscles' demand for oxygen. Meanwhile, your muscles are responding to the signals from your brain, which is telling them to keep moving.

As you maintain an exercise program for several weeks, you will begin to notice a change. What once seemed virtually impossible now becomes easier. The same exercises put less strain on your heart, lungs, and other muscles because they have become more efficient and you have become more fit. What has happened? Your body has adapted to stress.

The same can happen with psychological stresses. Many people become more resilient and stronger emotionally after experiencing emotional challenges and learning to adapt to them.

Recognizing When You Feel Stressed

Everyone needs a certain amount of stress. It helps your life run more efficiently. And most of us can tolerate more stress on some days than on others. But sometimes you can go beyond your breaking point and feel that your life is out of control. Often it is difficult to recognize when you are under too much stress. The following are some of the warning signs:

- Biting your nails, pulling your hair, tapping your foot, or other repetitive habits
- Grinding your teeth or clenching your jaw
- Tension in your head, neck, or shoulders
- Feeling anxious, nervous, helpless, or irritable
- Frequent accidents
- Forgetting things you usually don't forget
- Difficulty concentrating
- Fatigue and exhaustion

Some of these are also signs of chronic pain. That's why chronic pain is like a type of chronic stress.

Of course, there are many things that can make you feel stressed, not just your pain. Sometimes you may catch yourself when you are behaving or feeling stressed. When you do, take a few minutes to think about what is making you feel tense. Take a few deep breaths and try to relax. Also, a quick body scan can help you recognize stress in your body. You will learn how to perform a body scan and other good ideas for coping with stress in Chapter 5.

Dealing with Stress

Dealing effectively with stress doesn't have to be complicated. In fact, it can start with a simple three-step process:

1. **Identify your stressors by making a list.** Consider every area of your life: family, relationships, health, financial security, living environment, and so on.

2. **Sort your stressors.** For each stressor, ask yourself two things: Is it important or unimportant? Is it changeable or unchangeable? Then place each of your stressors in one of four categories:

   - Important and changeable
   - Important and unchangeable
   - Unimportant and changeable
   - Unimportant and unchangeable

   For example, the need to quit smoking is changeable and, for most people, important. Loss of a loved one or a job is important and unchangeable. The bad record of your favorite sports team, a traffic jam, or bad weather is unchangeable and may or may not be important. What really counts is what you think about each stressor.

3. **Match your strategy to each stressor.** Different strategies work for different stressors. The following are some strategies to help manage the different types of stressors more effectively.

   - **Important and changeable stressors.** These stressors are best managed by taking action to change the situation and to reduce the stress associated with them. Useful problem-solving skills include planning and goal setting (see Chapter 2); imagery (see page 85); positive, healthy thinking (see page 84), effective communication (see Chapter 10), and seeking social support.

   - **Important and unchangeable stressors.** These stressors are often the most difficult to manage. They can make you feel helpless and hopeless. No matter what you do, you cannot make another person change, bring someone back from the dead, or delete traumatic experiences from your life. Even though you may not be able to change the situation, you may be able to use one or more of the following strategies to deal with it:

1. **Change the way you think about the problem.** For example, consider how much worse it could be, focus on the positive and practice gratitude (see page 94), ignore the problem, distract yourself (see page 82), or simply accept what you can't change.

2. **Find some part of the problem that you can reclassify as changeable.** You can't stop a hurricane, but you can take steps to prepare for it, or you can rebuild if it's already struck.

3. **Reassess how important the problem is in light of your overall life and priorities.** Maybe your neighbor's criticism isn't so important after all.

4. **Change your emotional reactions to the situation.** You can't change what happened, but you can help yourself feel less distressed about it. Write your deepest thoughts and feelings in a journal (see page 95), seek social support, help others, practice relaxation techniques, use imagery, enjoy humor, or exercise.

◆ **Unimportant and changeable stressors.** If the stressor is unimportant, first try just letting it go. But if you can control it with relatively little effort, go ahead and deal with it. Solving small problems helps build your skills and confidence to tackle bigger ones. You can use the same strategies to address unimportant and changeable stressors that you use for important and changeable problems.

◆ **Unimportant and unchangeable stressors.** These are common hassles, and everybody has their share of them. The best solution for these problems is to ignore them. Starting now, you are given permission to let go of unimportant concerns. Don't let them bother you. Distract yourself with humor, relaxation, imagery, or focusing on more pleasurable things.

Also, it is important to know that certain chemicals you ingest can increase stress responses in your body. These include nicotine, alcohol, and caffeine. Some people smoke a cigarette, drink a glass of wine or beer, eat sugary candy, or drink a cup of coffee to soothe their tension, but this may actually increase stress. Eliminating or cutting down on these chemicals can help you feel less stressed.

Managing Stress and Problem Solving

Consider some situations that you recognize as stressful, such as being stuck in traffic, traveling, or preparing a meal. First, look at what it is about the particular situation that is stressful. Do traffic jams bother you because you hate to be late? Are trips stressful because of uncertainty about your destination? Does meal preparation involve too many steps and demand too much energy?

Once you have determined what the problem is, begin looking for possible ways to reduce the stress. When you travel by car, can you leave earlier or let someone else drive? Before a trip, can you contact someone at your destination and ask about wheelchair access, local mass transit, and other concerns? When you need to cook a meal, can you prepare food in the morning or take a short nap in the early afternoon?

If you know that certain situations make you stressed, develop ways to deal with them before they happen. Try to rehearse, in your mind, what you will do when the situation arises so you will be ready. After you have identified some possible solutions, select one to try the next time you face the situation. Then evaluate the results. (Recall that this is the problem-solving approach that was discussed in Chapter 2.)

Earlier in this chapter, we discussed how you can successfully manage some types of stress by modifying the situation. But sometimes stress sneaks up on you when you don't expect it. Dealing with unexpected stress involves problem solving just as dealing with other stressful situations does. As noted earlier, important tools for dealing with stress include getting enough sleep, exercising, and eating well. But sometimes stress is so overwhelming that these tools are not enough. These are times when good self-managers turn to consultants such as counselors, social workers, psychologists, or psychiatrists.

In summary, stress, like every other symptom, has many causes and can therefore be managed in many different ways. It is up to you to examine the problem and try to find solutions that meet your needs and suit your lifestyle.

Memory Problems

Many people worry about changes in their memory, particularly as they age. Although we all forget things, some people with chronic pain have memory problems that are not a normal part of aging. For people with chronic pain, memory problems may be caused by medications, other symptoms like depression, or other illnesses like dementia. But changes in memory and in thinking can also be a symptom of the pain condition itself. Scientists think this happens because of multiple changes in the brain caused by the constant barrage of pain signals. People with fibromyalgia seem especially prone to problems of memory and concentration. This is commonly referred to as "fibro fog."

Fibro fog and memory problems related to other chronic pain conditions make it more difficult to complete everyday tasks. You might feel confused. It may be challenging to think clearly, pay attention, remember new information, or concentrate on new things. Although this can be upsetting and frustrating, there are things you can do to manage this symptom.

As mentioned, memory problems can be a sign of other disorders, such as depression or disease, or they may result from some of the medications you take for your pain. Be sure to talk with your doctor openly about your problems with memory, concentration, or thinking. He or she will be able to assess your situation and help you manage your memory-related symptoms.

Self-management Tips for Memory and Thinking Problems

- Talk to your family about this problem. If you do, they will better understand your behavior and support you.

- Give yourself enough time to finish a task. Try not to rush. Don't let others hurry you.

- Don't try to accomplish too many things at the same time. Do one task at a time. If a task is complex, break it down into smaller steps. See Chapter 6 on pacing for other suggestions. The important thing is not to take on more than you can handle comfortably.

- Be physically active. This will increase the flow of blood and oxygen to the brain, which can help you think more clearly.

- Practice relaxation techniques on a regular basis. Make relaxation part of your daily routine. Relaxation can quiet the nervous system and, like physical activity, it can improve the quality of your thinking.

- Reduce distractions. When you are trying to concentrate or pay attention to something, turn down the radio, shut off the TV, or find some place quiet.

- Reduce clutter in your home. Assign a regular place for things like your keys or cell phone and get in the habit of putting things back in their place after you use them. This will help keep you more organized.

- Use reminders to stay on track. Place sticky notes in different locations in the house, or make lists in a calendar, notebook, or on your computer or cell phone so that you remember important appointments or tasks you want to do.

- Take a family member or friend with you to important appointments. That way you won't miss out on important information if you are having trouble paying attention or remembering new information.

Coping with Unemployment

Not being able to work at one's occupation is not a symptom like fatigue or depression, but it can be a consequence of chronic pain. A change in your employment status may be one more change in your life that requires major readjustment.

Questions like "What do you do for a living?" or "Are you back to work yet?" are commonly asked in everyday social conversation. When we are not working due to a problem like chronic pain, questions about employment, however well meaning, can be awkward, discouraging, and even infuriating. It's natural for others to be interested in your work life, but it's also natural if you become sensitive about the frequent inquiries.

For most people, work is how we define ourselves. Telling others where we work and what we

Causes of Unemployment

Most causes of unemployment are beyond an individual's control and unemployment affects millions of people each year. Restructuring, downsizing, work shortages, the changing labor force, regional or global issues, as well as disability or injury are all causes of unemployment and impact people with and without chronic pain alike.

But there are special concerns for people with health problems such as chronic pain. Chronic pain can affect your energy, concen-tration, and physical tolerances. It can be-come difficult to maintain expected productiv-ity levels or to perform work duties in general. The challenge faced by people with chronic pain who've lost a job is not to blame them-selves or be consumed by blaming others for their change in employment status. If you are one of these people, it is important that you utilize problem-solving skills and pain man-agement strategies to regain as much control as possible.

---

do has become a standard way to introduce our-selves and communicate who we are. For exam-ple, someone may introduce himself by saying, "My name is Joe and I'm the manager of Ace Busi-ness Products." In this scenario, Joe's roles and interests as husband, father, scout leader, com-puter enthusiast, and gardening expert are treated as secondary information. When not working we are forced to redefine our lives more broadly, not just by our place or type of employment.

Impact of Job Loss

Your reaction to losing employment depends on a number of factors.

■ **How did you feel about the job?** Did you like or dislike the work and environment?

■ **How attached were you to a particular workplace?** How long did you work there? Did you plan to remain there long term? How positive were your relationships with coworkers and superiors?

■ **Do you have prior experience coping with crisis?** Have you successfully coped with previous periods of unemployment or other obstacles in life?

■ **What is the nature or degree of your physi-cal limitation?** Are you able to assume dif-ferent responsibilities or change positions within the workplace or company?

■ **Do you have advanced or special educa-tion or transferable skills?** Are you able to utilize related skills in another position or organization?

■ **What is your financial status?** Were you in a short-term or permanent position? Did it have disability benefits or a pension? What are your current financial demands?

Regardless of your reaction to or even the cause of your unemployment, the impact is sig-nificant on many levels. Unemployment chal-lenges your well-being in three areas of your life: emotional, financial, and social.

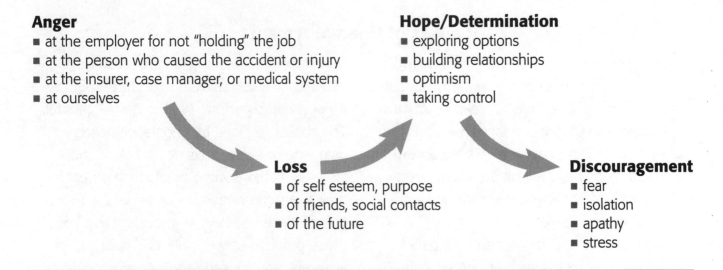

Anger
- at the employer for not "holding" the job
- at the person who caused the accident or injury
- at the insurer, case manager, or medical system
- at ourselves

Hope/Determination
- exploring options
- building relationships
- optimism
- taking control

Loss
- of self esteem, purpose
- of friends, social contacts
- of the future

Discouragement
- fear
- isolation
- apathy
- stress

Figure 4.2 **The Emotional Impact of Unemployment**

Emotional Impact

Unemployment has been described as an "emotional roller coaster." It's a time when people may struggle with many issues such as anger, loss, hopelessness, and discouragement, as illustrated in Figure 4.2.

The stages and emotions in Figure 4.2 are common to anyone who experiences job loss. It's a time of challenge and, for some, defeat. Therefore, it is no wonder that emotional reactions are even more complex when chronic pain is part of the equation. Job loss for someone with chronic pain might be a major contributor to anger and stress—key symptoms that we discussed earlier in this chapter. However, by identifying the specific factors that are affecting your emotions, you can become empowered to manage what you can and to learn to live positively with the rest.

Financial Impact

The impact of reduced or lost income depends on individual circumstances. Financial constraints may prevent you from providing for basic needs. Car payments, rent or mortgage payments, heating bills, medical bills, and children's expenses can become great stressors. Or financial loss may affect your ability to accomplish your life goals, ambitions, and dreams. It may create a dependency on family, friends, and systems that you have not relied on in the past, thereby affecting your relationships and your self-esteem.

Social Impact

Changes in employment can alter your interactions with others. When you are working, you are in contact with coworkers, customers, and clients. A large network generally develops through daily conversation, service provision, committee work, and social activities related to work. It is natural to miss this contact when you are no longer able to work. It may become a challenge to avoid isolation and remain socially connected when you no longer are working every day.

Unemployment can also affect family roles and responsibilities. When a parent or spouse is "at home", the expectations of everyone in the household can change. This is not necessarily negative; it may be an opportunity to redefine roles in a positive way (e.g., you can spend more time with family or be more involved in household tasks, if you pace yourself appropriately).

Self-Management during Unemployment

Coping with unemployment requires a range of strategies. Many of the techniques to better manage pain and other symptoms can also help you take control of life while out of work. You can:

- Maximize physical functioning through pain management strategies such as exercise, relaxation techniques, improving sleep, and pacing your activities

- Work at maintaining personal relationships. Talk with friends and family and try to understand the reactions and expectations of others

- Make an effort to remain positive and to redefine yourself outside of work

- Commit to a daily routine

- Engage in volunteer work to reinforce or broaden your interests, build self-esteem, and gain skills and experience

- Seek financial counseling

- Develop new friends, hobbies, and interests

- Obtain employment counseling from an agency that assists persons with special considerations

- Consider a new career path, further education, part-time or contractual positions, or self-employment

Living without work, with all its uncertainty and turmoil, is a challenge faced by many in today's society. If you are out of work, you are not alone. However, being unemployed while living with chronic pain can be particularly difficult. The techniques and skills outlined in this book, along with support from family, friends, and your health care team, will help you meet this challenge.

In this chapter we have discussed some of the most common symptoms experienced by people with chronic pain. In addition, we have described some tools you can use to cope with your symptoms. Taking action to deal physically with your symptoms is necessary for coping with your condition on a day-to-day basis.

But these tools are just one part of managing chronic pain. Every day you will need to escape from your surroundings and experience "your time"—a time that allows you to clear your mind, calm your nervous system, and gain a fresh perspective. The following chapter presents different ways to complement your physical symptom management with thinking techniques—using the power of your mind—to help reduce and even prevent some of the symptoms you may experience.

Some Resources to Explore

American Chronic Pain Association: www.theacpa.org

Canadian Mental Health Association: www.cmha.ca

National Institute of Mental Health: www.nimh.nih.gov

National Library of Medicine: www.nlm.nih.gov

National Sleep Foundation: www.sleepfoundation.org

Suggested Further Reading

To learn more about the topics discussed in this chapter, we suggest that you explore the following resources:

Bourne, Edmund. *Coping with Anxiety: 10 Simple Ways to Relieve Anxiety, Fear, and Worry.* Oakland, Calif.: New Harbinger, 2003.

Carter, Les. *The Anger Trap: Free Yourself from the Frustrations That Sabotage Your Life.* San Francisco: Jossey-Bass, 2004.

Casarjian, Robin. *Forgiveness: A Bold Choice for a Peaceful Heart.* New York: Bantam Books, 2010.

Caudill, Margaret. *Managing Pain Before It Manages You,* 3rd ed. New York: Guilford Press, 2009.

David, Martha, Elizabeth Robbins Eshelman, and Matthew McKay. *The Relaxation and Stress Reduction Workbook.* Oakland, Calif.: New Harbinger, 2008.

DePaulo, J. Raymond, and Leslie Alan Horvitz. *Understanding Depression: What We Know and What You Can Do About It.* New York: Wiley, 2003.

Donoghue, Paul J., and Mary E. Siegel. *Sick and Tired of Feeling Sick and Tired: Living with Invisible Chronic Illness,* 2nd ed. New York: Norton, 2000.

Foreman, Judy. *A Nation In Pain: Healing Our Biggest Health Problem.* New York: Oxford University Press, 2014.

Gardner-Nix, Jackie. *The Mindfulness Solution to Pain: Step-by-Step Techniques for Chronic Pain Management.* Oakland, Calif.: New Harbinger, 2009.

Gordon, James S. *Unstuck: Your Guide to the Seven-Stage Journey Out of Depression.* New York: Penguin, 2008.

Hankins, Gary, and Carol Hankins. *Prescription for Anger,* 3rd ed. Newberg, Ore.: Barclay Press, 2000.

Jacobs, Gregg D. *Say Good Night to Insomnia.* New York: Holt, 2009.

Kabat-Zinn, Jon. *Full Catastrophe Living: Using the Wisdom of Your Body and Mind to Face Stress, Pain, and Illness.* New York: Bantam Books, 2013.

Kabat-Zinn, Jon. *Mindfulness for Beginners: Reclaiming the Present Moment—and Your Life.* Louisville, Colo.: Sounds True, 2011.

Klein, Donald F., and Paul H. Wender. *Understanding Depression: A Complete Guide to Its Diagnosis and Treatment,* 2nd ed. New York: Oxford University Press, 2005.

Kleinke, Chris L. *Coping with Life Challenges,* 2nd ed. Pacific Grove, Calif.: Brooks/Cole, 2002.

McGonigal, Kelly. *The Willpower Instinct: How Self-Control Works, Why It Matters, and What You Can Do to Get More of It.* New York: Avery, 2012.

McKay, Matthew, Peter D. Rogers, and Judith McKay. *When Anger Hurts: Quieting the Storm Within,* 2nd ed. Oakland, Calif.: New Harbinger, 2003.

Natelson, Benjamin H. *Facing and Fighting Fatigue: A Practical Approach.* New Haven, Conn.: Yale University Press, 1998.

Rosenberg, Robert S. *Sleep Soundly Every Night, Feel Fantastic Every Day: A Doctor's Guide to Solving Your Sleep Problems.* New York: Demos Medical Publishing, 2014.

Sobel, David, and Robert Ornstein. *The Healthy Mind, Healthy Body Handbook* (also published under the title *The Mind and Body Health Handbook*). Los Altos, Calif.: DRx, 1996.

Stahl, Bob, and Elisha Goldstein. *A Mindfulness-Based Stress Reduction Workbook.* Oakland, Calif.: New Harbinger, 2010.

Torburn, Leslie. *Stop the Stress Habit: Change Your Perceptions and Improve Your Health.* Bloomington, Ind.: iUniverse, 2008.

Turk, Dennis C., and Frits Winter. *The Pain Survival Guide: How to Reclaim Your Life.*

Washington, D.C.:, American Psychological Association, 2006.

Williams, Redford, and Virginia Williams. *Anger Kills: 17 Strategies for Controlling the Hostility That Can Harm Your Health.* New York: HarperCollins, 1998.

Williams, Virginia, and Redford Williams. *Lifeskills: 8 Simple Ways to Build Stronger Relationships, Communicate More Clearly, and Improve Your Health.* New York: Three Rivers Press, 1998.

CHAPTER 5

Using Your Mind to Manage Pain and Other Symptoms

THERE IS A STRONG LINK BETWEEN our thoughts, attitudes, and emotions and our mental and physical health. As one of our self-managers said: "It's not always mind over matter, but mind matters." And in chronic pain, mind matters a lot. Brain imaging studies have found that the emotional and thinking regions of the brain are connected not only to each other but to the part of the brain that detects body sensations. And all of these regions are connected to multiple pathways in the nervous system. What you think and feel can lessen or worsen your pain by opening or closing the gate in the spinal cord and influencing the complex network of nerve cells in the brain (see Chapter 1).

Although thoughts and emotions do not directly cause chronic health conditions, they can influence many symptoms beyond just pain. Research has shown that thoughts and emotions trigger certain hormones and other chemicals that send messages throughout the body. These messages affect how our bodies function; they can, for example, alter our heart rate, blood pressure, breathing, blood sugar levels, muscle responses, immune response, concentration, the ability to get pregnant, and even our ability to fight off other illnesses. Both pleasant and unpleasant thoughts and emotions can make our heart rate and breathing increase or slow down. When we feel a strong emotion, we often have a physical response. We may sweat, blush, tear up, and so on. All of us have experienced how the mind affects the body in this way.

Sometimes just a memory or an image can trigger these responses. For example, try this simple exercise: Imagine you are holding a big, bright yellow lemon slice. You hold it close to your nose and smell its strong citrus aroma. Now you bite into the lemon. It's juicy! The juice fills your mouth and dribbles down your chin. You begin to suck on the lemon and its tart juice. What happens when you imagine this scenario? Your body responds! Your mouth puckers and starts to water. You may even smell the scent of the lemon. All of these reactions are triggered by the mind and its memory of your experience with a real lemon.

This example illustrates the power the mind has over the body. It also gives you a good reason to develop your mental abilities to help manage your symptoms. The mind can greatly help relieve the unpleasantness caused by pain. With training and practice, you can learn to use the mind to relax your tense muscles, calm your nervous system, and improve your breathing. You can also learn to reduce stress, anxiety, and other difficult emotions that are part of the chronic pain experience. Using the mind may even help you depend less on some medications.

In this chapter we describe several ways you can begin to use your mind to manage pain and associated symptoms. These are sometimes referred to as "thinking" or "cognitive" techniques because they involve the use of our thinking abilities to make changes in the body.

As you read, keep the following key principles in mind:

- **Symptoms have many causes.** This means there are many ways to manage most symptoms. When you understand the nature and causes of your symptoms, you are better able to manage them.

- **Not all management techniques work for everyone.** It is up to you to find out what works best for you. Be flexible. Experiment. Try different techniques and check the results to determine which management tool is most helpful for which symptoms and under what circumstances.

- **Learning new skills and gaining control of the situation take time.** Give yourself several weeks to practice before you decide if a new tool is working for you.

- **Don't give up too easily.** As with exercise and other new skills, using your mind to manage your health condition requires both practice and time. It may be awhile before you notice the benefits. Even if you feel you are not accomplishing anything, don't give up. Be patient and keep on trying.

- **These techniques should not have negative effects.** If you become frightened, angry, or depressed when using one of these tools, do not continue to use it. Try another tool instead.

Relaxation Techniques

Although you may have heard and read about relaxation as a pain management technique, you may still be confused as to what relaxation is, its benefits, and how to achieve it. Simply stated, relaxation involves using thinking or cognitive techniques to reduce or eliminate tension from both the body and the mind. Relaxation usually results in improved sleep quality, better breathing, and less stress, anxiety, and pain. It often also instills a feeling of calm and well-being.

There are different types of relaxation techniques, each with specific guidelines and uses. Some techniques are used mostly to achieve muscle relaxation, while others are aimed at reducing anxiety and emotional stress or diverting your attention from your symptoms. All of this helps with pain and symptom management.

Relaxation means different things to different people. We can all identify things we do that help us relax. For example, we may walk, watch TV, listen to music, knit, or garden. These methods, however, are different from most of the techniques discussed in this chapter because they include some form of physical activity or require a stimulus such as music that is outside of the mind. The relaxation tools we focus on in this chapter involve using your mind to help relax your body.

The goal of relaxation is to turn off the outside world so that the mind and body are at rest. This allows you to reduce the tensions that can increase the intensity or severity of symptoms.

The following guidelines will help you successfully practice relaxation.

■ **Pick a quiet place and time.** Find a time and place where you will not be disturbed for at least 15 to 20 minutes. If this seems too long, start with five minutes. (By the way, in some homes the only quiet place is the bathroom. That is just fine.)

■ **Try to practice the technique twice daily and not less than four times a week.** These are new techniques, and new techniques take repetition to master.

■ **Don't expect miracles or immediate results.** Sometimes it takes three to four weeks of consistent practice before you start to notice benefits.

■ **Relaxation should be helpful.** At worst, you may find it boring, but if practicing any technique is an unpleasant experience or makes you more nervous or anxious, switch to one of the other symptom management tools described in this chapter.

Relaxation Quick and Easy

Some types of relaxation are so easy, natural, and effective that people do not think of them as "relaxation techniques."

■ Take a nap or a warm, soothing bath.

■ Curl up and read or listen to a good book.

■ Watch a funny movie.

■ Make a paper airplane and sail it across the room.

■ Get a massage.

■ Enjoy an occasional glass of wine.

- Start a small garden or grow a beautiful plant indoors.
- Do some crafts such as knitting, pottery, or woodworking.
- Watch a favorite TV show.
- Read a poem or an inspirational saying.
- Go for a walk.
- Start a collection (coins, folk art, shells, or something in miniature).
- Listen to your favorite music.
- Sing around the house.
- Crumble paper into a ball and use a wastebasket as a basketball hoop.
- Watch water move (ocean waves, a lake, or a fountain).
- Watch the clouds in the sky.
- Put your head down on your desk and close your eyes for five minutes.
- Rub your hands together until they're warm, and then cup them over your closed eyes.
- Vigorously shake your hands and arms for ten seconds.
- Call up a friend or family member to chat.
- Smile and introduce yourself to someone new.
- Do something nice and unexpected for someone else.
- Play with a pet.
- Go to a vacation spot in your mind.

Relaxation Tools That Take 5 to 20 Minutes

The relaxation techniques we discuss in this section, body scan and relaxation response, take a bit longer but are quite effective.

Body scan

To relax muscles, you need to know how to scan your body and recognize where you are tense. Once you know how to do this, you can learn to release the tension.

The first step is to become familiar with the difference between the feeling of tension and the feeling of relaxation. This exercise allows you to compare those feelings and, with practice, spot and release tension anywhere in your body. It is best done lying on your back, but you can use any comfortable position. You will find a body scan script on page 81.

Relaxation response

In the early 1970s a physician named Herbert Benson studied what he calls the "relaxation response." According to Benson, our bodies have several natural states. One example is the "fight or flight" response experienced by people when faced with a great danger. Another is the body's natural tendency to relax after feeling tense. This is the relaxation response. As our lives become more and more hectic, our bodies tend to stay tense for long periods of time. We lose our ability to relax. The relaxation response helps change this.

To achieve the relaxation response, find a quiet place where there are few or no distractions; then find a comfortable position. You should be comfortable enough to remain in the same position for 20 minutes.

Choose a pleasant word and a tranquil object or feeling. For example, repeat a word or sound (such as the word *one*) while gazing at a symbol (perhaps a flower) or concentrating on a feeling (such as peace).

Adopt a passive attitude. This is of the utmost importance. Empty all thoughts and distractions

Body-Scan Script

As you get into a comfortable position, allowing yourself to begin to sink comfortably into the surface below you, you may perhaps begin to allow your eyes gradually to close . . . From there, turn your attention to your breath . . . Breathing in, allowing the breath gradually to go all the way down to your belly, and then breathing out . . . And again, breathing in . . . and out . . . noticing the natural rhythm of your breathing . . .

Now allow your attention to focus on your feet. Starting with your toes, notice whatever sensations are there—warmth, coolness, whatever's there . . . simply feel it. Using your mind's eye, imagine that as you breathe in, the breath goes all the way down into your toes, bringing with it new refreshing air . . . And now notice the sensations elsewhere in your feet. Not judging or thinking about what you're feeling, but simply becoming aware of the experience of your feet as you allow yourself to be fully supported by the surface below you . . .

Next focus on your lower legs and knees. These muscles and joints do a lot of work for us, but often we don't give them the attention they deserve. So now breathe down into the knees, calves, and ankles, noticing whatever sensations appear . . . See if you can simply stay with the sensations . . . breathing in new fresh air, and as you exhale, releasing tension and stress and allowing the muscles to relax and soften . . .

Now move your attention to the muscles, bones, and joints of the thighs, buttocks, and hips . . . breathing down into the upper legs, noticing whatever sensations you experience. It may be warmth, coolness, a heaviness or lightness. You may become aware of the contact with the surface beneath you, or perhaps the pulsing of your blood. Whatever's there . . . what matters is that you are taking time to learn to relax . . . deeper and deeper, as you breathe . . . in . . . and out.

Move your attention now to your back and chest. Feeling the breath fill the abdomen and chest . . . noticing whatever sensations are there . . . not judging or thinking, but simply observing what is right here right now. Allowing the fresh air to nourish the muscles, bones, and joints as you breathe in, and then exhaling any tension and stress.

Now focus on the neck, shoulders, arms, and hands. Inhaling down through the neck and shoulders, all the way down to the fingertips. Not trying too hard to relax, but simply becoming aware of your experience of these parts of your body in the present moment . . .

Turning now to your face and head, notice the sensations beginning at the back of your head, up along your scalp, and down into your forehead . . . Then become aware of the sensations in and around your eyes and down into your cheeks and jaw . . . Continue to allow your muscles to release and soften as you breathe in nourishing fresh air, and allow tension and stress to leave as you breathe out . . .

As you drink in fresh air, allow it to spread throughout your body, from the soles of your feet all the way up through the top of your head . . . And then exhale any remaining stress and tension . . . and now take a few moments to enjoy the stillness as you breathe in . . . and out . . . Awake, relaxed, and still . . .

Now as the body scan comes to a close, come back into the room, bringing with you whatever sensations of relaxation . . . comfort . . . peace, whatever's there . . . knowing that you can repeat this exercise at any appropriate time and place of your choosing . . . And when you're ready, open your eyes.

▶ To order the Relaxation for Mind & Body CD, go to www.bullpub.com/catalog/relaxation-for-mind-and-body

from your mind. You may become aware of thoughts, images, and feelings, but don't concentrate on them. Just allow them to pass on.

To elicit the relaxation response take the following steps:

- Sit quietly in a comfortable position.

- Close your eyes.

- Relax all your muscles, beginning at your feet and progressing up to your face. Keep them relaxed.

- Breathe in through your nose. Become aware of your breathing. As you breathe out through your mouth, say the word you chose silently to yourself. Try to empty all thoughts from your mind; concentrate on your word, symbol, or feeling.

- Continue this for 10 to 20 minutes. You may open your eyes to check the time, but do not use an alarm. When you finish, sit quietly for several minutes, at first with your eyes closed. Do not stand up for a few minutes.

- Maintain a passive attitude, and let relaxation occur at its own pace. When distracting thoughts occur, ignore them by not dwelling on them, and return to repeating the word you chose. Do not worry about whether you are successful in achieving a deep level of relaxation.

- Practice this once or twice daily.

Distraction/Attention Refocusing

Our minds have trouble focusing on more than one thing at a time. Therefore, we can lessen the intensity of symptoms by training our minds to focus attention on something other than our bodies and their sensations. This technique, called distraction or attention refocusing, is particularly helpful for people with chronic pain conditions.

Research has shown that when a person focuses on pain, several areas of the brain show more intense pain-related activity than when a person is distracted from the pain. Many studies have found that people who constantly direct their attention to pain and think about it all the time are more likely to expect the worst from their pain problem and to feel helpless about controlling it. Consciously redirecting attention away from pain can help you feel better. (It is important to mention that with distraction/attention refocusing you are not ignoring your pain or other symptoms. Instead, you are *choosing* not to dwell on them.)

Sometimes it may be difficult to put pain or other anxious thoughts out of your mind. When you try to suppress any thought, you may end up thinking more about it. For example, try not thinking about a tiger charging at you. Whatever you do, don't let the thought of a tiger enter your mind. You'll probably find it nearly impossible not to think about the tiger.

Although you can't easily stop thinking about something, you can distract yourself and redirect your attention elsewhere. For example, think about the charging tiger again. Now stand up suddenly, slam your hand on the table, and shout *"Stop!"* What happened to the tiger? Gone—at least for the moment.

Distraction is especially good for short activities or times when symptoms may be anticipated. For example, if you know climbing stairs will cause discomfort or that falling asleep at night is difficult, you might try one of the following distraction techniques:

■ Make plans for exactly what you will do after the unpleasant activity passes. For example, if climbing stairs is uncomfortable or painful, think about what you will do once you get to the top. If you have trouble falling asleep, try making plans for some future event, being as detailed as possible.

■ Think of a person's name, a bird, a brand of car, or whatever, for every letter of the alphabet. If you get stuck on one letter, go on to the next. (This is a good distraction technique for pain as well as for sleep problems.)

■ Challenge yourself to count backward from 100 by threes (100, 97, 94 . . .).

■ To get through unpleasant daily chores such as sweeping, mopping, or vacuuming, imagine your floor as a map of a country or continent. Try naming all the states, provinces, or countries, moving east to west or north to south as you work. If geography does not appeal to you, imagine your favorite store and where each department is located.

■ Try to remember words to favorite songs or the events in an old story.

■ Try the *"Stop!"* technique. If you find yourself worrying or entrapped in endlessly repeating negative thoughts, stand up suddenly, slap your hand on the table or your thigh, and shout *"Stop!"* With practice, you won't have to shout out loud. Just whispering *"Stop!"* or tightening your vocal cords and moving your tongue as if saying *"Stop!"* will often work. Some people imagine a large stop sign. Others put a rubber band on their wrist and snap it hard to break the chain of negative thought. Or just pinch yourself. Do anything that redirects your attention.

■ Redirect your attention to a pleasurable experience:

  ◆ Look outside at something in nature.

  ◆ Try to identify all the sounds around you.

  ◆ Massage your hand.

  ◆ Smell a sweet or pungent odor.

There are, of course, many variations to these examples, all of which can help you refocus attention away from your problem.

So far we have discussed short-term refocusing strategies that involve using only the mind for distraction, but long-term projects also work well. In these cases, the mind is focused not internally but externally on some type of activity. Find an activity that interests you and distracts you from the pain or other symptoms you might have. It can be almost anything, from gardening to cooking to reading or going to a movie, even doing volunteer work. One of the marks of a successful self-manager is that he or she has a variety of interests and always seems to be involved in something.

Positive Realistic Thinking and Self-Talk

We all talk to ourselves all the time. For example, when waking up in the morning, we might think, "I really don't want to get out of bed. I'm tired and don't want to go to work today." Or at the end of an enjoyable evening, we think, "Gee, that was fun. I should get out more often." What we think or say to ourselves is our "self-talk." The way we talk to ourselves is influenced by how we think about ourselves. Our self-image can be positive or negative, and so is our self-talk. Self-talk can be an important self-management tool when it's based on positive thinking or a weapon that hurts or defeats us when it's habitually negative.

Negative self-statements usually begin with something like, "I just can't do . . . ," "If only I could . . . ," "If only I didn't . . . ," or "I just don't have the energy . . ." This type of negative thinking represents the doubts and fears you have about yourself in general. This translates into doubts and fears about your abilities to deal with your pain condition and its symptoms.

Negative self-talk has no place in pain management. It damages your self-esteem, attitude, and mood. It makes your pain worse by opening the pain gate and makes your other symptoms worse as well. What you say to yourself plays a major role in determining your success or failure in becoming a good self-manager. Negative thinking limits your abilities and actions. If you tell yourself "I'm not very smart" or "I can't" all the time, you probably won't try to learn new skills because positive change just doesn't fit with how you think about yourself. Soon you become a prisoner of your own negative beliefs.

Fortunately, self-talk is not fixed in our biological makeup, and therefore it is often within our control. You can learn new, healthier ways to think about yourself so your self-talk can work for you instead of against you. By changing the negative, self-defeating statements to more positive, realistic ones, you can manage symptoms more effectively. This change, like any habit, requires practice and includes the following steps:

1. **Listen carefully to what you say about yourself, both out loud and silently.** If you find yourself feeling anxious, depressed, or angry, try to identify some of the thoughts you were having just before these feelings started. Then write down all the negative self-talk statements. Pay special attention to the things you say during times that are particularly difficult for you. For example, what do you say to yourself when getting up in the morning with pain, while doing those exercises you don't really like, or when you are feeling blue? Challenge these negative thoughts by identifying what is really true or not true about the statement. For example, are you exaggerating the situation, generalizing, worrying too much, or assuming the worst? Are you thinking in terms of black and white? Could there be gray? Maybe you are making an unrealistic or unfair comparison, assuming too much responsibility, taking something too personally, or expecting perfection. Are you making assumptions about what other people

think about you? What do you know for a fact? When you look at the evidence in this way, you will be better able to change these negative thoughts and statements.

2. **Next, work on changing each negative statement to a more positive one.** For example, you might find yourself saying negative statements such as:

   ◆ "My pain is just terrible."

   ◆ "My pain will never get better."

   ◆ "Nothing will ever be the same."

   ◆ "I can't stand it anymore."

   ◆ "I'm good for nothing."

   But these statements can be turned into more positive messages, such as:

   ◆ "My pain is really bad today but I know it's only temporary."

   ◆ "By relaxing and taking a warm bath, I can make my pain more bearable. I just have to take things one day at a time."

   ◆ "Everything changes—I need to consider new ways of doing the things I enjoy."

   ◆ "I'm going to call a friend for lunch to take my mind off the pain."

   ◆ "Other people need and depend on me; I'm worthwhile."

   Notice that these comments do not suggest that everything is rosy and the pain is all gone. Instead they express a more realistic and positive outlook that can have a real effect on your pain experience. More positive self-talk tends to produce more positive emotions that close the pain gate.

3. **Write down and rehearse these positive statements, mentally or with another**

person. This conscious repetition of the positive self-talk will help you replace those old, habitual negative statements.

4. **Practice new statements in real situations.** This practice, along with time and patience, can help the new patterns of thinking become automatic.

5. **Rehearse success.** When you aren't happy with the way you handled a particular situation, try this exercise:

   ◆ Write down three ways it could have gone better.

   ◆ Write down three ways it could have gone worse.

   ◆ If you can't think of alternatives to the way you handled it, imagine what someone whom you greatly respect would have done.

   ◆ Or think about what advice you would give to someone else facing a similar situation.

Remember that mistakes aren't failures; they're good opportunities to learn. Mistakes give you the chance to rehearse other ways of handling things. This is great practice for future crises.

At first, you may find it hard to change negative statements into more positive ones. A shortcut is to use either a thought stopper or a positive affirmation. A thought stopper can be anything that is meaningful to you—for example, a puppy, a polar bear, or a beautiful sunrise. When you have a negative thought, replace it with your thought stopper. We know it sounds silly, but try it.

Getting Professional Help

Sometimes negative self-talk is so automatic and intrusive that you cannot seem to control it even with your best efforts. When this happens, you might feel stuck, unmotivated, or helpless to change these thoughts. If you find you are constantly focused on your pain, feel overwhelmed by negative thoughts about your pain, or consistently have trouble distracting yourself, seek help from a professional such as a psychologist or therapist. Getting help with understanding and changing your negative thought pattern could be a breakthrough for you and your pain management. Research has found that people with chronic pain who continually expect the worst are more disabled than those who have a more positive outlook. So working on changing thoughts and attitudes is very important. Also, discuss your concerns with your health care provider. Be open about how you are feeling. You may have an underlying depression that is stopping you from moving forward, which needs to be evaluated and treated (see Chapter 4, page 57).

A positive affirmation is a positive phrase that you can use over and over. For example, "I am getting better every day" or "I can do this" or "I'm a good person." Use this phrase to replace negative thoughts.

Imagery

You may think that "imagination" is all in your mind. But the thoughts, words, and images that flow from your imagination can have very real effects on your body. Your body often cannot distinguish whether you are imagining something or if it is really happening. Perhaps you've had a racing heartbeat, rapid breathing, or tension in your neck muscles while watching a movie thriller. These sensations were all produced by images and sounds on a film. During a dream, your body may have responded with fear, joy, anger, or sadness—all triggered by your imagination. If you close your eyes and vividly imagine yourself by a still, quiet pool or relaxing on a warm beach, your body responds to some degree as though you were actually there.

Guided imagery and visualization allow you to use your imagination to relieve symptoms. These techniques will help you focus on healing images and suggestions.

Guided Imagery

This tool is like a guided daydream. Guided imagery allows you to refocus your mind away from your pain and other symptoms by transporting you to another time and place. It has the added benefit of helping you achieve deep relaxation by picturing yourself in a peaceful environment.

In guided imagery, the images are suggested to you by a script like the one included in this book on page 90. With guided imagery, you focus your mind on a particular image. This usually begins with your sense of sight, focusing on something visual. Adding other senses—smells, tastes, and sounds—makes the guided imagery even more vivid and powerful.

Some people are highly visual and easily see images with their "mind's eye." But if your images aren't as vivid as scenes from a great movie, don't worry; it's normal for the intensity of imagery to vary. The important thing is to focus on as much detail as possible and to strengthen the images by using all your senses. Adding real background music can also increase the impact of guided imagery.

With guided imagery, you are always completely in control. You're the movie director. You can project whatever thought or feeling you want onto your mental screen. If you don't like a particular image, thought, or feeling, you can redirect your mind to something more comfortable. You can use other images to get rid of unpleasant thoughts; for example, you might put them on a raft and watch them float away, sweep them away with a large broom, or erase them with a giant eraser. Or you can just open your eyes and stop the exercise.

The guided imagery scripts presented on pages 90 and 91 can help take you on this mental stroll. Here are some ways to use these scripts:

- Read the script several times until it is familiar. Then sit or lie down in a quiet place and try to reconstruct the scene in your mind. The script should take 15 to 20 minutes to complete.

- Have a family member or friend slowly read the script to you, pausing for about 10 seconds wherever there is a series of periods (. . .).

- Make a recording of the script and play it to yourself whenever convenient.

- Use a prerecorded tape, CD, or digital audio file that has a similar guided imagery script (see the "Other Resources" section at the end of this chapter).

Visualization

Visualization allows you to create your own images, which is different from guided imagery, where the images are suggested to you. Visualization is another way to use your imagination and create a picture of yourself in any way you want, doing the things you want to do.

All of us use a form of visualization every day—when we dream, worry, read a book, or listen to a story. In all these activities the mind creates images for us to see. We also use visualization intentionally when making plans for the day, considering the possible outcomes of a decision we have to make, or rehearsing for an event or activity.

One way to use visualization to manage symptoms is to remember pleasant scenes from your past. Try to remember every detail of a special holiday or party that made you happy. Who was there? What happened? What did you do or talk about? Or you can remember a vacation or some other memorable and pleasant event.

Visualization also can be used to plan the details of some future event or to fill in the details of a fantasy. For example, how would you spend a million dollars? What would be your ideal romantic encounter? What would your ideal home or garden look like? Where would you go and what would you do on your dream vacation?

Another form of visualization involves thinking of symbols that represent the discomfort or pain you feel. For example, a painful joint might be red, or a tight chest might have a constricting band around it. After forming these images, you then change them in your mind. The red color might fade until there is no more color, or the constricting band will stretch and stretch until it falls off. These new images transform the way you think of the pain or discomfort.

Visualization helps build confidence and skill and therefore is a useful technique to help you set and accomplish personal goals (see Chapter 2). After you write your weekly action plan, take a few minutes to imagine yourself taking a walk, doing your exercises, or making a healthy meal. Visualization is a way to rehearse the steps you need to take in order to achieve your goal successfully.

Imagery for Different Conditions

You have the ability to create special imagery to help ease (though not cure) your specific symptoms or illnesses. Use any image that is strong and vivid for you—this often involves using all your senses to create the image—and one that is meaningful to you. The image does not have to be accurate for it to work. Just use your imagination and trust yourself. Here are examples of images that some people have found useful to help them deal with various situations:

For Tension and Stress

A tight, twisted rope slowly untwists.

Hard wax softens and melts.

Tension swirls out of your body and down the drain.

For Pain

You grasp the TV remote control and slowly turn down the pain volume until you can barely hear it; then it disappears entirely.

A cool, calm river flowing through your entire body washes away the pain.

A radiant white light finds the areas of pain and tension in your body and dissolves them. As the light leaves your body, you feel warm and relaxed in its glow.

All of your pain is placed in a large, strong metal box that is closed, sealed tightly, and locked with a huge padlock. The box is placed on the deck of a ship that is heading out to sea.

For Depression

Your troubles and feelings of sadness are attached to big, colorful helium balloons and float off into a clear blue sky.

A strong, warm sun breaks through dark clouds.

You feel a sense of detachment and lightness, enabling you to float easily through your day.

For Healing of Cuts and Injuries

Plaster covers over a crack in a wall.

Cells and fibers stick together with very strong glue.

A shoe is laced up tight.

Jigsaw puzzle pieces come together.

For Arteries and Heart Disease

A miniature Roto-Rooter truck speeds through your arteries and cleans out the clogged pipes.

Water flows freely through a wide, open river.

A crew in a small boat rows in sync, easily and efficiently pulling the slender boat across the smooth surface of the water.

For a Weakened Immune System

Sluggish, sleepy white blood cells awaken, put on protective armor, and enter the fight against the virus.

White blood cells rapidly multiply like millions of seeds bursting from a single ripe seedpod.

For an Overactive Immune System (arthritis, psoriasis, etc.)

Overly alert immune cells in the fire station are reassured that the allergens have triggered a false alarm, and they go back to playing a game of poker.

The civil war ends with the warring sides agreeing not to attack their fellow citizens.

Use any of these images, or make up your own. Remember, the best ones are vivid and have meaning to you. Use the power of your personal imagination for health and healing.

Prayer and Spirituality

There is strong evidence in the medical literature of the relationship between spirituality and health. According to the American Academy of Family Physicians,* spirituality is a way to find meaning, hope, comfort, and inner peace in our lives. Many people find spirituality through religion. Some find it through music, art, or a connection with nature. Others find it in their values and principles.

Many people are religious and like to share their religion with others. Others do not practice a specific religion but do have spiritual beliefs. Our religion and beliefs can bring a sense of meaning and purpose to our lives. They can help us put things into perspective, set priorities, and find comfort during difficult times. Strong belief systems can help us with acceptance and motivate us to make difficult changes. Being part of a spiritual or religious community offers a source of support when needed and the opportunity to help others.

Recent studies find that people who belong to a religious or spiritual community or who regularly engage in religious activities such as prayer or study have improved health. There are many types of prayer, any of which may contribute to improved health. Asking for help, direction, or forgiveness is one form of prayer. Offering words of gratitude, praise, and blessing is another. In addition, many religions have a tradition of contemplation or meditation. Prayer and mediation are probably the oldest of all self-management tools. We encourage you to explore your own beliefs about what makes life meaningful and gives you hope. If you are religious, try engaging in prayer consistently. If you are not religious, consider adopting some form of reflection or meditative practice.

Also, if you are religious, consider telling your doctor and care team. Although they won't ask, it is helpful for them to understand the importance of your beliefs in managing your health and life. Most hospitals have chaplains or pastoral counselors. Even if you are not in the hospital, these spiritual leaders will probably

---

*Adapted from the American Academy of Family Physicians: www.aafp.org/afp/2001/0101/p89.html and www.aafp.org/afp/2006/0415/p1336.html

Guided-Imagery Script: A Walk in the Country

You're giving yourself some time to quiet your mind and body. Allow yourself to settle comfortably, wherever you are right now. If you wish, you can close your eyes. Breathe in deeply, through your nose, expanding your abdomen and filling your lungs; and, pursing your lips, exhale through your mouth slowly and completely, allowing your body to sink heavily into the surface beneath you . . .

And once again breathe in through your nose and all the way down to your abdomen, and then breathe out slowly through pursed lips—letting go of tension, letting go of anything that's on your mind right now and just allowing yourself to be present in this moment . . .

Imagine yourself walking along a peaceful old country road. The sun is gently warming your back . . . the birds are singing . . . the air is calm and fragrant . . .

With no need to hurry, you notice your walking is relaxed and easy. As you walk along in this way, taking in your surroundings, you come across an old gate. It looks inviting and you decide to take the path through the gate. The gate creaks as you open it and go through.

You find yourself in an old, overgrown garden—flowers growing where they've seeded themselves, vines climbing over a fallen tree, soft green wild grasses, shade trees.

You notice yourself breathing deeply . . . smelling the flowers . . . listening to the birds and insects . . . feeling a gentle breeze cool against your skin. All of your senses are alive and responding with pleasure to this peaceful time and place . . .

When you're ready to move on, you leisurely follow the path out behind the garden, eventually coming to a more wooded area. As you enter this area, your eyes find the trees and plant life restful. The sunlight is filtered through the leaves. The air feels mild and a little cooler . . . You savor the fragrance of trees and earth . . . and gradually become aware of the sound of a nearby stream. Pausing, you allow yourself to take in the sights and sounds, breathing in the cool and fragrant air several times . . . And with each breath, you notice how refreshed you are feeling . . .

Continuing along the path for a while, you come to the stream. It's clear and clean as it flows and tumbles over the rocks and some fallen logs. You follow the path easily along the creek for a way, and after a while, you come out into a sunlit clearing, where you discover a small waterfall emptying into a quiet pool of water.

You find a comfortable place to sit for a while, a perfect niche where you can feel completely relaxed. You feel good as you allow yourself to just enjoy the warmth and solitude of this peaceful place . . .

After a while, you become aware that it is time to return. You arise and walk back down the path in a relaxed and comfortable way, through the cool and fragrant trees, out into the sun-drenched overgrown garden . . . One last smell of the flowers, and out the creaky gate.

You leave this country retreat for now and return down the road. You notice you feel calm and rested. You feel grateful and remind yourself that you can visit this special place whenever you wish to take some time to refresh yourself and renew your energy.

And now, preparing to bring this period of relaxation to a close, you may want to take a moment to picture yourself carrying this experience of calm and refreshment with you into the ordinary activities of your life . . . And when you're ready, take a nice deep breath and open your eyes.

▶ To order the Relaxation for Mind & Body CD, go to www.bullpub.com/catalog/relaxation-for-mind-and-body

Guided-Imagery Script: A Walk on the Beach

Begin by getting into a comfortable position, whether you are seated or lying down. Loosen any tight clothing to allow yourself to be as comfortable as possible. Uncross your legs and allow your hands to fall by your sides or rest in your lap, and if you are at all uncomfortable shift to a more comfortable position.

When you are ready, you may allow your eyes gradually to close and turn your attention to your breathing. Allow your belly to expand as you breathe in, bringing in fresh new air to nourish your body. And then breathing out. Notice the rhythm of your breathing—in . . . and out . . . without trying to control it in any way at all. Simply attend to the natural rhythm of your breath . . .

And now in your mind's eye, imagine yourself standing on a beautiful beach. The sky is a brilliant blue, and as some fluffy white clouds float slowly by, you drink in the beautiful colors . . . The temperature is not too hot and not too cold. The sun is shining, and you close your eyes, allowing the warmth of the sun to wash over you . . . You notice a gentle breeze caressing your face, the perfect complement to the sunshine.

Then you find yourself turning and looking out over the vastness of the ocean . . . You become aware of the sound of the waves gently washing up on shore . . . You notice the firmness of the wet sand beneath your feet, or if you decide to take off your shoes, you may enjoy the feeling of standing in the cool, wet sand . . . perhaps you allow the surf to roll up and gently wash across your feet, or perhaps you stay just out of its reach . . .

In the distance you hear some seagulls calling to one another and look out to see the birds gracefully gliding through the air. And as you stand there, notice how easy it is to be here, perhaps noticing some sensations of relaxation, comfort, or peace—whatever's there . . .

Now take a walk along the shore. Turn and begin to stroll casually along the beach, enjoying the sounds of the surf, the warmth of the sun, and the gentle massage of the breeze. As you move along, taking your time, your stride becomes lighter, easier . . . you notice the scent of the ocean . . . you pause to take in the freshness of the air . . . And then you continue on your way, enjoying the peacefulness of this place.

After a time, you decide to rest a while, and find a comfortable place to sit or lie down . . . and simply allow yourself to take some time to enjoy this, your special place . . .

And now, when you feel ready to return, you stand and begin walking back down the beach in a comfortable, leisurely way, taking with you any sensations of relaxation, comfort, peace, joy—whatever's there . . . Noticing how easy it is to be here. Continuing back until you reach the place where you began your walk . . .

And now pausing to take one last long look around. Enjoying the vibrant colors of the sky and the sea . . . The gentle sound of the waves washing up on the shore. The warmth of the sun, the cool of the breeze . . .

And as you prepare to leave this special place, taking with you any sensations of joy, relaxation, comfort, peace, whatever's there. Knowing that you may return at any appropriate time and place of your choosing.

And now bringing your awareness back into the room, focusing on your breathing . . . in and out . . . Taking a few more breaths . . . and when you're ready, opening your eyes.

▶ To order the Relaxation for Mind & Body CD, go to www.bullpub.com/catalog/relaxation-for-mind-and-body

make time to talk with you. Choose someone you feel comfortable with. Their advice and counsel can supplement your medical and psychological care.

Additional Ways You Can Use Your Mind to Manage Symptoms

Consider employing these additional valuable techniques to clear your mind, calm your nervous system, positively shift your emotional state, and reduce your tension and stress.

Mindfulness

Mindfulness involves keeping your attention in the present moment, without judging it as happy or sad, good or bad. It encourages living each moment—even painful ones—as fully and as mindfully as possible. Mindfulness is more than a relaxation technique; it is an attitude toward living. It is a way of calmly and consciously observing and accepting whatever is happening, moment to moment.

This may sound simple enough, but our restless, judging minds make it surprisingly difficult. As a restless monkey jumps from branch to branch, our mind jumps from thought to thought.

To practice mindfulness, focus on the present moment. The "goal" of mindfulness is simply to observe—with no intention of changing or improving anything. But people are positively changed by the practice. Observing and accepting life just as it is, with all its pleasures, pains, frustrations, disappointments, and insecurities, enables you to become calmer, more confident, and better able to cope with whatever comes along.

To develop your capacity for mindfulness, follow the instructions below:

■ Sit comfortably on the floor or on a chair with your back, neck, and head straight, but not stiff.

■ Concentrate on a single object, such as your breathing. Focus your attention on the feeling of the air as it passes in and out of your nostrils with each breath. Don't try to control your breathing by speeding it up or slowing it down. Just observe it as it is.

■ Even when you resolve to keep your attention on your breathing, your mind will quickly wander off. When this occurs, observe where your mind went: perhaps to a memory, a worry about the future, a bodily ache, or a feeling of impatience. Then gently return your attention to your breathing.

■ Use your breath as an anchor. Each time a thought or feeling arises, momentarily acknowledge it. Don't analyze it or judge it. Just observe it and return to your breathing.

■ Let go of all thoughts of getting somewhere or having anything special happen. Just keep stringing moments of mindfulness together, breath by breath.

■ At first, practice this for just five minutes, or even one minute at a time. Eventually, you may wish to gradually extend the time to 10, 20, or 30 minutes.

Because the practice of mindfulness is simply the practice of moment-to-moment awareness, you can apply it to anything: eating, showering, working, talking, running errands, or playing with your children. Mindfulness takes no extra time. According to new scientific studies, the practice of mindfulness is linked to positive changes in areas of the brain associated with memory, learning, and emotion. Considerable research has demonstrated the benefits of mindfulness practice in relieving stress, easing pain, improving concentration, and relieving a variety of other symptoms.

Quieting Reflex

The quieting reflex technique was developed by a physician named Charles Stroebel. It will help you deal with short-term stress such as the urge to eat or smoke, succumb to road rage, or react to other annoyances. By activating what's called the sympathetic nervous system, this technique relieves muscle tightening, jaw clenching, and stops you from holding your breath. It should be practiced frequently throughout the day, whenever you start to feel stressed. It can be done with your eyes opened or closed.

To engage in the quieting reflex exercise, follow the steps outlined below:

1. Become aware of what is annoying you: a ringing phone, an angry comment, the urge to smoke, a worrisome thought—whatever.

2. Repeat the phrase "alert mind, calm body" to yourself.

3. Smile inwardly with your eyes and your mouth. This stops facial muscles from

making a fearful or angry expression. The inward smile is a feeling. It cannot be seen by others.

4. Inhale slowly to the count of three, imagining that the breath comes in through the bottom of your feet. Then exhale slowly. Feel your breath move back down your legs and out through your feet. Let your jaw, tongue, and shoulder muscles go limp.

With several months' practice the quieting reflex becomes an automatic skill.

Nature Therapy

Many of us suffer from what has been called "nature deficit disorder," but it can be readily cured with regular doses of the outdoors. For thousands of years, exposure to natural environments has been recommended for healing. Taking a break from artificial lighting, excessive computer and TV screen time, and indoor environments can be restorative. A brief walk in a park or a longer visit to a beautiful outdoor environment can restore the mind and body. When the weather is poor, visit a garden nursery to inhale the fragrance of the flowers and see the color and beauty. Or bring nature indoors with plants, pets, and nature photography. Even a few minutes of playing with or stroking a pet can lower blood pressure and calm a restless mind.

Worry Time

Worrisome negative thoughts feed anxiety. But we can't ignore negative thoughts forever. Ignored problems have a way of thrusting themselves back into our consciousness. You'll find it easier to set aside worries if you make time to deal with them.

Set aside 20 to 30 minutes a day as your "worry time." Whenever a worry pops into your mind, write it down and tell yourself that you'll deal with it during worry time. Jot down the little things (Did Linda take her lunch to school?), the not-so-little things (What will I do if my pain gets worse and I can't make my granddaughter's birthday party?), and the big ones (Will our children be able to find jobs?).

Sometimes you can relieve stress and break the cycle of negative thoughts by shifting your perspective. If you find yourself upset, ask, "How important will this be in an hour, a day, a month, or a year?" This reframing can help you differentiate between things that are really important and need action versus the more minor annoyances that capture your attention.

During your scheduled worry time, don't do anything except worry, brainstorm, and write down possible solutions. For each of your worries, ask yourself the following questions:

- What is the problem?
- How likely is it that the problem will occur?
- What's the worst that could happen?
- What's the best that could happen?
- How would I cope with the problem if it does occur?
- What are possible solutions?
- What is my plan of action?

Be specific. Instead of worrying about what might happen if you lose your job, ask yourself how likely it is that you will lose your job. And if you do lose it, brainstorm about what you will do, with whom, and by when. Write a job search plan.

If you're anxious about getting seasick on a boat trip and not making it to the bathroom in time, imagine how you would manage the situation. Ask yourself if any of this is really unbearable. Tell yourself you might feel uncomfortable or embarrassed, but you'll survive. Research ways to mitigate or avoid seasickness.

Remember, if a new worry pops up after your scheduled worry time, just jot it down for your next session. Then distract yourself by refocusing intently on whatever you are doing.

Scheduling a specific worry time can cut the amount of time you spend worrying by at least a third. If you look at your list of worries later, you'll find that the vast majority of them never materialized. Or they were not nearly as bad as you had anticipated.

Practice Gratitude

One of the most effective ways to improve your mood and overall happiness is by focusing your attention on what's going well in your life. For what are you grateful? Psychologists have done research to demonstrate that people can increase their happiness by practicing gratitude exercises. We encourage you to try these three:

- **Write a letter of thanks.** Write and then deliver a letter of gratitude to someone who had been especially kind to you but had never been properly thanked. Perhaps it's a teacher, a mentor, a friend, or a family member. In the letter, express your appreciation for the person's kindness. The letter will have more impact if you include some specific examples of what the recipient has done for you. Describe how the actions made you feel. Ideally, read your letter to the person, face-to-face if possible. Be aware of how you feel, and watch the other person's reaction.

- **Acknowledge at least three good things every day.** Each night before bed, write down at least three things that went well today. No event or feeling is too small to note. By putting your gratitude into words, you increase appreciation and memory of your blessings. Knowing that you will need to write each night changes your mental filters during the whole day. You will tend to seek out, look for, and specially note the good things that happen. If doing this daily is too much or begins to seem like a routine chore, do it once a week.

- **Make a list of the things you take for granted.** For example, if your chronic pain has affected your knees, you can still be grateful that your elbows and hands are unaffected. Perhaps you can celebrate a day in which you don't have a headache or backache. Counting your blessings can add up to a better mood and more happiness.

Compile a List of Strengths

Make a personal inventory of your talents, skills, achievements, and positive qualities, big and small. Celebrate your accomplishments. When something goes wrong, consult your list of positives to put the problem in perspective. It then becomes just one specific experience, not something that defines your whole life.

Put Kindness into Practice

This world is plagued by violence and suffering. When something bad happens, it's front-page news. As an antidote to this misery, despair, and cynicism, practice acts of kindness. Look for opportunities to give without expecting any-thing in return. Here are some examples of kind actions:

- Hold the door open for the person behind you.
- Give an unexpected gift of movie or concert tickets.
- Send an anonymous gift to a friend who needs cheering up.
- Help someone with a heavy load.
- Relate positive stories about helping and kindness.
- Cultivate an attitude of gratefulness for kindness you have received.
- Plant a tree.
- Smile and let people cut ahead of you in line or on the freeway.
- Pick up litter.
- Give another driver your parking space.

Be creative. Acts of kindness are contagious, and have a ripple effect. In one study, the people who were given an unexpected treat (cookies) were later more likely to help others.

Write Away Stress

It's hard work to keep our deep negative feelings hidden. Over time, this cumulative stress undermines our body's defenses and seems to weaken our immunity. Confiding our feelings to others or writing them down puts them into words and helps us sort them out. Words help us understand and absorb a traumatic event and eventually put it behind us. Sharing our feelings gives us a sense of release and control.

In his book *Opening Up*, the psychologist Jamie Pennebaker described a series of studies about healing effects of confiding or writing.

One group was asked to express their deepest thoughts and feelings about something bad that had happened to them. Another group wrote about ordinary matters such as their plans for the day. Both groups wrote for 15 to 20 minutes a day for three to five consecutive days. No one read what either group had written.

The results were surprisingly powerful. When compared with the people who wrote about ordinary events, the ones who wrote about their bad experiences reported fewer symptoms, fewer visits to the doctor, fewer days off from work, improved mood, and a more positive outlook. Their immune function was enhanced for at least six weeks after the writing exercise. This was especially true for those who expressed previously undisclosed painful feelings.

Try the "write thing" when something is bothering you. It could be when you find yourself thinking (or dreaming) too much about an experience, when you avoid thinking about something because it is too upsetting, or when there's something you would like to tell others but don't for fear of embarrassment or punishment.

The following guidelines can help you use writing as a way to deal with negative experiences:

- Set a specific schedule for writing. For example, you might write 15 minutes a day for four consecutive days, or one day a week for four weeks.

- Write in a place where you won't be interrupted or distracted.

- Don't plan to share your writing—that could stop your honest expression. Save what you write or destroy it, as you wish.

- Explore your very deepest thoughts and feelings and analyze why you feel the way you do. Write about your negative feelings such as sadness, hurt, hate, anger, fear, guilt, or resentment.

- Write continuously. Don't worry about grammar, spelling, or making sense. If clarity and coherence come as you continue to write, so much the better. If you run out of things to say, just repeat what you have already written in different words.

- Even if you find the writing awkward at first, keep going. It gets easier. If you just cannot write, try talking into a tape recorder for 15 minutes about your deepest thoughts and feelings.

- Don't expect to feel better immediately. You may feel sad or depressed when your deepest feelings begin to surface. This usually fades within an hour or two or a day or two. The overwhelming majority of people report feelings of relief, happiness, and contentment soon after writing for a few consecutive days.

- Writing may help you clarify what actions you need to take. But don't use writing as a substitute for taking action or as a way of avoiding things.

Relaxation, imagery, and positive, more realistic thinking can be some of the most powerful tools you can add to your self-management toolbox. They will help you manage pain and other symptoms as well as master the other skills discussed in this book.

As with exercise and other acquired skills, using your mind to manage your health

Other Resources to Explore

American Psychological Association (APA): www.apa.org

Association of Cancer Online Resources (ACOR): www.acor.org

Canadian Psychological Association (CPA): www.cpa.ca

Darnall, Beth. *Enhanced Pain Management: Binaural Relaxation* [audio CD]: Boulder, Colo.: Bull, 2014. www.bullpub.com

Gardner-Nix, Jackie. *Meditations for the Mindfulness Solution to Pain* [audio CD]: www.shopneuronova.com

Greater Good Science Center: www.greatergood.berkeley.edu

The Happiness Project: www.gretchenrubin.com

Mental Health America: www.liveyourlifewell.org

Naparstek, Belleruth. *Health Journeys Guided Imagery* [audio CDs]: www.healthjourneys.com

National Center for Complementary and Alternative Medicine: www.nccam.nih.gov

National Institute of Mental Health: www.nimh.nih.gov

Regan, Catherine, and Rick Seidel. *Relaxation for Mind and Body: Pathways to Healing* [audio CD]: Boulder, Colo.: Bull, 2012. www.bullpub.com

StressStop: www.stressstop.com

WebMD: www.webMD.com

Weil, Andrew, and Martin Rossman. *Self-Healing with Guided Imagery* [audio CD]: Louisville, Colo.: Sounds True, 2006

condition requires both practice and time before you begin to notice the benefits. If you feel you are not accomplishing anything, don't give up. Be patient and keep on trying. However if symptoms get worse, don't postpone seeing a health care provider. Be sure to tell him or her about any of the techniques you are trying. Give a full picture of what you do to manage your pain condition and your health. This will help ensure safe, coordinated care.

Suggested Further Reading

To learn more about the topics discussed in this chapter, we suggest that you explore the following resources:

Ben-Shahar, Tal. *Happier: Learn the Secrets to Daily Joy and Lasting Fulfillment.* New York: McGraw-Hill, 2007.

Benson, Herbert, and Miriam Z. Klipper. *The Relaxation Response.* New York: HarperCollins, 2000.

Benson, Herbert, and Eileen M. Stuart. *The Wellness Book: The Comprehensive Guide to Maintaining Health and Treating Stress-Related Illness.* New York: Fireside, 1993.

Boroson, Martin. *One Moment Meditation.* New York: Winter Road Publishing, 2009.

Borysenko, Joan. *Inner Peace for Busy People: 52 Simple Strategies for Transforming Your Life.* Carlsbad, Calif.: Hay House, 2003.

Burns, David D. *The Feeling Good Handbook,* rev. ed. New York: Plume, 1999.

Caudill, Margaret. *Managing Pain Before It Manages You.* New York: Guilford Press, 2008.

Cousins, Norman. *Head First: The Biology of Hope and the Healing Power of the Human Spirit.* New York: Penguin, 1990.

Craze, Richard. *Teach Yourself Relaxation,* 3rd ed. New York: McGraw-Hill, 2009.

Darnall, Beth. *Less Pain, Fewer Pills: Avoid the Dangers of Prescription Opioids and Gain Control over Chronic Pain.* Boulder: Bull Publishing, 2014.

Davis, Martha, Elizabeth Eshelman, and Matthew McKay. *The Relaxation and Stress Reduction Workbook.* Oakland, Calif.: New Harbinger, 2008.

Diener, Ed, and Robert Biswas-Diener. *Happiness: Unlocking the Mysteries of Psychological Wealth.* Malden, Mass.: Blackwell, 2008.

Dossey, Larry. *Prayer Is Good Medicine.* New York: HarperCollins, 1996.

Emmons, Robert A. *Thanks! How the New Science of Gratitude Can Make You Happier.* New York: Houghton Mifflin, 2007.

Funk, Mary Margaret. *Tools Matter for Practicing the Spiritual Life.* New York: Continuum, 2004.

Gardner-Nix, Jackie. *The Mindfulness Solution to Pain: Step-by-Step Techniques for Chronic Pain Management.* Oakland, CA: New Harbinger Publications. 2009.

Grenville-Cleave, Bridget. *Introducing Positive Psychology: A Practical Guide.* London: Totem Books/Icon Books, 2012.

Kabat-Zinn, Jon. *Coming to Our Senses: Healing Ourselves and the World Through Mindfulness.* New York: Hyperion, 2005.

Kabat-Zinn, Jon. *Full Catastrophe Living: Using the Wisdom of Your Body and Mind to Face Stress, Pain, and Illness.* New York: Bantam Books, 2013.

Kabat-Zinn, Jon. *Wherever You Go, There You Are: Mindfulness Meditation in Everyday Life.* New York: Hyperion, 2005.

Keating, Thomas. *Open Mind, Open Heart: The Contemplative Dimension of the Gospel.* New York: Continuum, 2006.

Keating, Thomas, Basil Pennington, Gustave Reininger, et al. *Centering Prayer in Daily Life and Ministry.* New York: Continuum, 1998.

Lyubomirsky, Sonia. *The How of Happiness: A New Approach to Getting the Life You Want.* New York: Penguin, 2008.

McKay, Matthew, Martha Davis, and Patrick Fanning. *Thoughts and Feelings: Taking Control of Your Moods and Your Life,* 4th ed. Oakland, Calif.: New Harbinger, 2011.

Ornstein, Robert, and David Sobel. *Healthy Pleasures.* Cambridge, Mass.: Perseus, 1989.

Peale, Norman V. *Positive Imaging: The Powerful Way to Change Your Life.* New York: Ballantine Books, 1996.

Remen, Rachel Naomi. *Kitchen Table Wisdom: Stories That Heal.* New York: Riverhead Books, 2006.

Seligman, Martin. *Authentic Happiness.* New York: Atria Books, 2004.

Seligman, Martin. *Flourish: A Visionary New Understanding of Happiness and Well-Being.* New York: Free Press, 2011.

Siegel, Bernie S. *Help Me to Heal: A Practical Guidebook for Patients, Visitors, and Caregivers.* Carlsbad, Calif.: Hay House, 2003.

Sobel, David, and Robert Ornstein. *The Healthy Mind, Healthy Body Handbook* (also published under the title *The Mind and Body Health Handbook*). Los Altos, Calif.: DRx, 1996.

Stahl, Bob, and Elisha Goldstein. *A Mindfulness-Based Stress Reduction Workbook.* Oakland, Calif.: New Harbinger, 2010.

Turk, Dennis C., and Frits Winter. *The Pain Survival Guide: How to Reclaim Your Life.* Washington, D.C.: American Psychological Association, 2006.

Wiseman, Richard. *59 Seconds: Think a Little, Change a Lot.* New York: Anchor Books, 2009.

CHAPTER 6

Pacing: Balancing Activity and Rest

*I*T CAN BE DIFFICULT TO STRIKE THE RIGHT BALANCE between activity and rest when you have chronic pain. In part, this is because it seems like you should stop an activity if it hurts. That's what we do with acute pain because from long experience, we know that acute pain is nature's way of telling us to pay attention, to rest, and to heal. Because we have responded to pain this way our whole lives, it's difficult to get out of the mind-set of "pain = stop activity."

But chronic pain is different from acute pain, as we discussed in Chapter 1. If you have a type of idiopathic chronic pain condition (that is, pain that should have gone away but didn't), damaged tissues have healed after three to six months. Being active is not going to impact healing because healing has already occurred.

If you have a well-understood progressive disease such as arthritis, stopping activity will only make your condition worse. With chronic pain, you have to think differently about activity. Being active can help you be healthier and live a fuller life. And that is very important. Even in the face of chronic pain, you still want to enjoy and be involved in life and do the things that are important to you.

Activity Patterns

People with chronic pain typically display one of three activity patterns: avoiding activity, overdoing activity, and pacing activity. Let's talk about each of these separately.

Avoiding Activity

Some people with chronic pain rest almost all the time. They avoid activity. They started resting a lot when their pain was in the early stages thinking that rest would help, but it didn't. Now, they have become so out of shape that movement of any kind hurts—not so much because of their chronic pain but because their muscles have become shortened and are tight and tense because they haven't exercised. Or, they find that they don't have the stamina to keep at a task for even short periods of time. This is largely due to poor muscle strength. Fear of pain leads people to avoid activity, but avoiding activity actually leads to more pain. It's a vicious cycle, as shown in Figure 6.1.

Resting too much has many other negative effects that can lead to further disability, additional depression, and more pain. Dr. Walter Bortz, who has studied the effects of inactivity, has coined the term "disuse syndrome." His research shows that physical inactivity leads to deterioration of your heart, bones, and even your mental state. Did you know that you can lose 10 to 20 percent of your muscle mass and muscle strength by being inactive for just one week? Resting too much is not good for your health and well-being. It is also not good for your chronic pain and other symptoms.

Overdoing Activity

The flip side of resting too much is forcing yourself to continue a task until you complete it. This is a common activity pattern for some people on the days when they might be feeling good. They decide that all the chores are going to get done "today," no matter what. They push on despite their pain and then they collapse in terrible pain at the end of the day. To get through the day, they may have taken extra pain medication, and they may have been irritable and unpleasant to be around. They may accomplish their goal, but they often have to take time off to recover. Recovery can be slow and depressing.

Like the people who rest too much, the people who push themselves and overdo activity are also in a vicious cycle, as shown in Figure 6.2. But as this cycle continues, recovery takes even longer. They may become discouraged and begin to do less and less.

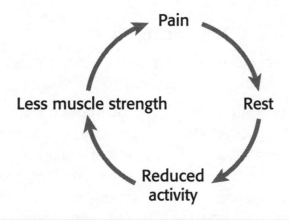

Figure 6.1 **Vicious cycle of underdoing activity**

Pacing Activity

Both the "too much rest" group and the "big push" group can improve their situation with a technique called pacing. Pacing is strategically balancing activity and rest. This allows you to accomplish the things you want to on most days, while keeping your pain under control.

Pacing is not about avoiding activity. It's about regulating activity. For the inactive group, pacing involves gradually increasing activity to more normal levels. Chapters 7, 8, and 9 are all about how to become more physically active while keeping safety in mind. For the people who tend to overdo it, it's about learning to moderate activities. This may involve taking short breaks, changing body position, alternating tasks, and other strategies. People who pace their activities tend to be more satisfied with what they accomplish. They also report feeling more in control of their pain. The box on page 104 lists pacing tips of successful self-managers.

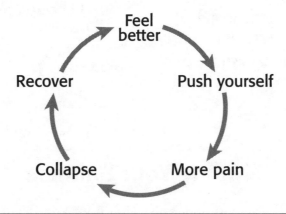

Figure 6.2 **Vicious cycle of overdoing activity**

Ten Pacing Tips

The goal of pacing is to gradually increase your activity to levels that are as near normal as possible on most days. This will allow you to accomplish the things you want to.

- **Determine how you spend your time.** Monitor your daily activities, including your rest periods, to find out how you spend your time. Keep a diary for a couple of days. Choose a typical weekday and a day on the weekend. Note what activities you do and how long you can do them before you are bothered by pain. Note your rest periods and how long you rest. (You can use the example activity and rest diary at the end of this chapter.)

- **Make a schedule.** Develop an activity schedule that includes rest breaks and stick to your schedule. For example, take 5 minutes of rest for every 20 minutes of activity. This is very individual, depending on the type of activity.

- **Be time oriented, not pain oriented.** Knowing how long you can do an activity before your pain gets worse means you can schedule specific activities for a certain number of minutes before taking a rest for a specified period of time. This keeps you, not the pain, in control.

- **Rest before your pain starts to get worse.** So many times we want to complete activities and push through the pain. Keep to your schedule. Stop. Take a rest.

- **Incorporate change into your activity routine.** A change may be as good as a rest. If you are in a situation where you can't take a rest break, alternate activities frequently, change body position, stretch, or go for a short walk.

- **Use a timer to signal rest breaks.** Then you don't have to worry about trying to remember when to take your break.

- **Break tasks into smaller, more manageable pieces.** Take breaks between the smaller tasks, or schedule some smaller tasks on different days.

- **Avoid rushing.** Slow down. Plan ahead. Rushing can increase your stress. Planning can save you energy and reduce frustration.

- **Don't overschedule activities.** Work on developing realistic expectations of yourself. Sometimes, you just have to say no.

- **Prioritize your activities.** Some days, you may not be able to get everything done. Determine the most important thing you want to accomplish today and then work on that.

Finding Your Balance

Hitting the right balance between activity and rest sounds like it should be easy, but it can be tricky. Balance is very individual. A balanced schedule for one person may be overdoing it or underdoing it for another. That's why you have to spend some time trying to sort out what is right for you. Through trial and error, you can find out what activities you can do and how long you can do

Rest	Find your balance	Activity

them without a significant increase in pain. For example, you may find you can work at a certain activity for half an hour if you take off 10 minutes after every 30 minutes. Maybe you need five minutes of rest for every 15 minutes of activity. Or maybe you need five minutes of rest after every five minutes of a particularly difficult activity for you. The goal is to find a reasonable comfort level while still being active. Set a timer to help you remember rest periods.

Your rest periods might be a time for you to get up and walk around, stretch, practice relaxation techniques, call a friend, listen to music, or read the paper. At the end of the day you may discover that you were active for a total of four or five hours without significantly increasing your pain. In contrast, if you had pushed yourself to work three hours straight without a break, you might have increased pain to the point where you had to stop. In this way, you can accomplish more if you build in breaks.

Planning rest breaks *before* pain forces you to stop an activity is a key technique of pacing. This technique is called working to schedule. This is in contrast to working to tolerance. When you work to tolerance, you push yourself to your limit. Pain begins to escalate, becoming significantly worse. This does not need to happen if you systematically plan bouts of your activity and rest periods. When you plan and stick to your schedule, *you* are in control, not your pain!

Managing Your Activity

What activities do you do in the normal course of a day? The best way to find out is to keep a diary of your activities for a couple of days. See the sample Activity and Rest Diary on page 108 of this chapter. This diary will help you to establish your baseline. Be sure to track at least one weekday and one weekend day. You can use the form at the end of this chapter, or simply list each hour on a piece of paper and jot down all your activities as you go about your day. Be sure to include your rest times. Note the amount of time you spend doing each activity or resting. Also note whether your pain stays the same, increases, or decreases when doing the activity. This can be done with a pain intensity scale, with 0 representing no pain at all and 10 the worst pain imaginable. (See Chapter 11, page 184 for more instructions.) Once you have your diary notes, you will get a sense of how you actually spend your time—the activities you do, how long you do them—and how activity affects your pain. Then, you will be able to see whether you are resting so much that you accomplish very little in your day, or whether you push yourself too much, spending too long at an activity before taking a rest.

Dr. David Corey, the clinical director of the Function and Pain Program at Mount Sinai Hospital in Toronto, has spent almost four decades working with people who have pain. He suggests a three-part program for self-managing and pacing. Why not give the following suggestions a try? (Dr. Corey's book is available free on the Internet. See Suggested Further Reading at the end of this chapter.)

Prepare a Daily Schedule

Each evening, prepare a schedule for the following day. Each night, decide what time you will get up the following morning and what your activities will be. Establish realistic goals. Ask yourself, "What do I really want to get done tomorrow?"

It is important not to overschedule your activities. For each one activity, think about how certain you are that you can accomplish that task even on a "bad" day. If you are not at least 70 percent sure you can do the activity, you may be taking on too much. In that case, cut back so you will be able to meet your activity schedule. Over time, you will be able to do more. This process follows the same principles as action planning, discussed in Chapter 2.

Chapter 2 also discusses problem solving and decision making, two other critical self-management skills for pacing. Think about how you can use those skills for pacing your activity and rest. Also, you might find it helpful to purchase an inexpensive daily planner at a business supply store or local drug store. It will list the hours of the day for each day of the week, with space for writing in activities and rest periods. This can make planning easier.

Build in Rest Periods

Schedule rest periods during the day, and take them at the specified times. You should be able to figure out from your diary how long you can do an activity before your pain increases. Learn to listen to your body. Often, our bodies let us know when pain is going to get worse. You might feel an extra tightness, muscle twinge, or spasm in an area of the body that hurts. A cue like this is almost like a yellow warning sign telling us that pain is on the way up—that it's going to go from a 4 to a 6 out of 10 on the pain intensity scale. Learn to stop and take your rest break before you get this warning sign.

For example, you may be able to peel vegetables for supper for only 10 minutes before feeling that extra tightness in your neck and shoulders. With this in mind, schedule a rest period after every eight or nine minutes of meal preparation. On the other hand, you might be able to sit at a computer or drive a car for 30 minutes before feeling muscle twinges in your back. Schedule rest after 25 minutes of these activities. The idea is to plan your day so you get up and change activities before the pain forces you to stop what you are doing. Always plan ahead so you are preventing pain from getting significantly worse. That keeps you in control.

Taking a break is not a sign of weakness or failure; it is a wise move to allow you to gradually build up your stamina. As you improve, you may be able to reduce the number and duration of your rest periods. For those of you who go to work every day, it may not always be possible to schedule a rest. In that case, can you do a different task that allows you to change your body position for a few minutes? Can you get up and stretch or take a short walk around the worksite? Sometimes a change is as good as a rest. Make use of your coffee and lunch breaks to relax.

Account for Every Hour of the Day

When you plan your day, make sure all the time periods are filled with activities and rest breaks. Account for every hour of the day. This encourages you to be time-oriented (working to schedule) rather than pain-oriented (working to tolerance). You will tend to concentrate on your activity rather than on your discomfort, knowing that a rest break is coming up. Set a timer to signal your breaks so you don't have to remember to look at your watch all the time. Take full advantage of rest breaks. You can spend the time productively in relaxation. Do gentle exercise, take a short walk, read, or call a friend. The one thing you should not do is worry!

When people first develop a schedule, they tend to overschedule activities. Resist this urge. Be realistic about what you can accomplish. Take it slow and build in rest periods throughout the day. Set your timer and take the breaks you built into your schedule. Scheduling is a skill that takes time to perfect. You probably won't get it exactly right the first few times you do it. But be persistent and stick with it. It may seem tedious but once scheduling is a habit, it gets easier and faster and the results are worth it.

Suggested Further Reading

To learn more about the topics discussed in this chapter, we suggest that you explore the following resources:

Caudill, Margaret A. *Managing Pain Before It Manages You.* New York: Guilford Press, 2009 (see especially Chapter 4).

Corey, David. *Pain: Learning to Live Without It.* Toronto: Macmillan Canada, 1993, 2004. Available as a free download in two parts at www.healthrecoverygroup.com/pmp/pain_handbooks.htm:

Part 1: *Why We Hurt: The Human Body and Pain.*

Part 2: *Towards Solutions: Strategies for Overcoming Pain* (see especially Chapter 7).

Turk, Dennis C., and Frits Winter. *The Pain Survival Guide: How to Reclaim Your Life.* Washington, D.C.: American Psychological Association, 2006 (see especially Chapter 2).

Activity and Rest Diary

Complete the diary for a typical weekday and for a typical day on the weekend.

Time	Activity and Rest Periods	Time spent on each activity/rest period	Pain level 0 = no pain to 10 = extreme pain
7 A.M.			
8 A.M.			
9 A.M.			
10 A.M.			
11 A.M.			
12 noon			
1 P.M.			
2 P.M.			

Time	Activity and Rest Periods	Time spent on each activity/rest period	Pain level 0 = no pain to 10 = extreme pain
3 P.M.			
4 P.M.			
5 P.M.			
6 P.M.			
7 P.M.			
8 P.M.			
9 P.M.			
10 P.M.			

The weakest and oldest among us can become some sort of athlete, but only the strongest can survive as spectators. Only the hardiest can withstand the perils of inertia, inactivity, and immobility.

—J. H. Bland and S. M. Cooper,
Seminars in Arthritis and Rheumatism (1984)

CHAPTER 7

Exercise and Physical Activity for Every Body

ACTIVE PEOPLE ARE HEALTHIER AND HAPPIER than people who are not active. This is true for people of all ages and conditions, including chronic pain. Not moving enough can cause or worsen pain, disability, and other illness. In order to better manage your chronic pain, you need to learn how to balance activity and rest. Chapter 6 explained the importance of planning for appropriate rest periods throughout the day. Equally important is planning for regular activity and exercise.

Physical activity keeps you fit so you have the strength, stamina, and energy to do the things you want to do in life. Being more fit can improve your chronic pain over the long run. Scientific research conducted over the past 30 years has consistently shown that increasing physical activity helps chronic pain, improves functioning, and boosts overall health and well-being. In fact, exercise is most often the largest part of rehabilitation programs for people with chronic pain.

The bottom line: *keep moving!*

You probably know that regular physical activity is important, but when you have chronic pain it can be difficult to know what you can do and how to do it. The good news is that there is plenty of information available to help you get started and be successful. For example, there are government guidelines that explain the importance of physical activity and offer programs to get going. These guidelines spell out what kinds of exercise or physical activities are best and how much you need. In this and the following two chapters, you will learn about these guidelines and about how to make wise exercise choices.

Of course, learning what to do is not enough. You also have to do it! It is up to you to make your life more enjoyable, more comfortable, and healthier through physical activity. As is the case in every chapter, the information about exercise in this book is not intended to take the place of medical or other health professional advice. If you already have a prescribed exercise plan that differs from the suggestions here, be sure to share this book with your health care provider or therapist before beginning this program.

Why Exercise?

Decades of research confirm that regular exercise is key to a healthier life. It can prevent and help in the management of heart disease and diabetes. It improves blood pressure, blood sugar, and blood fat levels. Exercise can help you to maintain a good weight, which takes stress off your weight-bearing joints. It is also part of keeping bones strong and treating osteoporosis. There is evidence that regular exercise can help prevent blood clots, which is one of the reasons it can be of particular benefit to people with heart and vascular diseases. Regular exercise improves levels of strength, energy, and self-confidence and lessens feelings of stress, anxiety, and depression. It can help you sleep better and feel more relaxed and happy.

In addition, regular exercise has consistently been shown to be the single most important thing you can do to manage chronic pain. It improves the ability to do normal activities; reduces pain, tenderness, and fatigue; and increases muscle strength in people with various types of widespread pain, including fibromyalgia. It also lessons pain and improves function in people with chronic back pain. Strengthening and stretching exercises improve chronic neck pain and some types of headache. Strong muscles help people with arthritis protect their joints by improving stability and absorbing shock. Regular exercise also helps nourish joints and keeps cartilage and bone healthy. Many people with leg pain from poor circulation or other causes can walk farther and more comfortably with a regular exercise program.

That is all good news. The better news is that it doesn't take hours of painful, sweaty exercise to achieve health benefits. Studies have shown that even short periods of moderate physical activity can improve health and fitness, lessen pain and improve everyday functioning, reduce disease risks, and boost mood. Being active also helps you feel more in control of your life and less at the mercy of your chronic pain.

Developing an Exercise Program

If you are not already active, starting a regular exercise program means making room for a new habit or routine in your life. This involves setting aside a period of time on most days of the week to make exercise a part of your routine. Recommended exercise programs focus on four types of fitness:

- **Flexibility.** Being flexible means you can move comfortably to do everything you need and want to do. Limited flexibility can cause pain, lead to injury, and make muscles work harder and tire more quickly. You lose flexibility when you are inactive and as a result of some chronic pain conditions, but you can increase flexibility by doing gentle stretching exercises like those described in Chapter 8.

- **Strength.** Muscles need to be exercised to maintain their strength. When inactive, muscles weaken and atrophy (shrink). When your muscles are not strong, you feel weak and get tired quickly. Much of the disability and lack of mobility for people with chronic pain is due to muscle weakness. Exercise programs that ask muscles to do more work (such as lifting a weight) strengthen muscles.

- **Endurance (aerobics).** Feeling energetic depends on the fitness of your heart, lungs, and muscles. The heart and lungs must work efficiently to send oxygen-rich blood to the muscles. The muscles must be fit enough to use the oxygen. Aerobic ("with oxygen") exercise engages the large muscles of your body in continuous activity such as walking, swimming, dancing, mowing the lawn, and riding a bike. Aerobic exercise improves cardiovascular fitness, lessens heart attack risk, and helps control weight. Aerobic exercise also promotes a sense of well-being, eases depression and anxiety, promotes restful sleep, and improves mood and energy levels.

- **Balance.** Good balance helps prevent falls. Strong and coordinated muscles in your trunk and legs are an important part of good balance. Flexibility, strength, and endurance also contribute to balance. Of course, there are other reasons people fall (poor vision, poor lighting, dizziness, tripping over rugs), but being strong and coordinated are crucial preventive measures. Certain exercises are especially good for improving balance.

Setting Your Exercise Goals

A complete exercise program improves all four aspects of fitness: flexibility, strength, endurance, and balance. The material in this book can help you develop just such a program. Chapter 8 includes a gentle flexibility program and some specific exercises for your posture and balance. Chapter 9 explains and gives examples of aerobic exercise for improving endurance and your overall health.

If you haven't exercised regularly in some time, talk with a health care provider such as your doctor, nurse practitioner, or physical therapist before beginning a new program of physical activity. Because everyone's chronic pain is different, you need to identify the specific exercises that are right for you, how to modify exercises if needed, and the precautions you need to take when starting an exercise program. You especially need to talk to your doctor before starting any new activity, if, in addition to your chronic pain, you have experienced any of the following symptoms or have the following problems: heart disease, pains in your chest, high blood pressure, faintness, severe dizziness, or shortness of breath.

Certified fitness trainers, sometimes called kinesiologists, are another group of knowledgeable people who can help you. Employed at fitness or rehabilitation centers, these trainers can help design a safe fitness program for you, keeping your chronic pain in mind. Some fitness centers have special programs available for people with pain. When talking to these experts, always let them know about your pain problem.

One way to begin thinking about an exercise program is to choose a goal that exercise can help you achieve. For example, you might want to be able to take your new grandchild for a walk in her stroller, or be able to sit comfortably at a monthly breakfast with old friends, or get back to playing a sport you used to enjoy.

Once you have a goal in mind, it is much easier to plan an exercise program that makes sense to you. If you can see how exercise can be helpful, it is easier to get excited about adding yet another task to your day.

Overcoming Your Exercise Barriers

Health and fitness make sense. Yet when people with chronic pain are encouraged to become more physically active, they often have many fears, concerns, and worries. These barriers can prevent you from taking the first step. The following are some common barriers and possible solutions:

"Exercise will harm me." It is important to understand that "hurt" does not equal "harm." If you have been inactive for a while, your muscles may be weak and shortened, and joints may be stiff because they haven't been used to their full range. So beginning an exercise program, even a gentle one, may cause some muscle soreness for a short time. But this is normal—it will not harm you or cause your condition to worsen. A safe program of exercise, if started slowly and gradually, should produce minimal muscle soreness. Keep in mind this important rule of thumb: start where you are now—and go slow.

"I don't have enough time." We all have the same amount of time; we just use it differently. It's a matter of priorities. Some people find time to watch television but not to exercise. Exercise doesn't take a lot of time. Just 15 minutes a day is a good start, and even this minimum investment is much better than nothing. You may be

Choose Your Goal and Make a Plan

1. **Choose something that you want to do but don't do now because of some physical reason.** For example, you might want to enjoy a shopping or fishing trip with your friends, mow your own lawn, or take a family vacation.

2. **Think about why you don't do it or don't enjoy doing it now.** It might be that you get tired before everybody else, or it's too hard to get up from a low chair or bench. Maybe climbing steps is painful or makes your legs tired, or your shoulders are too weak or stiff to cast your fishing line or stow your carry-on bag.

3. **Decide what makes it difficult to do what you want.** For example, if getting up from a low seat is difficult, it may be because your hips or knees are stiff and your leg muscles are weak. In this case, flexibility and strengthening exercises for hips and knees will be helpful. If you tire easily when climbing stairs, then you need to work on your aerobic fitness to build endurance.

4. **Design your exercise plan.** Read Chapter 8 and review the Moving Easy Program (MEP). The MEP is a gentle, safe flexibility exercise program designed for people with chronic pain. It's a great way to start moving all parts of your body, and it feels good. Listen to the audio CD provided with this book and follow the instructions and photographs on page 126. As you get more comfortable moving your body, you can start doing more. If you want to improve your endurance, read Chapter 9 about aerobic exercise. Start exercising for short intervals and build up gradually. Health and fitness take time to build, but every day you exercise you are becoming healthier and more successful at controlling your life. That's why it's so important to make sure you keep it up.

able to work exercise into your established routine: you could, for example, watch television while pedaling a stationary bicycle or arrange a "walking meeting" to discuss business or family matters. If you add three 10-minute walks to your daily routine, you will have completed 30 minutes of exercise for the day!

"I'm too tired." When you're out of shape or depressed, you may feel tired. You have to break out of this cycle. Try an experiment: next time you feel "too tired," take a short walk (walk for five minutes, or even two). You may be surprised to discover that walking gives you energy. As you get into shape, you will recognize the difference between feeling listless and feeling physically tired.

"I'm too old." You're never too old for physical activity. In fact, fitness is especially important as we age. No matter what your age or level of fitness, you can always find ways to increase your activity, energy, and sense of well-being.

"I get enough exercise." This may be true, but for most people, their jobs and daily activities do not provide enough sustained exercise at a moderate level to keep them fit and energetic.

"Exercise is boring." You can make it more interesting and fun. Exercise with other people. Entertain yourself with a headset and musical tapes, or listen to the radio. Vary your activities or your venues. For example, if you choose walking as a form of exercise, try different routes. You might find exercise time good thinking time.

"Exercise will cause my pain to flare up." Health benefits come from moderate-intensity physical activity. For some chronic pain conditions, exercise actually reduces pain. If you feel more pain when you finish than before you started, take a close look at what you are doing. The old saying "no pain, no gain" is simply wrong. You may be exercising improperly or overdoing it. Talk with your instructor, therapist, or doctor. You may simply need to be less vigorous or change the type of exercise you're doing.

"I'm too embarrassed." For some people the thought of donning a skin-tight designer exercise outfit and trotting around in public is delightful, but for others it is downright distressing. The options for physical activity range from exercise in the privacy of your own home to group social activities. You will be able to find something that suits you. And, no, you don't have to wear any exotic clothing to do it!

"I'm afraid I might fall." Check where you will exercise for fall safety (good lighting, well-maintained parking lots and walkways, handrails, and uncluttered floors). Choose exercises that feel safe—chair exercise, water exercise, or recumbent bicycling provide a lot of support

as you get started. Remember, strong and flexible legs and ankles and coordination reduce the risks of falls. Staying active helps you prevent falls by keeping you strong and coordinated. Your doctor or therapist may recommend a cane, walking stick, or walker to enhance your balance, but it is important to have a therapist fit it to you and to learn how to use it safely. Using a cane or walker that doesn't fit or is used improperly can cause a fall.

"I'm afraid I'll have a heart attack." In most cases, the risk of a heart attack is greater for people who are not physically active than for those who exercise regularly. But if you are worried about your heart health, check with your doctor. Especially if your illness is under control, it's probably safer to exercise than not to exercise. If you have angina pain or coronary artery disease, read Chapter 19 for more information.

"It's too cold (hot, dark, etc.)." If you are flexible and vary your type of exercise, you can generally work around the changes in weather that make certain types of exercise more difficult. Consider indoor activities such as stationary bicycling, swimming, or mall walking when weather is a barrier.

"I'm afraid I won't be able to do it right or won't be successful." Many people don't start a new project because they are afraid they will fail. If you feel this way, remember two things. First, whatever activities you are able to do— no matter how short or "easy"—are much better than doing nothing. Be proud of what you have done, not guilty about what you haven't done. Second, new projects often seem overwhelming—until we get started and learn to enjoy each day's adventures and successes.

Better Balance

Sometimes people decide that the best way not to fall is to spend more time sitting. After all, if you are not up walking around, you won't be at risk for falling. However, inactivity causes weakness, stiffness, slower reflexes, slower muscles, and even social isolation and depression. All of these harm your balance and increase your risk of falling. If you are inactive, even simple things such as getting up or sitting down in a chair, going to the bathroom, or going down a step can cause problems.

Other physical conditions such as weakness, dizziness, stiffness, poor eyesight, loss of feeling in feet, or inner ear problems can cause a fall, as can the side effects of some medications. Falls can also be caused by the conditions of the space around you: poor lighting, uneven ground, rugs, and cluttered floors. To avoid falls, reduce all these risks and keep yourself strong, flexible, and coordinated. Research shows that people have less fear of falling and actually fall less if they have strong legs and ankles, are flexible, and do things that require them to maintain balance

If you have fallen or are afraid you may fall, talk with your health care provider and get your balance checked to make sure there are no vision, inner ear, or medication problems that need to be fixed. Make sure your home is safe. Exercising keeps you strong, flexible, and active and also helps protect you from falling. Look in Chapter 8 for the better balance exercises marked BB 1 to BB 6 on pages 143–146.

Perhaps you have some other barriers. Be honest with yourself about your worries. Talk to yourself and others to develop positive thoughts about exercise. If you get stuck, ask others for suggestions, or try some of the positive thinking suggestions in Chapter 5.

Preparing to Exercise

Committing to regular exercise is a big deal for anyone. If you have a chronic pain condition, you may also have many daily challenges and special exercise needs. You may need to adapt exercise to your particular type of chronic pain. If you have been inactive for more than six months, or if you have questions about starting an exercise program, it is best to check with your health care provider or therapist. Take this book with you and discuss your exercise plans, or make a list of your questions. If, for example, you have chronic stable angina pain, you will need to pay special attention to potentially serious symptoms such as chest pain, palpitations (irregular heartbeat), shortness of breath, or excessive fatigue. You should notify your health care provider if these, or new symptoms, appear. Read more in Chapter 19.

The goal of this chapter is to encourage you to explore the benefits of physical activity. Start by knowing your own needs and limits, and respect your body. Talk to other people like you who exercise. Talk with your doctor and other health professionals who understand your kind of chronic condition. Always pay attention to your own experience. That helps you know your body and make wise choices.

Putting Your Program into Action

The best way to enjoy and stick with your exercise program is to suit yourself! Choose what you want to do, a place where you feel comfortable doing it, and an exercise time that fits your schedule. If you want to have dinner on the table at 6 o'clock, don't choose an exercise program that requires you to attend a 5 o'clock class. If you are retired and enjoy lunch with friends and an afternoon nap, choose an early or midmorning exercise time.

Pick two or three activities that you think you will enjoy, will be comfortable and safe for you, and you can fit into your daily routine. If an activity is new, try it out before going to the expense of buying equipment or joining a special facility. By doing more than one type of exercise, you can keep active and work around vacations, seasons, and your changing condition. Variety also helps prevent overuse injuries and keeps you from getting bored.

Having fun and enjoying yourself are benefits of exercise that often go unmentioned. Too often we think of exercise as serious business. However, most people who stick with a program do so because they enjoy it and because it makes them feel good. People who stay committed to an exercise program think of their exercise as recreation or a positive part of life rather than a chore. Start off with success in mind. Allow yourself time to get used to something new and meeting new people. You'll probably find that you look forward to exercise.

Experience, practice, and success help build a habit. Follow the self-management steps from Chapter 2 to make it easier to start your program. The following tips will help you be successful as you expand your life to include activity:

- **Keep your exercise goal in mind.** Review "Choose Your Goal and Make a Plan" on page 24.

- **Choose exercises you want to do.** Select exercises and activities from Chapters 8 and 9 to get started. Combine activities that help you achieve your goal with those recommended by your health professionals.

- **Choose the time and place to exercise.** Tell your family and friends about your plan. Making your commitment known makes you more likely to follow through and stick with your program.

- **Commit to an action plan.** Decide how long you'll stick with these particular exercises; six to eight weeks is a reasonable time for any new program.

- **Start your program as soon as you can.** Remember to begin doing what you can and proceed slowly, especially if you haven't exercised in a while.

- **Keep an exercise diary or calendar.** A diary or journal is good for people who enjoy having a more detailed record of what they did and how they felt. Others like keeping a simple calendar on which they note each exercise session.

- **Repeat self-tests at regular intervals.** It is important to monitor changes (both positive and negative) in your health and fitness.

■ **Revise your program.** At the end of six to eight weeks, decide what you liked, what worked, and what made exercising difficult. Make changes in response to your findings and draw up an action plan for another few weeks. You may decide to change some exercises, the place or time you exercise, or your exercise partner or group.

■ **Reward yourself for a job well done.** Rewards come not only from improved health and endurance but you will be rewarded from your ability to partake in enjoyable activities such as family outings, refreshing walks, trips to a concert or museum, or a day of fishing. Pats on the back and a new exercise shirt can be fun too.

Maintaining Your Program

If you haven't exercised recently, you'll probably experience some new feelings and even discomfort when you begin to exercise. It's normal to feel sore muscles and tender joints and to be more tired in the evenings after starting a new fitness program. But if you experience muscle or joint pain that lasts more than two hours after the exercise or you feel tired into the next day, you probably did too much too fast. Don't stop; just don't work so hard the next day, or exercise for a shorter time.

During aerobic exercise, it's natural to feel your heart beat faster, your breathing speed up, and your body get warmer. However, if you experience chest pain, feel sick to your stomach or dizzy, or are severely short of breath, stop exercising until you check with your doctor (see Table 7.1 on the next page).

People who have a chronic pain problem often have additional sensations to sort out when they exercise. It can be difficult to separate if it is pain, exercise, or anxiety that is causing concern and discomfort. You can learn a lot from talking to someone with your condition who has already started an exercise program. Once you've sorted out the new feelings, you'll be able to exercise with more confidence.

Expect setbacks. During the first year, people often have two to three interruptions in their exercise schedule. These interruptions may result from family needs, minor injuries, or illnesses not related to exercise. You may benefit from an occasional rest, a different schedule, or different activities. If you get off track for a while, don't be discouraged. When you are feeling better or have more time and are ready to start again, begin at a lower, more gentle level. And be patient. If you miss three weeks, it may take at least that long to get back to your previous level. Go slowly. Be kind to yourself. You're in this for the long haul.

Think of your head as the coach and your body as your team. For success, all parts of the team need attention. Be a good coach. Encourage and praise yourself. Design "plays" you feel your team will enjoy. Choose places to exercise that you like and are safe. A good coach knows his or her team, sets good goals, and helps the team succeed and gain confidence. A good coach is loyal. A good coach does not belittle, nag, or make anyone feel guilty. Be a good coach to your team—your body!

Besides a good coach, everyone needs a good cheerleader or two. Of course, you can be your own cheerleader, but being both coach and

Table 7.1 **If Exercise Problems Occur**

Problem	Advice
Irregular or rapid heartbeat. Pain, tightness, or pressure in the chest, jaw, arms, or neck. Shortness of breath lasting past the exercise period.	Stop exercising. Talk with your doctor right away. Don't resume exercise until your doctor clears your exercise program.
Light-headedness, dizziness, fainting, cold sweat, or confusion.	Lie down with your feet up or sit down with your head between your knees. Seek medical advice immediately.
Shortness of breath or calf pain from circulation or breathing problems.	Warm up by going slowly at first. Take short rests to recover and resume exercise.
Excessive tiredness or muscle soreness after exercise, especially if you are still tired or sore the next day.	Exercise less strenuously next time. If tiredness lasts, check with your doctor.

cheerleader is a lot to do. Successful exercisers usually have at least one family member or close friend who encourages them. Your cheerleader can exercise with you, help you get other chores done so you can exercise, praise you, or just take your exercise time into account when making plans. Sometimes cheerleaders pop up by themselves, but don't be bashful about asking for a hand.

With exercise experience, you develop a sense of control over yourself and your illness. You learn how to choose your activity to fit your needs. You know when to do less and when to do more. You know that a change in symptoms or a period of inactivity is usually only temporary and doesn't have to feel like a disaster. You know you have the tools to get back on track. Give yourself a chance to succeed. Sticking with it and doing it your way makes you a sure winner.

Physical Activity Guidelines

Many countries now have guidelines for what kinds of physical activity, and how much, people should do to be healthy. The guidelines are pretty much the same all over the world and are geared toward adults with and without chronic conditions and disability. It is important to remember that these guidelines are goals to work toward; they are not the starting point.

Physical Activity Guidelines

Perform moderate aerobic (endurance) exercise for at least 150 minutes (2½ hours) a week or vigorous-intensity activity for at least 75 minutes (1¼ hour) a week.

Engage in aerobic activity at least 10 minutes at a time spread out through the week.

Perform moderate-intensity strengthening exercise of all major muscle groups at least two days a week.

If you cannot meet the guidelines, be as active as you can and avoid inactivity.

Examples of 150 Minutes a Week of Moderate Aerobic Activity

A 10-minute walk at moderate intensity three times a day, five days a week

A 20-minute bike ride at moderate intensity three days a week and a 30-minute walk three days a week

A 30-minute aerobic dance class at moderate intensity twice a week and three 10-minute walks three days a week

Gardening and yard work (digging, raking, lifting) 30 minutes a day, five days a week

Examples of Muscle-Strengthening Exercise

Do exercises for your arms, trunk, and legs (lifting weights, using bands, or just working against your own body weight)

Perform ten of the above exercises twice a week, eight to 12 repetitions each, with enough weight or resistance that you feel tired when you finish each exercise

Try yoga twice a week

On average, only about 25 percent of people in any country exercise enough to meet the guidelines. So don't worry that everyone else but you can do these. Your goal is to gradually and safely increase your physical activity to a level that is right for you. You may eventually be able to meet national exercise goals, but maybe you won't. The important point is to use the information to motivate you to be more active and healthier. Start by simply doing what you can. Even a few minutes of activity several times a day is a good beginning. Pick an exercise that works for you, make it a habit, and gradually increase your time or number of days a week as you are able.

The U.S. Department of Health and Human Services came out with its guidelines in 2008, which we include above. (Canadian physical activity guidelines published in 2010 are very similar.) Remember, they are a guide to where you could go, not where you should be now. Chapters 8 and 9 will give you more information to help you get started on your exercise plan.

Opportunities in Your Community

Many people who exercise regularly do so with at least one other person. Two or more people can keep each other motivated, and a whole class can become a circle of friends. On the other hand, exercising alone gives you the most freedom. You may feel there are no classes that would work for you, or there is no buddy with whom to exercise. If so, start your own program; as you progress, you may find that these feelings change.

Most communities offer a variety of fitness classes, including special programs for people over 50, adaptive exercises, mall walking, group hikes, water aerobics, tai chi, and yoga. Check with the local YMCA or YWCA, community and senior centers, parks and recreation programs, adult education classes, organizations for specific diseases (such as arthritis, diabetes, heart disease), and community colleges. By and large, classes are inexpensive, and the staff in charge of planning are responsive to people's needs. Public health offices also sponsor classes that are appropriate for a wide range of ages and needs.

Hospitals often have medically supervised classes for people with heart or lung disease (cardiac or pulmonary rehabilitation classes). Occasionally, people with other chronic conditions such as chronic pain can be included as well. These programs tend to be more expensive than other community classes, but they have the added benefit of medical supervision, if that's important to you.

Health and fitness clubs usually offer aerobic classes, weight training, cardiovascular equipment, and sometimes a heated pool. When you search for fitness club or community programs, ask the following questions:

- **Are classes appropriate for moderate- and low-intensity exercise and for beginners?** You should be able to observe classes and participate in at least one class before signing up and paying.

- **Do the classes include safe and effective endurance, strength, balance, and flexibility components that are tailored to meet your needs?** Again, observing a class usually will answer this question for you. If not, it's okay to approach the instructor after the class with any questions or concerns you may have.

- **Are there qualified instructors on staff who have experience working with people with chronic pain?** Knowledgeable instructors are more likely to understand special needs and be willing and able to work with you.

- **Do membership policies allow you to pay by the class or for a short series of classes or let you freeze your membership at times when you can't participate?** Some fitness facilities offer different rates depending on how many services you use.

- **Are the facilities easy to get to, park near, and enter?** Parking lots, dressing rooms, and exercise areas should be accessible and safe, with professional staff on site.

- **Is there a pool with "adult only" times when children are not allowed in the lanes?** Small children playing and making

Other Resources to Explore

Physical activity guidelines:

Australia: www.health.gov.au/internet/main/publishing.nsf/content/health-pubhlth-strateg-act-guidelines

Canada: www.phac-aspc.gc.ca/hp-ps/hl-mvs/pa-ap

United States: www.health.gov/paguidelines

Centers for Disease Control and Prevention: www.cdc.gov/physicalactivity

National Center for Injury Prevention and Control, *What You Can Do to Prevent Falls*: www.cdc.gov/HomeandRecreationalSafety/Falls/WhatYouCanDoToPreventFalls.htm

National Center on Health, Physical Activity, and Disability: www.nchpad.org

National Institute on Aging, *Exercise and Physical Activity: Your Everyday Guide from the National Institute on Aging*: www.nia.nih.gov/health/publication/exercise-physical-activity/introduction

noise in the pool may not be good for your needs.

■ **Are staff and other members friendly and easy to talk to?** You want to feel welcome in what may be a new environment for you.

■ **Is there an emergency management protocol, and are instructors certified in CPR and first aid?** The answer will be yes in most facilities, but it doesn't hurt to learn more and put any concerns you have to rest.

There are many excellent exercise videotapes and DVDs for use at home. These vary in intensity, from very gentle chair exercises to more strenuous aerobic exercise. Ask your health care provider or therapist for suggestions, or review tapes yourself. Many websites devoted to these video programs offer sample clips of the instruction so you can preview the content before you purchase. Nonprofit organizations devoted to your condition may also have good recommendations.

Suggested Further Reading

To learn more about the topics discussed in this chapter, we suggest that you explore the following resources:

Dahm, Diane, and Jay Smith, eds. *Mayo Clinic Fitness for Everybody*. Rochester, Minn.: Mayo Clinic Health Information, 2005.

Foreman, Judy. *A Nation in Pain: Healing Our Biggest Health Problem*. New York: Oxford University Press, 2014 (see Chapter 13, Exercise: The Real Magic Bullet).

Moffat, Marilyn, and Steve Vickery. *The American Physical Therapy Association Book of Body Maintenance and Repair*. New York: Henry Holt, 1999.

Nelson, Miriam E., and Sarah Wernick. *Strong Women Stay Young*, rev. ed. New York: Bantam Books, 2005.

Vernikos, Joan. *Sitting Kills, Moving Heals: How Everyday Movement will Prevent Pain, Illness and Early Death*. Fresno, CA: Linden Publishing, 2011.

White, Martha. *Water Exercise: 78 Safe and Effective Exercises for Fitness and Therapy*. Champaign, Ill.: Human Kinetics, 1995.

CHAPTER 8

Exercising for Flexibility, Balance, and Strength

*I*N CHAPTERS 6 AND 7 WE TALKED ABOUT the importance of keeping physically active when you have chronic pain. This chapter is your guide to a gentle set of 26 range of motion and flexibility movements called the Moving Easy Program (MEP). Once you have learned the sequence of moves, you can include the MEP in your exercise routine as a warm-up or cool-down to aerobic exercise, or you can do the MEP by itself to promote relaxation and relieve stress and tension. This chapter also includes six exercises that improve your balance and a short introduction to water fitness, tai chi, and yoga exercises.

There is an old adage: use it or lose it. If you don't use your body—by moving your muscles and joints and being active—you will start to lose strength and flexibility. A common problem with chronic pain is that you often stop using your body the way you used to. You aren't as active and you don't exercise as much. You tend to hold your muscles in tension, which leads to restricted movement, and your joints become stiff.

125

As a consequence, you become less flexible and have limited range of motion of your joints. This becomes a vicious cycle because the less flexible you are, the less you do and the more your muscles shorten and weaken, which leads to even less flexibility and so on.

Flexibility refers to the ability of muscles and joints to move comfortably through a full range of motion. As an example, think of your wrist. You can make a circle with your wrist going clockwise and counterclockwise. You can extend your wrist back and flex it forward. Holding your forearm straight in front of you, you can move your hand to the right and to the left by using your wrist. These moves put your wrist through its range of motion, which involves gently stretching the muscles that act on the joint. Doing these kinds of range of motion and gentle stretching exercises for all your joints helps keep you flexible.

Flexibility exercises, like the ones in the MEP, help loosen tight muscles and joints and reduce stiffness so it's easier to get going in the mornings. They are gentle so they can be done every day, even on days when you are not feeling your best. They can help with relaxation by promoting body awareness, which leads to improved posture and better breathing. And because they increase circulation to muscles and joints, flexibility exercises are a great way to warm up or cool down before and after aerobic exercise.

The Moving Easy Program

The Moving Easy Program is an enjoyable way to safely improve your flexibility. It gently loosens muscles and joints and increases circulation. It incorporates the whole body and is not meant to be strenuous. The MEP consists of 26 movements that take less than 15 minutes to do. Flexibility exercises and gentle strength training combine with better breathing to reduce stress and tension. The program is safe for almost all people with chronic pain. To help you get started, an audio CD of the 26 moves is included in this book. Use the CD and the photographs on pages 128–142 as your guide when doing the MEP at home. The box on the next page lists important tips to keep in mind as you get started with the MEP.

Precautions and Suggestions for Individuals with Pain

1. The MEP program contains gentle neck and back exercises. If you have neck or back pain or are not sure if these exercises are right for you, check with your doctor, physical therapist, or other health care provider before doing these exercises.

2. If there are some moves in the MEP you know are not right for you, don't do them. Instead, modify the moves (see suggestion 7 below) or just imagine you are doing them. Scientific evidence suggests that imagining moving an area of the body actually activates areas of the brain and stimulates nerves that connect to that part of the body.

MEP Tips

Preparation

- Clear your mind of any worries or unnecessary thoughts. Focus your mind on the present.

- Monitor your breathing. Take deep, relaxed breaths.

- Be aware of your posture. Maintain good posture by imagining a string at the top of your head being gently tugged up toward the ceiling.

Movements

- Pay attention to your joints as you move. Move gently but with purpose.

- Move slowly—don't jerk or bounce.

- Relax as you move, paying special attention to your shoulders. They should be soft and relaxed.

- Keep breathing as you move. Don't hold your breath.

- Never force beyond what is comfortable.

3. Loosen your joints and relax your muscles with the MEP before proceeding to aerobic exercise.

4. You can do the MEP even on days when you don't feel up to par because it is not a strenuous program. However, modify the movements to avoid any increased pain or stress on days when you are not at your best.

5. Although your long-term goal is to be able to do the MEP routine to the full range of motion, always avoid straining or forcing beyond your current comfort level. Your goal is not to achieve perfection but to reach a level of flexibility and fitness where moving feels good!

6. When moving from sitting to standing positions, avoid tipping your trunk backwards, which may strain your lower back.

7. You may modify any of the MEP movements if you are not able to perform specific moves. If you are unable to stand, you can modify most of the moves so you can do them while sitting.

8. To gently increase the active range of motion of a specific joint, move the joint to the point of comfort, pause and relax, and then move it again without straining.

Moving Easy Program Sequence Instruction and Illustration

Begin by placing a stable chair in an area where you have enough space to move freely. Sit down and get comfortable. Take a few moments to clear your mind. Now, start by focusing on your breathing . . . take a few deep, relaxing breaths before beginning. Remember to breathe naturally throughout the program and not to hold your breath.

1. Raise It Up

Inhale, lift your arms, raising them as high as you can, very gently and slowly, and if you can past your shoulders. Bring your hands together and guide them down toward the center of your body. Let's repeat this . . . lifting up . . . hands together . . . and guiding them down. Let's finish by guiding your arms back down to the side of your body.

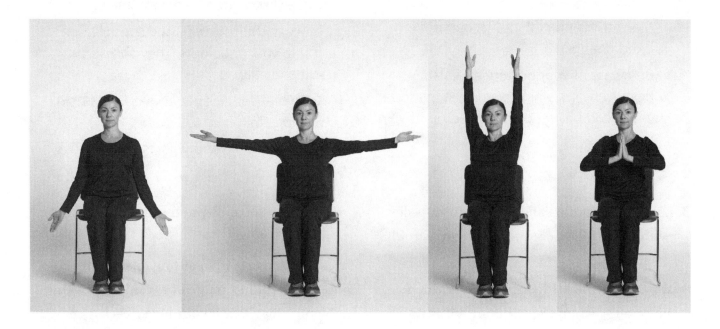

2. Ear to Shoulder

Focusing on your head, bring your ear a little closer to your shoulder . . . Hold this stretch . . . and return to center. Let's repeat to the other side, gently dropping your ear to your shoulder. Hold this stretch . . . and return to center.

(*Note:* For every move in the MEP, "return to center" means "go back to the starting position.")

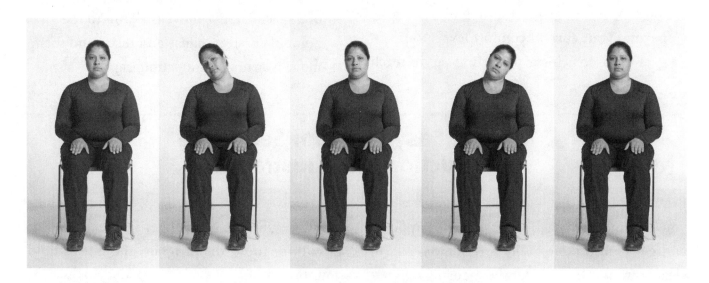

Special thanks to Ned Pratt for the photographs in this section.

3. Side Look

Gently turn your head and look to the side. You may feel a stretch or tension release . . . Return to center. Repeat, gently looking to the other side, holding your stretch . . . and return to center.

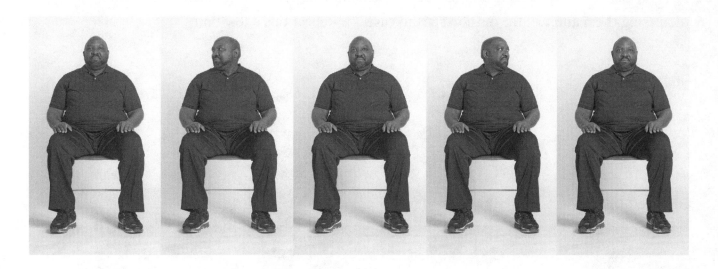

4. Head Bow

Drop your head gently to your chest and hold . . . feeling more tension leave that area . . . Return to center. Repeat . . . gently dropping your head forward . . . and return to center.

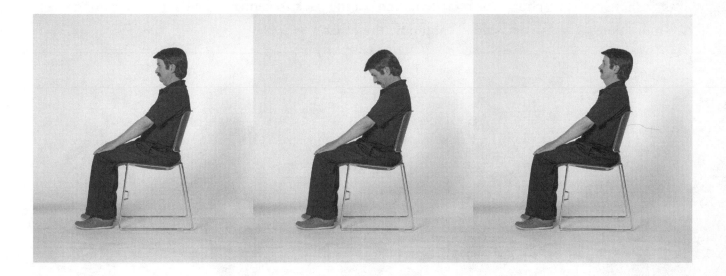

5. Shoulder Rolls

Bring your attention to your shoulders and think about making small gentle circles forward, starting with small circles and increasing them, remembering that even the smallest of movements can be beneficial . . . Now reverse this circular movement back . . . making small, gentle circles and increasing them and feel the tension start to ease . . . Repeat this a few times.

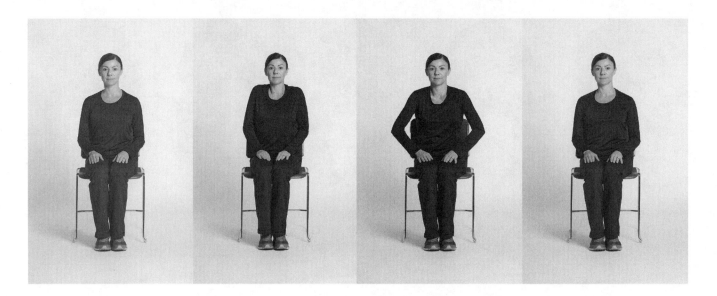

6. Side Turn

Placing both hands on one thigh and using your body's mid-section, gently look to the side turning your head, shoulders and chest . . . feeling a lengthening of your spine, and hold . . . Come back to center. Now place your hands on the other thigh, and gently turn your head, shoulders, and chest to the other side . . . feeling your body lengthen. Come back to center . . . Now repeat these moves two more times. First to one side . . . and now the other.

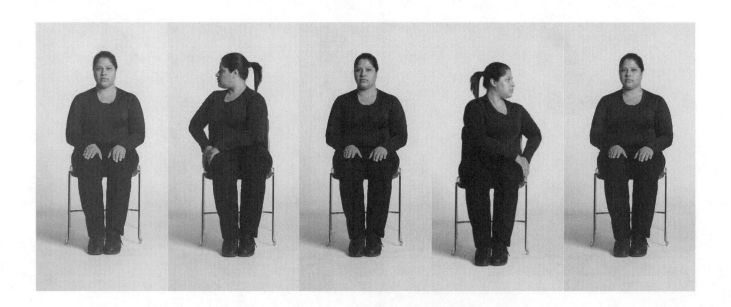

7. Scoop and Splash

With larger movements, reach your arms behind you, while you bend forward from the hips—keeping your back straight—reach down to the best of your ability, with comfort and no pain, and picture scooping water from beneath you . . . and slowly sit back up, splashing the water over your shoulders. Good . . . Let's do that two more times.

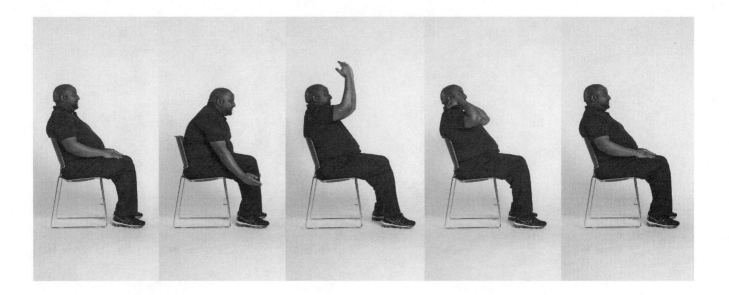

8. Squat Up

If you are able to stand, using your hands, lean forward and lift yourself out of the chair, focusing on the large muscle groups in the tops of your legs and stand up.
(*Note*: Avoid tipping your body backwards since this may strain your lower back.)

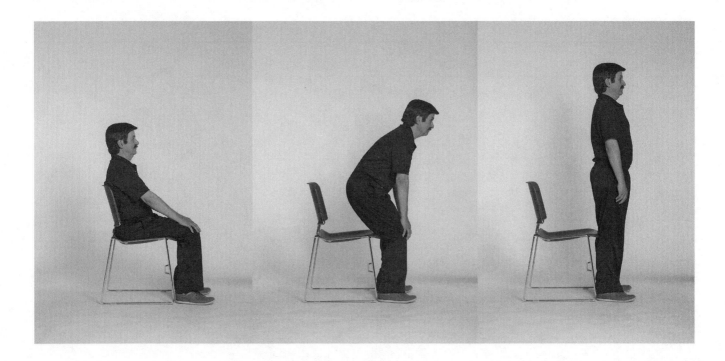

9. Leg Kicks

Now move to one side of the chair. Holding gently onto the chair for balance (or sitting in your chair), extend one leg forward as if moving your foot through a shallow pool of water . . . back and forth . . . back and forth . . . Repeat this a few more times.

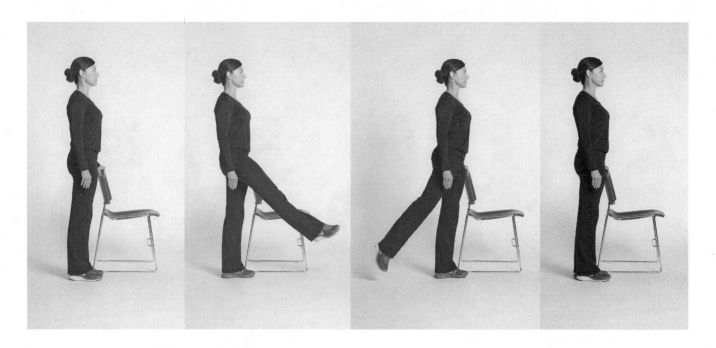

10. Leg Swing

Using the same leg, gently glide your leg through this shallow pool of water from side to side in front of you . . . Repeat with gentle, slow, easy movements a few more times.

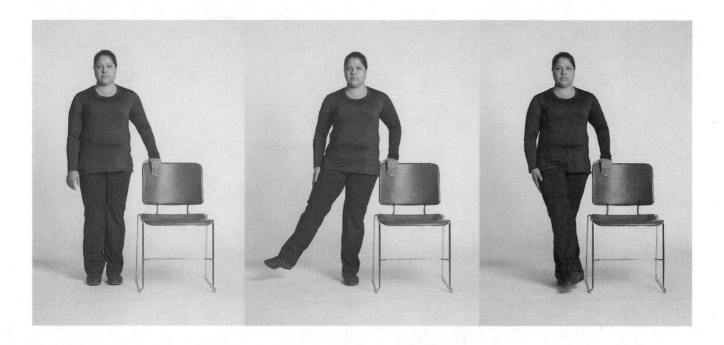

11. Flex and Point

Now, keeping this leg extended in front of you, flex your toes up . . . and point your toes down. Feeling the tension in your calf flexing up, and releasing by pointing down. Repeat this again . . . up . . . and down . . . up . . . and down.

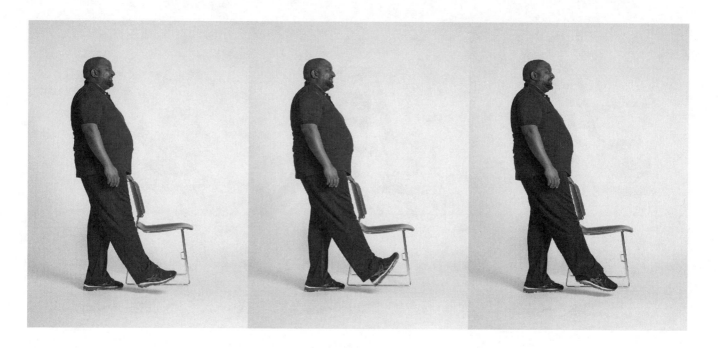

12. Leg Kicks (2)

Now move to the other side of the chair. Holding gently onto the chair for balance, extend your other leg forward as if moving your foot through a shallow pool of water . . . back and forth . . . back and forth . . . Repeat a few more times.

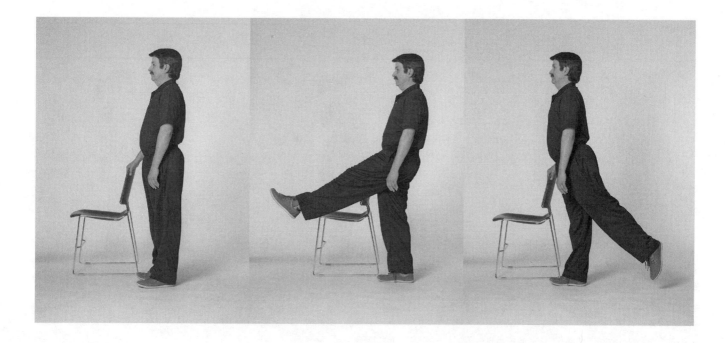

13. Leg Swing (2)

Now, using the same leg, glide your leg through this water from side to side in front of you. Repeat with gentle, slow, easy movements a few more times.

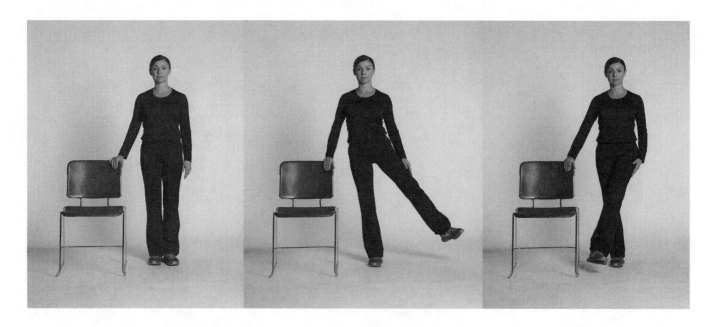

14. Flex and Point (2)

Keeping the same leg extended in front of you, flex your toes up . . . and point your toes down. Feel the tension in your calf, flexing up . . . and releasing by pointing down. Up . . . and down . . . Repeat a few more times.

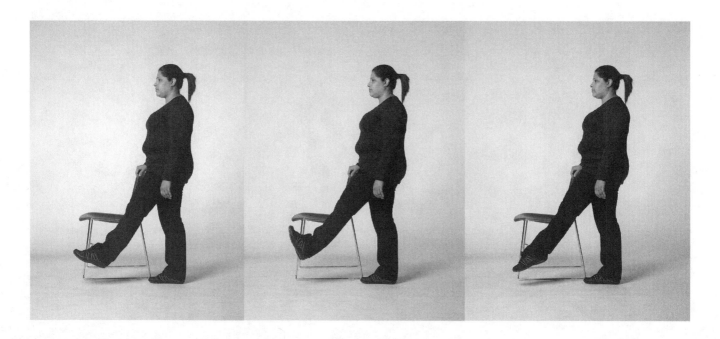

15. Squat Up and Down

Returning to the front of your chair, we're going to use the large muscles in the tops of our legs to squat up and down. Leaning slightly forward, slowly lower yourself into your chair, being mindful to let your weight sit in your heels as you lower yourself down . . . Now slightly leaning forward, lift yourself up out of your chair to a standing position, concentrating on your large muscle groups. Let's repeat that, slowly sitting back down . . . and raising yourself up . . . and sitting back down.

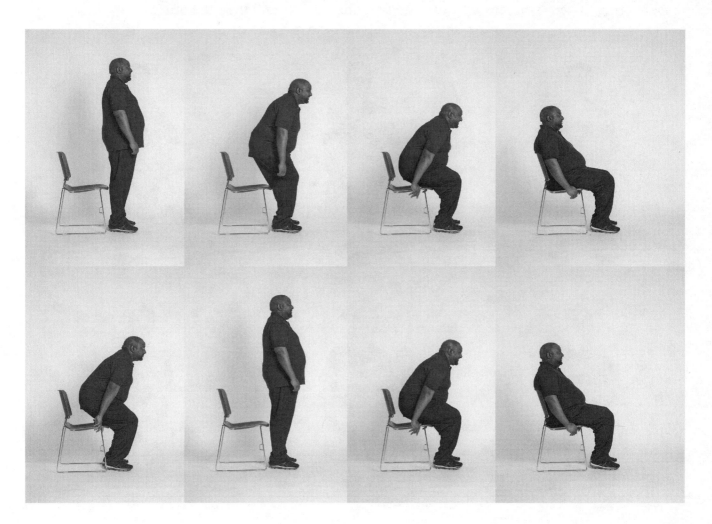

16. Knee to Chest

While sitting, place both hands under one knee, and gently bring your knee up toward your chest, while keeping an erect posture. (If you have a hip or back problem, you may want to just lift your knee without using your hands.) Feel a gentle stretch in your hip and buttock area. Hold for 2 or 3 seconds and then place your leg back on the floor. Change legs and put your hands under your other knee and lift up . . . and then place your leg back on the floor. Let's do this one more time, remembering to keep your erect posture . . . first one side . . . and then the other.

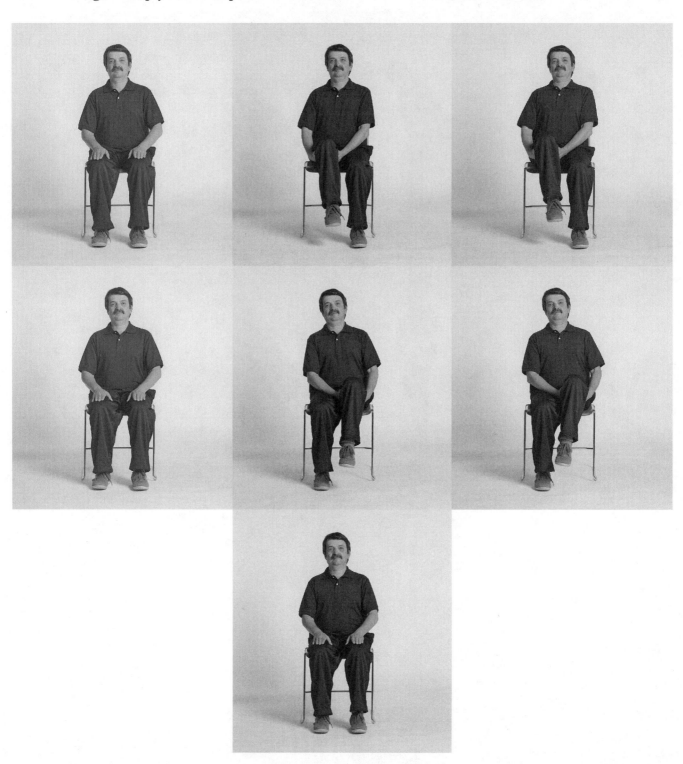

17. Abdominal Lean

Now, slide slightly forward in your chair. Crossing your arms in front of your chest, or holding onto the sides of your chair, lean back VERY SLOWLY, at about 45 degrees, using your abdominal muscles. Hold . . . and return to center. Repeat a few more times. Lean back VERY SLOWLY, about 45 degrees. You should feel your abdominal muscles tighten . . . but only go to what is comfortable. Abdominal work can be that easy!

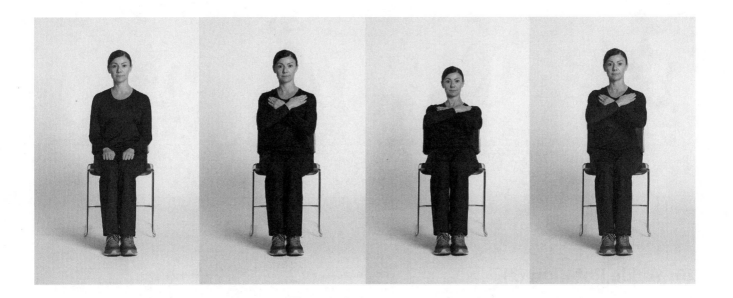

18. Ankle Rotation

Extending one foot in front of you, rotate your ankle in one direction. Feel the tension release . . . and now in the other direction.

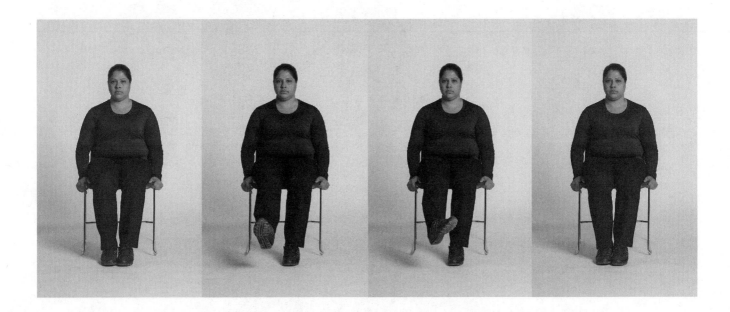

19. Hamstring Stretch

Placing your foot on the floor slightly in front of you, gently lean forward as if making a little bow and stretch the hamstrings in the back of your knee. Move slowly, gently, and comfortably. Hold this stretch for a few seconds . . . Return to center. Do this one more time, going a little deeper if you can . . . Return to center.

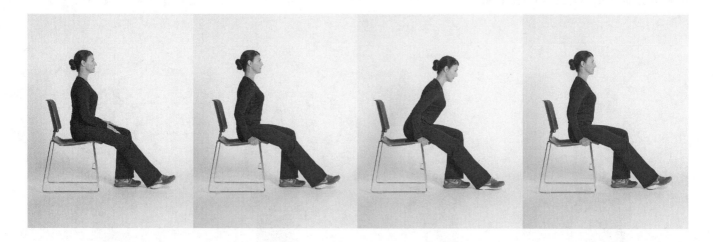

20. Ankle Rotation (2)

Now, extend your other leg in front of you for ankle rotations. Rotate your ankle in one direction . . . and now in the other direction.

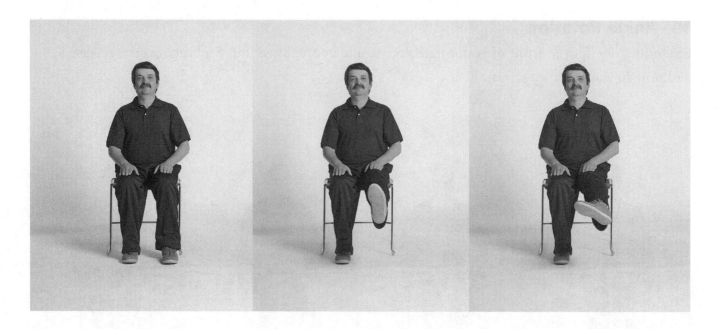

21. Hamstring Stretch (2)

Now do a hamstring bow by placing that foot slightly in front of you. Gently lean forward as if making a little bow. You should feel a stretch in the back of the knee. Move slowly, gently, and comfortably. Hold this stretch for a few seconds . . . Return to center. Try this one more time, and if you can, go a little deeper . . . and return to center.

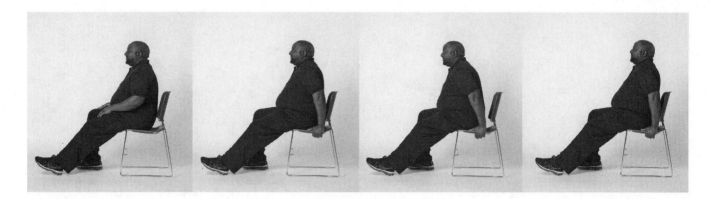

22. Side Stretch

Take a deep breath . . . in and out . . . Now lifting both arms up over your head if you can, drop one arm to your side. Take the lifted arm and move it toward the center of your body, giving you an added stretch. Hold . . . Good. Now, moving to the other side, lift the other arm up and move it toward the center . . . holding that stretch . . . return to center. Repeat this again on both sides . . . First one side . . . then the other . . . and return to center.

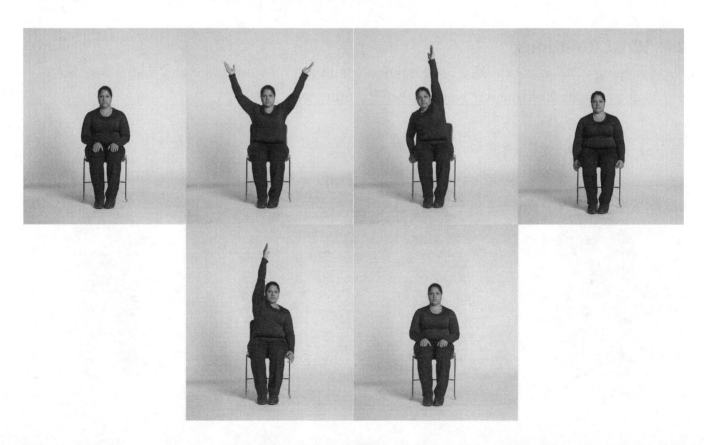

23. Bicep Curls/Wrist Flexion

Now, let's bring the arms in front of our body and bend your arms at the elbows, moving your arms toward your shoulders. Making a gentle fist, and curling your fist, extend your arms back out and hold this position . . . Feel that stretch in your forearms and the back of your hands. Let's repeat this a few more times . . . bringing your arms forward, curling your fists inward, and extending your arms out.

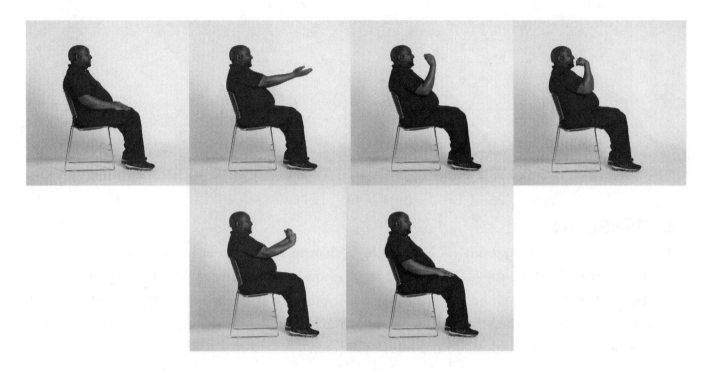

24. Wrist Rotations

Now, keeping your arms extended or dropping them to rest on your legs if you wish, rotate both wrists in a circular direction one way . . . then the other way.

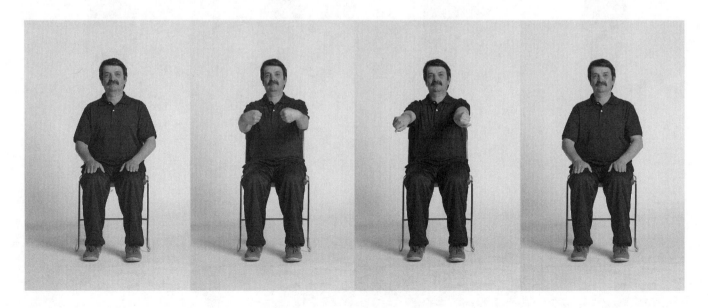

25. Wing Span Stretch

Now, lifting your arms out to the side of your body as if they were wings, move them back, opening your chest and holding this stretch for a few seconds, remembering to keep your shoulders soft and relaxed. Bring your arms to the front of your body, and repeat . . . Now release your arms down.

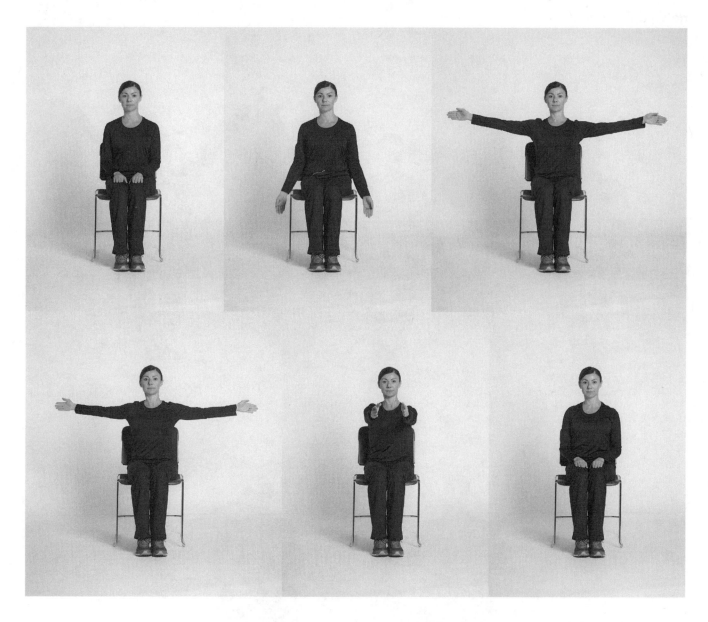

26. Raise It Up

Take a deep relaxed breath . . . in . . . and out . . . Lift your arms, raising them as high as is comfortable, very gently and slowly. Bring your hands together and guide them down toward the center of your body . . . and finish by bringing your arms down through the center, exhaling as you do. And now you're done!

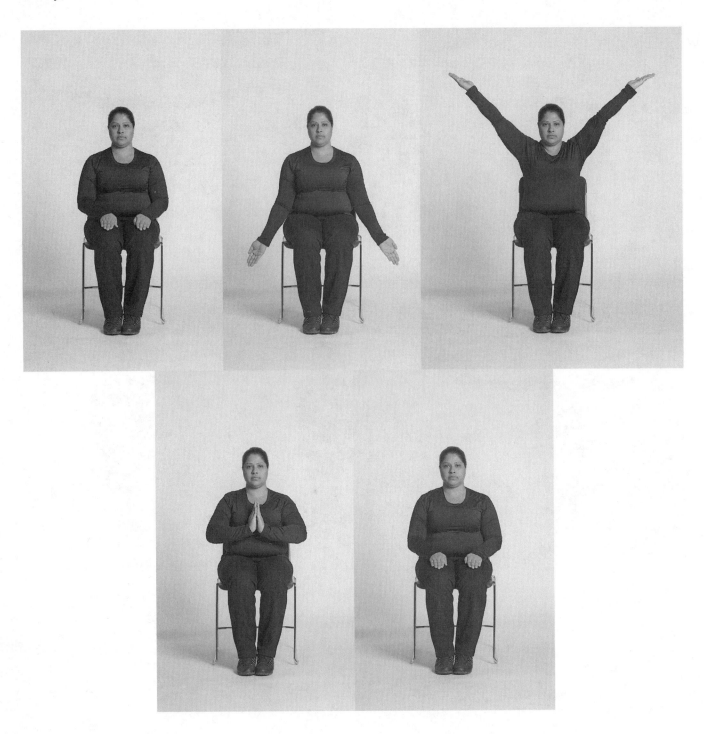

Balance Exercises

Similar to the MEP, the exercises in this section are designed so you can practice balance activities in a safe and progressive way. These better balance (BB) exercises are listed in order of difficulty. Start with the first exercises and work up to the more difficult ones as your strength and balance improve. If you feel that your balance is particularly poor, exercise with someone who can give you a supporting hand if needed. Always practice by a counter or stable chair that you can hold on to if necessary. Signs of improving balance include being able to hold a position longer or without extra support, or being able to do the exercise or hold the position with your eyes closed.

The National Institute on Aging, a division of the U.S. National Institutes of Health, offers an exercise guide and video that includes other balance exercises. There may also be some balance exercise classes in your community to help continue your progress. Tai chi is a wonderful program to help you work on balance and strength. (See more on tai chi later in this chapter.) It is low impact and gentle on your joints.

BB 1. Beginning Balance

Stand quietly with your feet comfortably apart. Place your hands on your hips and turn your head and trunk as far to the left as is comfortable and then to the right. Repeat 5 to 10 times. To increase the difficulty, do the same thing with your eyes closed.

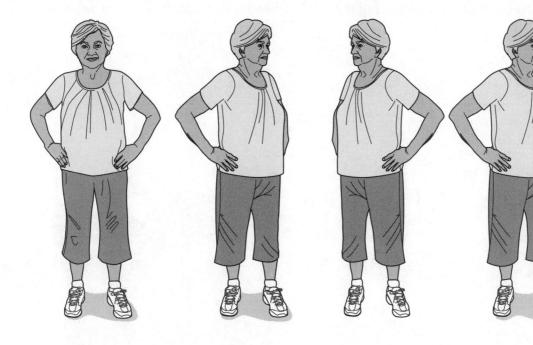

BB 2. Swing and Sway

Using a counter or the back of a stable chair for support, do each of the following five to ten times:

1. Rock back on your heels and then rise up on your toes.

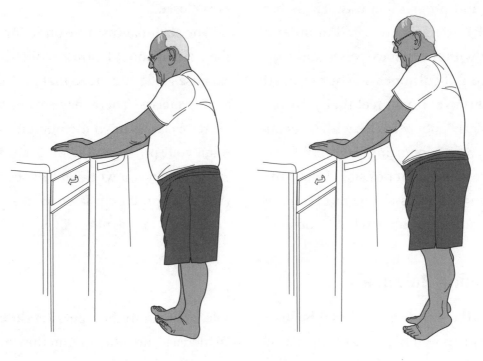

2. Do the box step (as if you were dancing the waltz).

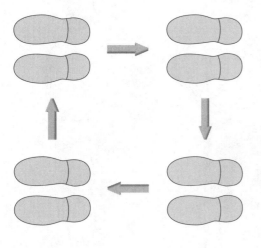

3. March in place, first with your eyes open and then with your eyes closed.

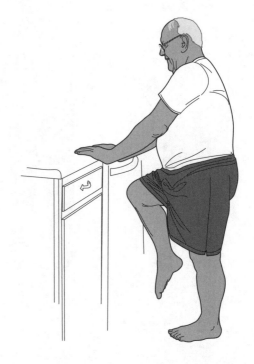

BB 3. Base of Support

Do these exercises standing close to a counter for support or with someone nearby for assistance. The purpose of this exercise set is to help you improve your balance by going from a larger to a smaller base of support. Work on being able to hold each position for 10 seconds. Once you can hold each position with your eyes open, practice with your eyes closed.

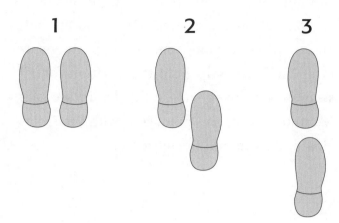

1. Stand with feet together.
2. Stand with one foot out in front and the other back.
3. Stand heel to toe.

BB 4. Toe Walk

The purpose of this exercise is to increase ankle strength and give you practice balancing on a small base of support while moving. Staying close to a counter for support, rise up on your toes and walk up and back along the counter. Once you are comfortable walking on your toes without support and with your eyes open, try it with your eyes closed.

BB 5. Heel Walk

The purpose of this exercise is to increase your lower leg strength and allow you to practice moving on a small base of support. Staying close to a counter for support, raise your toes and forefoot and walk up and back along the counter on your heels. Once you are comfortable walking on your heels without support and with your eyes open, try it with your eyes closed.

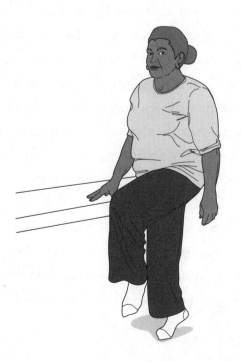

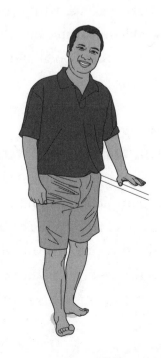

BB 6. One-Legged Stand

Holding on to a counter or chair, lift one foot completely off the ground. Once you are balanced, lift your hand from the supporting surface. The goal is to hold the position for 10 seconds. Once you can do this for 10 seconds without holding on, practice it with your eyes closed. Repeat with the other leg.

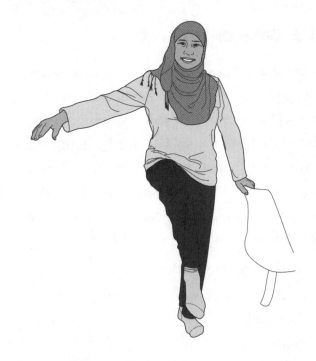

Is Your Balance Improving?

In order to determine if your balance is getting better, do Exercise BB 6 (one-legged stand) and record how long you can stand on each foot without needing to reach for support. Record how long you can stand with your eyes open and closed. When you are ready to test your balance again, see if you can stand without support longer or if you can balance with eyes closed. The goal is to be able to balance on one foot for 30 seconds with your eyes open and again for 30 seconds with your eyes closed.

Other Gentle Exercise: Water Fitness, Tai Chi, and Yoga

Exercise in the water, or aquacise, is another gentle way to be more active and introduce variety to your program of activities. The buoyancy of water takes the pressure off painful areas of the body such as the back, hips, knees, and feet. Shallow water fitness is a great way to improve your flexibility, strength, and endurance in a fun, relaxed environment. The nice thing is that you do not have to know how to swim to participate in water fitness classes.

In general, people with chronic pain should avoid jogging and hopping, whether on dry land or in water. Be sure to tell your water exercise instructor that you have chronic pain. He or she can modify exercises for you if needed. If you are a swimmer, know that certain swimming strokes may aggravate your pain problem, while other strokes may be ideal. Always consult with your health care provider to be sure that the exercise you choose is right for you. Read more about water exercise in Chapter 9, pages 158–160.

Tai chi and yoga are excellent forms of exercise that involve the mind and the body. Both combine strength and flexibility training with relaxation in order to reduce stress and tension.

Tai chi is suited to many people with chronic pain because it involves gentle, slow, relaxed movements that safely increase flexibility, build strength, and improve balance. In fact, it is often referred to as "moving meditation." It is a form of exercise done by young and old alike and by the healthy and those who have chronic health problems. Recent scientific studies have found that tai chi and a related practice from Eastern traditions called qigong are beneficial for those with fibromyalgia and osteoarthritis as well as for general health and well-being. For more information, go to the website of the National Center for Complementary and Alternative Medicine (nccam.nih.gov/health/taichi).

Yoga combines physical postures, breathing techniques, and relaxation. Recent studies found that people with lower back pain improved their ability to walk and move and had reduced pain after they practiced an adapted set of yoga poses. Other studies have found that yoga helps relieve anxiety and depression, may reduce blood pressure, and improves balance and reduces falls in older adults.

Be aware that there are many types of yoga practice, and some are more demanding of the body than others. If yoga is of interest to you, investigate the types available in your community. Contact instructors to find out if they have knowledge of chronic pain and how to adapt yoga poses for your specific problem. To get more general information about yoga's health benefits, a good place to start is the website of the National Center for Complementary and Alternative Medicine (nccam.nih.gov/health/yoga).

Again, always talk with your health care provider or physical therapist before starting a new movement or exercise program. Fill him or her in about any complementary or alternative practices you are using to manage your chronic pain and your overall health. This will help ensure you have the safest care possible.

A Word about Strength Training

Strength training is a critical component to an overall exercise program for men and women of all ages. Weight-bearing exercise helps you to build and maintain healthy bones. Strength training halts bone loss, improves balance, can help prevent bone fractures, helps control weight, and increases energy. Exercises discussed in this chapter are a first step to improving strength. Before you move to a more challenging strengthening program that may include weights or other resistance exercise, be sure to consult with a knowledgeable health professional such as a physical therapist or exercise specialist who understands your particular chronic pain problem. This person can work with you to identify a safe approach to a strengthening program suited specifically to you.

Other Resources to Explore

Centers for Disease Control and Prevention, *Growing Stronger: Strength Training for Older Adults* [free download]: www.cdc.gov/physicalactivity/downloads/growing_stronger.pdf

Exercise! Arthritis Self-Management [audio CDs]. Bull Publishing Company, 2006.

National Center for Complementary and Alternative Medicine: www.nccam.nih.gov/health/yoga and www.nccam.nih.gov/health/taichi

National Council on Aging: www.ncoa.org

National Institute on Aging: www.nia.nih.gov

Sit and Be Fit [DVDs]: www.sitandbefit.org

Yoga for People with Pain (online seminar): www.cirpd.org/resources/Webinars/Pages/YogaforPain.aspx

Suggested Further Reading

To learn more about the topics discussed in this chapter, we suggest that you explore the following resources:

Blahnik, Jay. *Full Body Flexibility*. Champaign, Ill.: Human Kinetics, 2010.

Hadjistavropoulos, Thomas, and Heather Hadjistavropoulos, eds. *Pain Management for Older Adults: A Self-Help Guide*. Seattle, Wash.: IASP Press, 2008 (see Chapter 6).

Keelor, Richard, ed. *Pep Up Your Life: A Fitness Book for Seniors*. AARP, 1990.

Knopf, Karl. *Core Strength for 50+*. Berkeley, Calif.: Ulysses Press, 2012.

Knopf, Karl. *Make the Pool Your Gym*. Berkeley, Calif.: Ulysses Press, 2012.

Knopf, Karl. *Stretching for 50+*. Berkeley, Calif.: Ulysses Press, 2005.

Knopf, Karl. *Weights for 50+*. Berkeley, Calif.: Ulysses Press, 2005.

Maccadanza, Roberto. *Stretching Basics*. New York: Sterling, 2004.

Martin, Margaret. *Exercise for Better Bones*. Raleigh, N.C.: Lulu, 2010.

Martin, Margaret. *Yoga for Better Bones*. Raleigh, N.C.: Lulu, 2011.

Torkelson, Charlene. *Get Fit While You Sit: Easy Workouts from Your Chair*. Alameda, Calif.: Hunter House, 1999.

There is a great need to increase the duration of moderate and vigorous activity in the chronic pain population, as few individuals accumulate the recommended number of minutes of physical activity at these intensities.

—E. J. Dansie, D. C. Turk, et al.
The Journal of Pain, 2014

CHAPTER 9

Exercising for Endurance and Fitness: Moderate to Vigorous Physical Activity

A RECENT NATIONAL STUDY OF PHYSICAL ACTIVITY in U.S. adults found that most people with chronic pain did just about the same amount of sedentary and light exercise as those without chronic pain. But women and especially men with chronic pain did much less moderate to vigorous physical activity than people without pain. As a result, people with painful conditions are at increased risk of developing heart problems, diabetes, and other chronic diseases.

This doesn't have to happen. People with chronic pain can increase the intensity of exercise gradually and safely and reap the health benefits of exercise.

In this chapter you will learn about exercise effort, various aerobic activities, and how to put together a program that works for you. Recall from Chapter 7 that aerobic ("with oxygen") exercise involves moving the large muscles of your body in continuous activity. Aerobic activities include walking, swimming, dancing, mowing the lawn, and riding a bike. Aerobic exercise is good for your cardiovascular fitness, lessens your heart attack risk, and helps you to control your weight. It promotes a sense of well-being, can lessen depression and anxiety, helps you to sleep, improves your mood and boosts your energy levels.

When thinking about stepping up an exercise program to include moderate to vigorous physical activity (called aerobic or endurance exercise), many people are confused about what to do and how much to do. Recall that the guidelines we discussed in Chapter 7 recommend that adults exercise at a moderate intensity for at least 150 minutes (2½ hours) spread out through the week. We also described the guidelines for aerobic, flexibility, and strengthening exercise in Chapters 7 and 8. Even with all this information at hand, figuring out your very own program can still be a challenge.

The most important point to embrace is that some activity is better than none. If you start off doing what is comfortable and increase your efforts gradually, you likely will build a healthy, lifelong exercise habit. You will learn how to stay active and get back on track even if changes in your condition may slow you down for a while. Generally, it is always better to begin your program by underdoing rather than overdoing.

Frequency, Time, and Intensity

To achieve your exercise goal, remember the three basic building blocks of any exercise program: frequency, time, and intensity.

- **Frequency** refers to how often you exercise. Most guidelines suggest engaging in at least some exercise most days of the week. For moderately intense aerobic exercise, three to five times a week is a good choice. Taking a day off gives your body a chance to rest and recover.

- **Time** refers to the length of each exercise period. It is best if you can exercise at least 10 minutes at a time. You can add up your 10-minute exercise periods all week to work toward meeting your 150-minute per week goal. For example, three 10-minute walks a day for five days gets you to 150 minutes for the week. If 10 minutes is too much at first, start with what you can do—even two minutes is a start—and work toward 10 minutes.

- **Intensity** refers to your exercise effort—how hard you are working. Aerobic exercise is safe and effective at a moderate intensity. When you exercise at moderate intensity, you'll feel warm, you'll breathe more deeply and faster than usual, and your heart will beat faster than normal. At the same time, if you are exercising at the appropriate intensity, you should feel that you can continue for a while longer. Exercise intensity is relative to your fitness. For an athlete, running a mile in 10 minutes is probably low-intensity exercise.

For a person who hasn't exercised in a long time, a brisk 10-minute walk may be moderate to high intensity. For someone with severe physical limitations, a slow walk may be high intensity. The trick, of course, is to figure out what is moderate intensity for you. In the following material, we discuss several easy ways to do this.

Talk Test

The talk test is an easy and quick way to recognize your effort and regulate intensity. When exercising, talk to another person or to yourself. You can also recite poems or the words of a song out loud. If you are engaged in moderate-intensity exercise, you should still be able to speak comfortably. If you can't carry on a conversation because you are breathing too hard or are short of breath, you're working at a high intensity. Slow down to a more moderate level.

Perceived Exertion

Another way to determine intensity is to rate how hard you're working on a scale of perceived exertion. This might be a better method than the talk test if you have chronic angina pain or other conditions that impact your breathing.

There are two scales: 0 to 10 and 6 to 20. On the 0 to 10 scale, 0 is equivalent to lying down, doing no work at all, and 10 is equivalent to working as hard as possible, i.e., very intense effort that you couldn't sustain for more than a few seconds. A good level for moderate aerobic exercise on this scale is between 4 and 5.

On the 6 to 20 scale, 6 is considered the same as sitting quietly and 20 as working as hard as possible. On this scale, moderate intensity is between 11 and 14. (See Chapter 19, pages 314–315 for more detail about the 6 to 20 scale.)

Use whichever scale suits you better.

Heart Rate

Unless you're taking heart-regulating medicine, checking your heart rate is another way to measure exercise intensity. The faster your heart beats, the harder you're working. (Your heart also beats fast when you are frightened or nervous, but in this case we're talking about how your heart responds to physical activity.) Endurance exercise at moderate intensity raises your heart rate to between 55 and 70 percent of your safe maximum heart rate. The safe maximum heart rate declines with age, so your safe exercise heart rate gets lower as you get older. Table 9.1 on page 152 lists the general guidelines for safe exercise heart rate by age, or you can calculate your own using the formula presented here.

Which ever method you choose to monitor your heart rate, you need to know how to take your pulse. Start by placing the tips of your index and middle fingers at your wrist below the base of your thumb. Move your fingers around lightly until you feel the pulsations of blood pumping with each heartbeat. Then, push down and count how many beats you feel in 15 seconds. Multiply this number by four to get your resting heart rate. Most people have a resting heart rate between 60 and 100 beats per minute. By taking your pulse whenever you think of it, you'll soon learn the difference between your resting and exercise heart rates.

Table 9.1 Moderate-Intensity Exercise Heart Rate, by Age

Age	Exercise Pulse (beats per minute)	Exercise Pulse (15-second count)
30s	105–133	26–33
40s	99–126	25–32
50s	94–119	24–30
60s	88–112	23–28
70s	83–105	21–26
80s	77–98	19–25
90 and above	72–91	18–23

Take the following steps to calculate your own exercise heart rate range:

1. Subtract your age from 220:

   Example: 220 − 60 = 160

   You: 220 − _____ = _____

2. To find the low end of your exercise heart rate range, multiply your answer to step 1 by 0.55:

   Example: 160 × 0.55 = 88

   You: _____ × 0.55 = _____

3. To find the upper end of your moderate intensity range, multiply your answer to step 1 by 0.7:

   Example: 160 × 0.7 = 112

   You: _____ × 0.7 = _____

In our example, the exercise heart rate range for moderate intensity is from 88 to 112 beats per minute. What is yours?

When checking your heart rate during exercise, you only need to count your pulse for 15 seconds, not a whole minute. To find your 15-second pulse range for exercise, divide both the lower-end and upper-end numbers by 4. The person in our example should be able to count between 22 (88 ÷ 4) and 28 (112 ÷ 4) beats in 15 seconds while exercising.

The most important reason for knowing your exercise heart rate range is so you can learn not to exercise too vigorously. After you've done your warm-up and five minutes of endurance exercise, take your pulse. If it's higher than the upper rate, don't panic; just slow down a bit. You don't need to work so hard.

If you are taking medicine that regulates your heart rate, have trouble feeling your pulse, or think that keeping track of your heart rate is a bother, use the talk test or a perceived exertion scale to monitor your exercise intensity.

Be FIT

You can design your own endurance and fitness exercise program using the FIT approach. FIT stands for how often you exercise (F = Frequency), how hard you work (I = Intensity), and how long you exercise each day (T = Time). Build your exercise program by varying frequency, time, and activities. Start slowly and increase frequency and time as you work toward or even beyond the recommended 150 minutes each week. You can use different kinds or combinations of exercises.

Almost everyone can reach the guideline goals for minimum physical activity and achieve important health benefits. An easy way to remember the guideline is that you should accumulate 30 minutes of moderate physical activity on most days of the week (30 minutes/day × 5 days/week = 150 minutes/week. Your moderate activity goals can be met by walking, stationary bicycling, dancing, swimming, or doing chores that require moderate-intensity activity (such as mowing the lawn or vacuuming).

The following are programs of moderate intensity that reach 150 minutes each week:

■ A 10-minute walk at moderate intensity three times a day, five days a week

■ A 20-minute bike ride at moderate intensity (outside mostly on level ground, or on a stationary bike) three days a week and a 30-minute walk three days a week

■ A 30-minute low-impact aerobic dance class at moderate intensity twice a week and three 10-minute walks three days a week

If you are just starting, you could begin like this:

■ Take a 5-minute walk around the house three times a day, six days a week (total = 90 minutes).

■ Take a water aerobics class for 40 minutes twice a week and two 10-minute walks a day on two other days a week (total = 120 minutes).

■ Take a low-impact aerobic class once a week (50 minutes), do yard work for 30 minutes, and take two 20-minute walks (total = 120 minutes).

It is important to remember that 150 minutes is a goal, not necessarily your starting point. If you begin exercising just two minutes at a time, you will likely be able to reach the recommended 10 minutes three times a day. If you have a setback and stop exercising for a while, restart your program by exercising for less time and less vigorously than when you stopped. It takes some time to work back up again; be patient with yourself.

> **Be FIT**
>
> Here's a quick way to remember the three building blocks of your exercise program:
>
> **F** = Frequency (how often)
> **I** = Intensity (how hard)
> **T** = Time (how long)

Warming Up and Cooling Down

If you are going to exercise at moderate intensity, it is important to warm up first and cool down afterward.

Warming Up

Before building your exercise to moderate intensity, you must prepare your body to do more strenuous work. This means doing at least five minutes of a low-intensity activity to allow your muscles, heart, lungs, and circulation to gradually increase their work. If you are going for a brisk walk, warm up with five minutes of slow walking. If you are riding a stationary bike, warm up with five minutes of easy pedaling. In an aerobic exercise class, you warm up with a gentle routine before getting more vigorous.

Warming up reduces the risk of injuries, soreness, and irregular heartbeat.

Cooling Down

A cool-down period after moderate-intensity exercise helps your body return to its normal resting state. Repeating the five-minute warm-up activity or taking a slow walk following more vigorous activity helps your muscles gradually relax and your heart and breathing slow down. Gentle flexibility exercises during the cool-down can be relaxing, and gentle stretching after exercise helps reduce muscle soreness and stiffness.

Remember that the MEP (see Chapter 8) is a great warm-up or cool-down routine that also increases your flexibility and range of motion of your joints.

Aerobic (Endurance) Exercises

Aerobic exercises use the large muscles of the body in a rhythmic, continuous fashion. The most effective exercises involve your whole body. In this section of the chapter, we examine a few common low-impact aerobic exercises. All of these exercises can condition your heart and lungs, strengthen your muscles, relieve tension, and help you manage your weight. Most of them can also strengthen your bones (swimming and water aerobics are the exceptions).

Walking

Walking is a moderate-intensity activity that most people with chronic pain can do safely. It's easy, inexpensive, and can be done almost anywhere. You can walk by yourself or with company. In fact, walking with someone else is good motivation. Walking is safer than jogging or running and puts less stress on the body. It is an especially good choice if you have been sedentary, have balance problems, or have chronic musculoskeletal pain such as lower back pain or neck or joint-related pain.

If you are able to go shopping, visit friends, and do household chores, then you can probably walk for exercise. Age is not a barrier. A cane or walker need not stop you from getting into a walking routine. If you are in a wheelchair or use crutches, there are other types of aerobic exercise you can do. Consult a physical therapist for help.

Be cautious the first two weeks of an exercise walking program. If you haven't been doing much for a while, even a few minutes may be enough for you. Do what you can do comfortably, and build up slowly. Alternate slow walks and brisk walks. Each week, increase the brisk walking interval by no more than five minutes until you are walking briskly for a total of 20 or 30 minutes. Remember that your goal is to walk most days of the week, at moderate intensity, for at least 10 minutes at a time. Many studies of people with back pain have found that walking fast does not increase pain and has the added benefit of improving mood.

Walking tips

- **Choose your ground.** Walk on a flat, level surface. Walking on hills, uneven ground, soft earth, sand, or gravel is hard work. Fitness trails, shopping malls, school tracks, streets with sidewalks, and quiet neighborhoods are good places to start.

- **Always warm up and cool down with a slower stroll.** Walk slowly for five minutes to prepare your circulation and muscles for a brisker walk. Finish up with the same slow walk to let your body calm down gradually and to avoid sore muscles. Experienced walkers know they can avoid shin and foot discomfort if they begin and end with a stroll.

- **Set your own pace.** It takes practice to find the right walking speed. To find your speed, start walking slowly for a few minutes, then increase your speed to a pace that is slightly faster than normal for you. After five minutes, check your exercise intensity by using a perceived exertion or talk test. If you are working too hard or feel out of breath, slow down. If you are below your desired intensity, try walking a little faster. Walk another five minutes and check your intensity again. If you are still below your target, keep walking at a comfortable speed and check your intensity in the middle and at the end of each walk.

- **Increase your arm work.** You can use your arms to raise your heart rate into the target exercise range. Bend your elbows a bit and swing your arms more vigorously. Another idea is to carry a 1- or 2-pound (0.5 or 1.0 kg) weight in each hand. You can purchase hand weights for walking, hold a small can of food in each hand, or put sand, dried beans, or pennies in two small plastic beverage bottles or socks. The extra work you do with your arms increases the intensity of exercise without requiring that you walk faster than you find comfortable. (If you have been told to avoid arm exercises because of your pain problem or not to carry weights for any reason, just hold the weights but keep your arms by your side.)

Walking shoes

Wear shoes of the correct length and width. You shouldn't feel pressure on the sides or tops of your toes. Make sure your shoes are big enough in the toe area. Make sure there is a thumb width between the tip of your longest toe and the end of the shoe. The back of the shoe should hold your heel firmly in place when you walk.

Be sure your shoes are in good repair. Shoes with laces let you adjust width and give more support than slip-ons. If you have problems tying laces, consider Velcro closures or elastic shoelaces. Shoes with leather soles and a separate heel don't absorb shock as well as athletic and casual shoes that have a continuous composite sole. Avoid shoes that are too heavy or that have very thick, rubbery, or sticky soles that may create a tripping hazard.

Many people like shoes with removable insoles that can be exchanged for more shock-absorbing ones. You can find special insoles in sporting goods stores and shoe stores. When you shop for insoles, take your walking shoes with you. Remove the original insole and try on the shoe with the new insole inserted. You want to make sure there's still enough room for your foot to be comfortable. Insoles come in different sizes and can be trimmed with scissors for a custom fit. To give your toes more room, try the three-quarter insoles that stop just short of your toes. If you wear prescribed inserts in your shoes already, ask your doctor about appropriate insoles for exercise.

Good shoes do not need to be expensive. Any shoes that meet the criteria we have just described will serve your purposes.

Possible walking challenges

If you feel pain around your shins when you walk, you may not be spending enough time warming up. Try some leg and ankle exercises before you start walking (see Chapter 8, MEP exercises 9 through 14, 18, and 20). Or complete the whole MEP program to warm up. Then, start your walk at a slow pace for at least five minutes. Keep your feet and toes relaxed.

Sore knees are another common problem. Fast walking puts more stress on knee joints. To keep your heart rate up at slower speeds, try doing more work with your arms. Add the two exercises in Figure 9.1, which help strengthen your knees and thigh muscles. An added benefit is that they can help improve your balance.

Knee Exercise 1 (BB)

Strong knees are important for walking and standing comfortably. This exercise strengthens the knee. Sitting in a chair, straighten the knee by tightening up the muscle on the upper surface of your thigh. Place your hand on your thigh and feel the muscle work. If you wish, make circles with your toes. As your knee strengthens, see if you can build up to holding your leg out for 30 seconds. Count out loud. Do not hold your breath.

Knee Exercise 2 (BB)

Stand with one leg slightly in front of the other with your heel on the floor as if ready to take a step with the front foot. Now tighten the muscles on the front of your thigh, making your knee firm and straight. Hold to a count of 10. Relax. Repeat with the other leg.

You can reduce cramps in the calf and pain in the heel by starting with the Achilles stretch shown in Figure 9.2. If you have circulation problems in your legs and get cramps or pain in your calves while walking, alternate between comfortably brisk and slow walking. Slow down and give your circulation a chance to catch up before the pain is so intense that you have to stop. As you will see, such exercises may even help you gradually walk farther with less

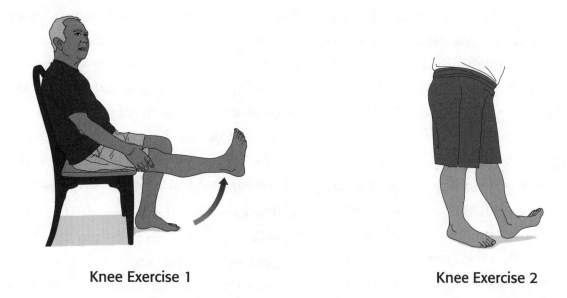

Knee Exercise 1   Knee Exercise 2

Figure 9.1 **Exercises to Strengthen Your Knees**

cramping or pain and the Achilles stretch can also help with balance (BB). If these suggestions don't help, check with your health care provider or physical therapist for other suggestions.

Achilles Stretch (BB)

This exercise helps maintain flexibility in the Achilles tendon, the large tendon at the back of your ankle. Good flexibility helps reduce the risk of injury, calf discomfort, and heel pain. The Achilles stretch is especially helpful for cooling down after walking or cycling and for people who get cramps in the calf muscles.

Stand at a counter or against a wall (see Figure 9.2). Place one foot in front of the other, toes pointing forward and heels on the ground. Lean forward, bend the knee of the forward leg, and keep the back knee straight, heel down. You will feel a good stretch in the calf. Hold the stretch for 10 seconds. Do not bounce. Move gently. You can adjust this exercise to reach the other large calf muscle by slightly bending your knee back while you stretch the calf. Can you feel the

difference? It's easy to get sore doing this exercise. If you've worn shoes with high heels for a long time, be particularly careful.

If you have trouble with standing balance or spasticity (muscle jerks), you can do a seated version of this exercise. Sit in a chair with feet flat on the floor. Keep your heel on the floor and slowly slide your foot (one foot at a time) back to bend your ankle and feel some tension on the back of your calf (lower leg).

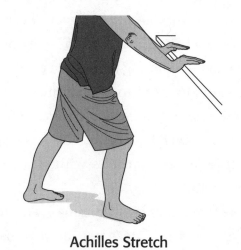

Achilles Stretch

Figure 9.2 **Exercise to Reduce Cramps**

One last but very important point: To help reduce neck and upper back discomfort, maintain good posture while you walk. Keep your head balanced over your neck and trunk, not in the lead, and keep your shoulders relaxed.

Swimming

Swimming is another aerobic exercise that can be done by people of all ages and ability levels. Because water is buoyant, it fully supports your whole body and takes the pressure off painful areas. It provides an excellent workout for your heart and lungs and challenges your muscles with the water's resistance. Be sure to check with a health care provider or fitness specialist about which strokes you should avoid, if any. Some strokes will get you stretching and increase your flexibility, but other strokes may aggravate a painful area of the body. If you have a heart condition like chronic stable angina, it is important to discuss whether swimming is right for you. People with heart disease who have severely irregular heartbeats and have had a defibrillator (AICD) implanted should avoid swimming. For most people with chronic pain conditions, however, swimming is excellent exercise. It is a whole-body workout. If you haven't been swimming for a while, consider a refresher course.

To make swimming an aerobic exercise, you will eventually need to swim continuously for 10 minutes. Try different strokes, changing strokes after each lap or two. This lets you exercise all joints and muscles without overtiring any one area.

Note that although swimming is an excellent aerobic exercise, it does not improve balance, nor does it provide weight-bearing exercise that builds and maintains healthy bones. (Recall from Chapter 8 that strength training halts bone loss and can help prevent bone fractures.) Incorporate swimming as one part of your overall fitness regime, and get your balance and weight-bearing workouts with other exercises recommended in this book.

The following tips can help you incorporate swimming into your exercise action plan:

- The breaststroke and freestyle (formally called the crawl) normally require a lot of neck motion and may be uncomfortable. To solve this problem, use a mask and snorkel so you can breathe without twisting your neck.

- Avoid the butterfly stroke if you suffer from chronic back, neck, or shoulder pain.

- Chlorine can be irritating to the eyes. Invest in a good pair of goggles. You can even have swim goggles made in your eyeglass prescription.

- A hot shower or soak in a hot tub after your workout helps reduce stiffness and muscle soreness. Remember not to work too hard or get too tired. If you're sore for more than two hours after your swim session, go easier next time.

- Always swim where there are qualified lifeguards, if possible, or with a friend. Never swim alone.

Aquacising

If you don't like to swim or are uncomfortable learning strokes, you can walk laps in the pool or join the millions who are "aquacising"—exercising in water. Recall that in Chapter 8 we discussed how water exercise can help you improve your flexibility. Exercising in the water is also a good way to improve your fitness and endurance.

Aquacise is comfortable, fun, and effective as a flexibility, strengthening, and aerobic activity. The buoyancy of the water takes weight off the hips, knees, feet, and back. Because of this, exercise in water is generally better tolerated than land-based exercise for people with various kinds of chronic pain. Exercising in a pool allows you a degree of privacy because no one can see much below shoulder level.

Joining a water exercise class with a good instructor is an excellent way to get started. Many community pools and private health centers offer water exercise classes, some geared to older adults. Organizations such as the Arthritis Foundation, Arthritis Society, and the Y sponsor water exercise classes and train instructors to teach them. Take the time to find out what is available in your local area and then ask if you can observe a class. If you have access to a pool and want to exercise on your own, there are many water exercise books and DVDs available that can guide you.

Water temperature is always a concern when people talk about water exercise. The Arthritis Foundation recommends a pool temperature of 84°F (29°C), with the surrounding air temperature in the same range. Except in warm climates, this means a heated pool. If you're just starting to aquacise, find a pool around this temperature. If you can exercise more vigorously and are not sensitive to cold, you can probably aquacise in cooler water. Many pools where people swim laps are about 80–83°F (27–28°C). It feels quite cool when you first get in, but starting off simply by walking in water or with another whole-body exercise helps you warm up quickly.

The deeper the water you stand in, the less stress there is on joints; however, water above the chest can make it hard to keep your balance. You can let shallower water cover more of your body just by spreading your legs apart or bending your knees a bit.

The following tips can help you incorporate aquacise into your exercise action plan:

- Wear something on your feet to protect them from rough pool floors and to provide traction in the pool and on the deck. There is footgear especially designed for water. Some styles have Velcro straps to make them easier to put on. Beach shoes with rubber soles and mesh tops also work well.

- If your hands are sensitive to cold or you have Raynaud's disease, wear a pair of disposable latex surgical gloves. You can purchase boxes of gloves at most pharmacies. The water trapped and warmed inside the glove seems to insulate the hand. If your core gets cold in the water, wear a T-shirt or full-leg Lycra exercise tights for warmth.

- If your condition affects your strength and balance, make sure you have someone to help you in and out of the pool. To add to your safety and security, find a position close to the wall or stay close to a buddy who can lend a hand if needed. You may even wish to sit on a chair in fairly shallow water as you do exercises. Ask the instructor to help you determine the best exercise program, equipment, and facilities for your specific needs.

- If the pool does not have steps and it is difficult for you to climb up and down a ladder, ask that pool staff position a three-step kitchen stool in the water by the ladder rails. This is an inexpensive way to provide steps for easier entry and exit, and the steps are easy to remove and store when not needed.

■ Wearing a flotation belt or life vest adds extra buoyancy and comfort by taking weight off hips, knees, and feet.

■ Moving slowly makes water exercise easier. Another way to regulate exercise intensity is to change how much water you push when you move. For example, when you move your arms back and forth in front of you under water, it is hard work if you hold your palms facing each other as if you were trying to clap. It is easier if you turn your palms down and slice your arms back and forth with only the narrow edge of your hands pushing against the water.

■ Be aware that additional buoyancy allows for greater joint motion than you are probably used to, especially if you are exercising in a warm pool. Start slowly and do not overextend your time in the pool even if it feels good. You need to learn how your body will react or feel the day after exercise before you increase the intensity level.

Stationary Bicycling

Stationary bicycles offer the fitness benefits of bicycling outdoors without the hazards. They're a good option for people who don't have the flexibility, strength, or balance to be comfortable pedaling and steering on the road. They are also a great alternative for people who live in a cold or hilly area. Stationary bicycles can be modified for various physical conditions. For example,

some people with paralysis of one leg or arm can exercise on stationary bicycles with special attachments for their paralyzed limb.

The stationary bicycle is a particularly good alternative for people with chronic pain. This form of cycling doesn't put excess strain on your hips, knees, feet, or spine. You can easily adjust how hard you work, and you can choose the most comfortable style of bicycle for you. Two general types of bicycles are recommended for people with chronic pain conditions. Some people feel more comfortable leaning slightly forward on an upright exercise bicycle, often called a "hybrid" or "town bike" style. Other people are more comfortable with a recumbent bicycle that has a long, low design with a full-size seat and backrest. You want to avoid a racing-style bicycle that requires you to curve your back excessively. Many fitness centers have both styles of stationary bicycles available and offer supervised indoor cycling classes. There are also many styles of bicycles to choose from if you decide to purchase one for home use. Like swimming, bicycling is not a weight-bearing exercise, so it does not improve balance or build healthy bones. Use the bicycle on days when you don't want to walk or do other weight-bearing exercise or when you can't exercise outside.

Making stationary bicycling interesting

The most common complaint about riding a stationary bike is that it's boring. If you ride while watching television, reading, or listening to music, you can become fit without becoming bored. One woman keeps interested by mapping out bike tours of places she would like to visit and then charts her progress on a map as she rolls off the miles. Other people get in

Stationary Bicycle Checklist

- The bicycle is steady when you get on and off.

- The resistance is easy to set and can be set to zero.

- The seat is comfortable and can be adjusted so your knee is close to full extension when the pedal is at its lowest point.

- The pedals are large enough and the pedal straps are loose enough to allow your feet to move slightly while pedaling.

- There is ample clearance from the frame for your knees and ankles.

- The handlebars allow good posture and comfortable arm position.

their bicycle time during the half hour of soap opera or news that they watch every day. There are also videocassettes and DVDs of exotic bike tours from a rider's perspective. Book racks that clip onto the handlebars make reading easy.

Stationary bicycling tips

- Stationary bicycling involves different muscles than walking does. Until your leg muscles get used to pedaling, you may be able to ride for only a few minutes at a time. Start off with no resistance. Increase resistance slightly as riding gets easier. Biking with increasing resistance resembles bicycling up hills. If you use too much resistance, your knees are likely to hurt, and you'll have to stop before you get the benefit of endurance.

- Pedal at a comfortable speed. For most people, 50 to 70 revolutions per minute (rpm) is a good place to start. Most bicycles have a monitor that states the rpm rate, or you can count the number of times your right foot reaches its lowest point in a minute. As you get used to bicycling, you can increase your speed. However, faster is not necessarily

better. Listening to music at the appropriate tempo makes it easier to pedal at a consistent speed. With experience you will figure out the best combination of speed and resistance.

- Set a goal of pedaling 20 to 30 minutes at a comfortable speed. Build up your time by alternating intervals of brisk pedaling with periods of less exertion. Use your heart rate, the perceived exertion scale, or the talk test (see page 151) to make sure you aren't working too hard. If you're alone, reciting poems or telling a story to yourself as you pedal can make the time pass more quickly. If you get out of breath, slow down.

- Keep a record of the times and distances of your bike trips. You'll be amazed at how far you can bicycle.

- On bad days, maintain your exercise habit by pedaling with no resistance, at a lower rpm, or for a shorter period of time.

- Make sure to warm up and cool down—pedal slowly with no resistance for five minutes before and after more vigorous exercise.

Using Other Exercise Equipment

In addition to stationary bicycles, there are many other types of exercise equipment. These include treadmills, self-powered and motor-driven rowing machines, cross-country skiing machines, stair-climbers, and elliptical machines. Most are available at fitness centers or for purchase for use at home. If you're thinking about any of these exercise options, take the time to be sure of what you want to achieve. For cardiovascular fitness and endurance, you want equipment that will help you exercise as much of your body at one time as possible. The motion should be rhythmic, repetitive, and smooth. The equipment should be comfortable, safe, and not stressful on joints. Be sure to consult your doctor, therapist, or a trained fitness instructor if you're interested in a new piece of equipment, then try it out for a week or two before committing to a health club membership or buying the equipment for home.

Exercise equipment that requires you to use weights usually does not improve cardiovascular fitness but does improve strength and build strong bones. Again, be sure to consult with your health care experts if you want to add weight machines or strengthening exercises involving weights to your program.

Low-Impact Aerobics

Most people find low-impact aerobic dance a fun and safe form of exercise. "Low impact" means that one foot is always on the floor and there is no jumping. However, low impact does not necessarily mean low intensity, nor do all the low-impact routines protect all your joints. If you participate in a low-impact aerobics class, you'll probably need to make some modifications to routines to suit your needs. You can also experience low-impact aerobic exercise in Zumba or Jazzercise classes. Regular dancing such as salsa, ballroom, and square dancing also provide good aerobic exercise.

To get started, let the instructor know about your condition. Tell her or him that you may need to modify some movements to meet your needs, and that you may need to ask for advice. It's easier to start off with a newly formed class than it is to join an ongoing class. If you don't know other people in the class, try to get acquainted. Be open about why you may sometimes do things a little differently. You'll be more comfortable and may find others who also have special needs.

Most instructors use music or count to a specific beat and do a set number of repetitions. You may find that the movement is too fast or that you don't want to do as many repetitions. Modify the routine by moving to every other beat or keeping up with the beat until you start to tire; then slow down or stop. If the class is doing an exercise that involves arms and legs and you get tired, try resting your arms and doing only the leg movements or just walking in place until you are ready to go again. Most instructors will be able to instruct you in chair aerobics if you need some time off your feet.

Some low-impact routines incorporate a lot of arm movements done at or above shoulder level to raise the heart rate. For people with shoulder, neck, or upper back pain or conditions like hypertension or lung problems, too much arm exercise above shoulder level can worsen shortness of breath, increase blood pressure, or cause pain. Modify the exercise by lowering your arms or taking a rest break as needed.

Doing things differently from the rest of the group in a room walled with mirrors takes courage, conviction, and a sense of humor. The most important thing you can do is choose an instructor who encourages everyone to exercise at her or his own pace and a class where people are friendly and having fun. Observe classes, speak with instructors, and participate in at least one class session before making any financial commitment.

The following tips can help you incorporate low-impact aerobics into your exercise action plan:

- **Wear shoes.** Many studios have cushioned floors and soft carpet that might tempt you to go barefoot. Don't! Shoes help protect the small joints and muscles in your feet and ankles by providing a firm, flat surface for support.

- **Protect your knees.** Stand with knees straight but relaxed. Many low-impact routines are done with bent, tensed knees and a lot of bobbing up and down. This can be painful and is unnecessarily stressful. Avoid this by remembering to keep your knees relaxed (aerobics instructors refer to this as "soft knees"). Watch in the mirror to see that you keep the top of your head steady as you exercise. Don't bob up and down.

- **Don't overstretch.** The beginning (warm-up) and end (cool-down) of the session will have stretching and strengthening exercises. Remember to stretch only as far as you comfortably can. Hold the position, and don't bounce. If the stretch hurts, don't do it. Instead, ask your instructor for a less stressful substitute, or choose one of your own.

- **Vary movements.** Do this often enough that you don't get sore muscles or joints. It's normal to feel some new sensations in your muscles and around your joints when you start a new exercise program. However, if you feel discomfort doing the same movement for some time, change movements or stop for a while and rest.

- **Alternate kinds of exercise.** Many exercise facilities provide a variety of exercise opportunities, including equipment rooms with cardiovascular machines, pools, and aerobics studios. If you have trouble with an hour-long aerobics class, see if you can join the class for the warm-up and cool-down and use a stationary bicycle or treadmill during the aerobics portion. Many people have found that this mixed routine gives them the benefits of both an individualized program and group exercise.

Self-Tests for Endurance (Aerobic Fitness)

For some people, just the feelings of increased endurance and well-being are enough to indicate progress. Others may need proof that their exercise program is making a measurable difference. You can use one or both of the following fitness tests. Not everyone will be able to do both tests. Pick the one that works best for you. Record your results. After four weeks of exercise, repeat the test and check your improvement. Measure yourself again after four more weeks of your exercise action plan.

Testing by Distance

- **Use a fitness monitor.** One of the least expensive pieces of exercise equipment is a pedometer. Because distance can be difficult to set, the best pedometers measure your steps. If you get in the habit of wearing a pedometer, it is easy to motivate yourself to add a few extra steps each day. You will be surprised at how these add up. A more expensive option is one of the new digital fitness wristbands that keeps track of step count, calorie burn, and other useful information.

- **Measure distance.** Find a place to walk, bicycle, swim, or water-walk where you can measure distance. A running track works well. On a street you can measure distance with the odometer in a car. A stationary bicycle or a treadmill with an odometer provides the same measurement. If you plan on swimming or water-walking, you can count lengths of the pool. After a warm-up, note your starting point and then bicycle, swim, or walk as briskly as you comfortably can for 5 minutes. Try to move at a steady pace for the full time. At the end of five minutes, mark your spot or note the distance or number of laps. Immediately take your pulse or rate your perceived exertion from 0 to 10. Continue at a slow pace for three to five more minutes to cool down. Record the distance, your heart rate, and your perceived exertion.

- **Repeat the test after several weeks of exercise.** There may be a change in as little as four weeks. However, it often takes eight to 12 weeks to see improvement.

  Goal: To cover more distance, to lower your heart rate, or to lower your perceived exertion.

Testing by Time

- **Set a time.** Measure a given distance to walk, bike, swim, or water-walk. Estimate how far you think you can go in one to five minutes. You can pick actual distance, a number of blocks, or lengths in a pool. Spend three to five minutes warming up. Start timing and begin moving steadily, briskly, and comfortably. At the finish line, record how long it took you to cover your course, your heart rate, and your perceived exertion.

- **Repeat the test** after several weeks of exercise, as you would for distance.

  Goal: To complete the distance in less time, at a lower heart rate, or at a lower perceived exertion.

Other Resources to Explore

In the search box on the following websites, enter such phrases as "chair exercises," "limited mobility fitness," or "fitness advice for wheelchair users."

HelpGuide.org: www.helpguide.org

National Health Service: www.nhs.uk/livewell

Sit and Be Fit (chair exercise): www.sitandbefit.org

Suggested Further Reading

To learn more about the topics discussed in this chapter, we suggest that you explore the following resources:

Fenton, Mark. *The Complete Guide to Walking for Health, Weight Loss, and Fitness.* Guilford, Conn.: Lyons Press, 2007.

Fortmann, Stephen P., and Prudence E. Breitrose. *The Blood Pressure Book: How to Get It Down and Keep It Down,* 3rd ed. Boulder, Colo.: Bull, 2006.

Karpay, Ellen. *The Everything Total Fitness Book.* Avon, Mass.: Adams Media, 2000.

Knopf, Karl. *Make the Pool Your Gym: No-Impact Water Workouts for Getting Fit,* *Building Strength, and Rehabbing from Injury.* Berkeley, Calif.: Ulysses Press, 2012.

Nelson, Miriam E., Alice H. Lichtenstein, and Lawrence Lindner. *Strong Women, Strong Hearts: Proven Strategies to Prevent and Reverse Heart Disease Now.* New York: Putnam, 2005.

White, Martha. *Water Exercise: 78 Safe and Effective Exercises for Fitness and Therapy.* Champaign, Ill.: Human Kinetics, 1998.

CHAPTER 10

Communicating with Family and Friends

"You just don't understand!"

Ow OFTEN HAS THIS STATEMENT summed up a frustrating discussion for you? Whenever you talk with someone, you want the person to understand. And you are understandably frustrated when you feel you have not been understood. Failure to communicate effectively can lead to anger, helplessness, isolation, and depression. Such feelings can be even worse when you have chronic pain.

Pain gets in the way of interaction with others. For example, pain can distract you so that you don't listen very well when others are talking to you. Pain can make you angry and irritable, and sometimes you may vent these feelings inappropriately—at family, friends, or coworkers. Pain can make you feel so overwhelmed that your world begins to shrink in size and revolve solely around you and your pain. Your communication with others can become self-centered. In the long run, these styles of communication turn off the people you care about most. The result: poor relationships with family members, friends, coworkers, or members of our health care team.

When communication breaks down, it affects your pain and symptoms. Your muscles tense, pain can increase, blood sugar and blood pressure levels may rise, and there is increased strain on the heart. Worry caused by conflict and misunderstanding can make you more irritable, further interfere with concentration, and sometimes lead to accidents. Clearly, poor communication is bad for your physical, mental, and emotional health.

For a self-manager, effective communication skills are essential. In this chapter we discuss tools to improve communication. These tools will help you express your feelings in a positive way. We give tips to help you minimize conflict, ask for help, and say no. We also discuss how to listen, how to recognize body language and different styles of communication, and how to get more information from others. In Chapter 11, we discuss how to more effectively communicate about your pain and other symptoms with your health care providers and how to work with the health care system.

Keep in mind that communication is a two-way street. As uncomfortable as you may feel about expressing your feelings or asking for help, chances are that others are also feeling the same way. It may be up to you to make sure the lines of communication are open.

Expressing Your Feelings

When communication is difficult, take the following steps. First, review the situation. Exactly what is bothering you? What are you feeling? Here is an example.

Bob and Jim had agreed to go to a football game. When Bob came to pick him up, Jim was not ready. In fact, he was not sure he wanted to go because he was having trouble with his back. The following conversation took place.

Jim: *"You just don't understand. If you had pain like I do, you wouldn't be so quick to criticize.*

Bob: *"Well, I can see that I should just go by myself."*

In this conversation, neither Bob nor Jim had stopped to think about what was really bothering him or how he felt about it. Each blamed the other for an unfortunate situation.

The following is the same conversation but with both people using more thoughtful communication.

Bob: *"When we have made plans and then at the last minute you are not sure you can go, I feel frustrated and angry. I don't know what to do—go on without you, stay here and change our plans, or just not make future plans."*

Jim : *"When this back pain acts up at the last minute, I am also confused. I keep hoping I can go and so I don't call you because I don't want to disappoint you and I really want to go. I keep hoping that my back will get better as the day wears on."*

Keys to Better Communication

- Do not assume that others know what you want because "they should know." People are not mind readers. If you want to be sure they know something, tell them.

- You cannot change the communication of others. What you can do is change *your* communication to be sure you are as clear as possible. (See Table 10.1, page 172).

Bob: *"I understand."*

Jim: *"Let's go to the game. You can let me off at the gate before parking so I won't have to walk as far. Then I can do the steps slowly and be in our seats when you arrive. I really want to go to the game with you. In the future, I will let you know sooner if I think my back is acting up."*

Bob: *"Sounds good to me. I really do like your company and knowing how I can help. It's just that being caught by surprise sometimes makes me angry."*

In this dialogue, Bob and Jim talked about the situation and how they felt about it. Neither blamed the other.

Unfortunately, people often use blaming communications in these situations. For example, maybe we are not listening, get caught, and then we blame the other person. Even then, thoughtful communication can be helpful. Consider the following example.

Jean: *"Why do you always spoil my plans? At least you could have called. I am really tired of trying to do anything with you."*

Cathy: *"I understand. When my fibromyalgia gets bad at the last minute, I am confused. I keep hoping I can go and so I don't call you because I don't want to disappoint you. I really want to go. I keep hoping that I will feel better as the day wears on."*

Jean: *"Well, I hope that in the future you will call. I don't like being caught by surprise."*

Cathy: *"I understand. If it is OK with you, let's go shopping now. If I start feeling too sore, I'll take a break in the coffee shop with my book while you continue to shop. I do want us to keep making plans. In the future, if I am not feeling good, I'll let you know sooner."*

In this example, only Cathy is using thoughtful communication. Jean continues to blame. The outcome, however, is still positive. Both people get what they want.

The following are some suggestions for using good communications and creating supportive relationships:

- **Show respect.** Always show respect and regard for the other person. Try not to preach or be excessively demanding. Avoid demeaning or blaming comments such as, "Why do you always spoil my plans?" The use of the word *you* is a clue that your communication might be blaming. Try to start sentences with the word "I" instead (we discuss this practice more in the pages that follow). A bit of tact and courtesy can defuse many of these situations (see the section on Anger in Chapter 4, page 63).

- **Be clear.** Describe a specific situation or your observations using the facts. Avoid words like *always* and *never.* Don't make or respond to unhelpful generalizations. For example, rather than react to Jean's accusation, Cathy responded by clearly explaining her last-minute pain, as well as her hopes for continuing to enjoy Jean's company despite the pain and fatigue.

- **Don't make assumptions.** Ask for more detail. Jean did not do this. She assumed that Cathy was rude because she did not call. It would have been better if she asked Cathy why she hadn't called earlier. Assumptions are the enemy of good communication. Many arguments arise from one person expecting the other person to be able to read his or her mind. Ask questions if you don't understand something.

- **Open up.** Try to express your feelings openly and honestly. Express your own needs directly and clearly. Don't make others guess what you are feeling or what you need—chances are they may be off base. Cathy did the right thing. She talked about wanting to go, not wanting to disappoint Jean, and hoping that her fibromyalgia symptoms would get better.

- **Accept the feelings of others.** Try to understand their perspective. This is not always easy. Sometimes you need to think about what was said instead of answering at once. You can always stall a bit by saying "I am

trying to understand" or "I'm not sure I understand; could you explain some more?"

- **Use humor—sparingly.** Sometimes gently introducing a bit of humor works wonders. But don't use sarcasm or demeaning humor, and know when to be serious.

- **Avoid playing the victim.** You become a victim when you do not express your needs and feelings or expect that someone else should act in a certain way. Unless you have done something to hurt another person, you should not apologize. Apologizing all the time is a sign that you view yourself as a victim. You deserve respect, and you have a right to express your wants and needs.

- **Listen first.** Good listeners seldom interrupt. Wait a few seconds when someone is finished talking before you respond. He or she may have more to say.

"I" Messages

Many of us are uncomfortable expressing our feelings, especially when it may seem as if we are being critical of someone else. But there are some guidelines to follow that can help us better express our feelings without making our listeners feel attacked or on the defensive.

If emotions are high and we feel frustrated, our communication may be full of "you" messages. "You" messages are sentences that begin with the word "you." In a heated discussion, "you" statements are often accusative and confrontational. They suggest blame, causing the other person to feel under attack. Once we start flinging "you" statements around, the other person is on the defensive, and barriers go up. The situation just escalates from there, leading to anger, frustration, and bad feelings.

"I" statements are direct, assertive expressions of your views and feelings. To craft "I" messages, avoid the word *you* and instead report your personal feelings using the word *I*. For example, say, "I try very hard to do the best work I can" rather than "You always criticize me." Or "I appreciate it when you turn down the television while I talk," not "You never pay attention." Here are some more examples:

"You" message: *"Why are you always late? We never get anywhere on time."*

"I" message: *"I get really upset when I'm late. It's important to me to be on time."*

"You" message: *"There's no way you can understand how lousy I feel."*

"I" message: *"I'm not feeling well. I could really use a little help today."*

Watch out for disguised or hidden "you" messages. These are "you" messages with "I feel . . ." stuck in front of them. For example, "I feel that you are not treating me fairly" is actually a disguised "you" statement. A true "I" statement

would be, "I feel angry and hurt." Here's another example:

"You" message: *"You always walk too fast."*

Hidden "you" message: *"I feel angry when you walk so fast."*

"I" message: *"I have a hard time walking fast."*

Of course, like any new skill, crafting "I" messages takes practice. Start by really listening, to yourself and to others. (Grocery stores are a good place to here lots of "you" messages as parents talk to their children.) In your head, turn some of the "you" messages into "I" messages. You'll be surprised at how fast "I" messages become a habit.

To get started, adopt the following format for your "I" message communication:

"I notice . . ." (state just the facts)

"I think . . ." (state your opinion)

"I feel . . ." (state what your feelings are)

"I want . . ." (state exactly what you'd like the other person to do)

For example, imagine you have baked a special bread to bring as a gift to a friend. A family

---

Exercise: "I" Messages

Change the following statements into "I" messages. (Watch out for hidden "you" messages.)

1. "You expect me to wait on you hand and foot!"

2. "You hardly ever touch me anymore. You haven't paid any attention to me since my car accident."

3. "You never have enough time for me. You're always in a hurry."

4. "Doctor, you didn't tell me the side effects of all these drugs or why I have to take them."

Table 10. 1 **Ensuring Clear Communication**

Words That Aid Understanding	Words That Hinder Understanding
I	You
Right now, at this time, at this point	Never, always, every time, constantly
Who, which, where, when	Obviously . . .
What do you mean, please explain, tell me more, I don't understand	Why?

member wanders into the kitchen, sees the bread on the counter, and cuts out a large slice. You're upset because, with a piece missing, the gift is ruined. You might say to the bread eater: "I see you cut into my special bread [fact], but I think you should have asked me about it first [opinion]. I'm really upset and disappointed because I can't give it as a gift now [feeling]. I'd like an apology, and I'd like you to ask me first next time [want]."

"I" messages are a great tool but there are some "I" message cautions to keep in mind. First, they are not a cure-all. They only work if the listener is able to really hear them. This can be a problem if the person is used to hearing blaming "you" messages. Even when you switch to "I" messages, your listener may be so accustomed to "you" messages, they may not be able to hear your new method of communication. If using "I" messages does not work at first, continue to use them. Things will change as you gain skill and old patterns of communication are broken.

Second, some people use "I" messages as a means of manipulation. They may often express that they are sad, angry, or frustrated in order to gain sympathy from others. If used in this way, problems can escalate. Effective "I" messages must report honest feelings, not be used as attention-seeking devices.

Finally, note that "I" messages are not just about conveying disappointment or upset. They are an excellent way to express positive feelings and compliments. For example, "I really appreciate the extra time you gave me today, doctor."

Good communication skills help make life easier for everyone, especially those with long-term health problems. Table 10.1 summarizes some words that can help or hinder this communication.

Minimizing Conflict

In addition to using "I" messages, the following are methods that you can use to reduce conflict.

- **Shift the focus.** If a discussion gets off topic and emotions are running high, shift the focus of the conversation. That is, bring the discussion back to the original topic. For example, you might say something like, "We're both getting upset now and drifting away from the topic we agreed to discuss," or "I feel like things other than what we agreed to talk about are coming up, and I'm getting upset. Can we discuss these other things later and just talk about the topics we originally agreed on?"

Effective Apologies

Rather than a sign of weak character, an apology shows great strength. To be effective, your apology should do all of the following:

- Admit the specific mistake and accept responsibility for it. You must name the offense; no glossing over with just, "I'm sorry for what I did." Be specific. You might say, for example, "I'm very sorry that I spoke behind your back." Explain the particular circumstances that led you to do what you did. Don't offer excuses or sidestep responsibility.

- Express your feelings. A genuine, heartfelt apology involves some suffering. Sadness shows that the relationship matters to you.

- Acknowledge the impact of wrongdoing. You might say, "I know that I hurt you and that my behavior cost you a lot. For that I am very sorry."

- Offer to make amends. Ask what you can do to make the situation better, or volunteer specific suggestions.

- **Buy time.** For example, you might say, "I think I understand your concerns, but I need more time to think about it before I can respond," or "I hear what you are saying, but I am too frustrated to respond now. I need to find out more about this before I can respond."

- **Make sure you understand each other's viewpoints.** Do this by summarizing what you heard and asking for clarification. You can also switch roles. Try arguing the other person's position as thoroughly and thoughtfully as possible. This will help you understand all sides of an issue, as well as convey that you respect and value the other's point of view. It will also help you develop tolerance and empathy for others.

- **Look for compromise.** You may not always find the perfect solution to a problem or reach total agreement. Nevertheless, it may be possible to compromise. Find something on which you can agree. For example, you may decide to do it your way this time and the other person's way the next time. Agree to part of what you want and part of what the other person wants. Or decide what adjustment you'll make and what the other person will do in return. These are all forms of compromise that can help you through some difficult times.

- **Say you're sorry.** We all say or do things that, intentionally or unintentionally, hurt others. Many relationships suffer—sometimes for years—because people have not learned the powerful social skill of apologizing. Often all it takes is a simple, sincere apology to restore a relationship. Apologizing is not fun, but it is an act of courage, generosity, and healing. It brings the possibility of a renewed and stronger relationship, and it can also bring peace within yourself.

Asking for Help

Getting and giving help are a part of life, but offering and requesting assistance can cause many problems. Even though most of us need help sometimes, few of us like to ask for it. We may not want to admit that we are unable to do things for ourselves. We may not want to be a burden on others. We may hedge or make a very vague request: "I'm sorry to have to ask this . . . ," "I know this is asking a lot . . . ," "I hate to ask this, but . . ." Hedging tends to put the other person on the defensive: "Gosh, what's he going to ask that's such a big deal, anyway?"

To avoid this sort of response, be specific when you ask for help. A general request can lead to misunderstanding. The person being asked to help may react negatively if the request is not clear. This leads to a further breakdown in communication and no help. A specific request is more likely to have a positive result.

> General request: *"I know this is the last thing you want to do, but I need help moving. Will you help me?"*
>
> Reaction: *"Uh . . . well . . . I don't know. Um . . . can I get back to you after I check my schedule?" (Probably next year!)*
>
> Specific request: *"I'm moving next week, and I'd like to move my books and kitchen stuff ahead of time. Would you mind helping me load and unload the boxes in my car Saturday morning? I think it can be done in one trip."*
>
> Reaction: *"I'm busy Saturday morning, but I could give you a hand Friday night."*

Refusing Help

People with chronic pain sometimes are given offers of help that are not needed or desired. In most cases, these offers come from important people in your life, such as friends, family, and coworkers. They can be overly sympathetic and try to do things for you that you can do yourself; it just might take a bit longer. These people care for you and genuinely want to help, but when other people take over activities that you can do yourself you may feel dependent and disabled. This may lower your self-esteem A well-worded "I" message allows you to decline the help without embarrassing the other person. You could say, "Thank you for being so thoughtful, but today I think I can handle it myself. I hope I can take you up on your offer another time."

Accepting Help

You may often hear, "How can I help?" Your answer may often be, "I don't know" or "Thank you, but I don't need any help." Meanwhile you are thinking, "They should know . . ." Be prepared to accept help by having a specific answer. For example, when general offers of help are made, respond with specifics such as, "It would be great if we could go for a walk together once a week," or "Could you please take out the garbage? I can't lift it."

Remember that people cannot read your mind, so you need to tell them what you want. Think about how each person can help. If possible, give people a task that they can easily accomplish. You are giving them a gift. People like being helpful and feel rejected when they cannot assist someone they care about. It is also beneficial to be grateful for the help you receive. When people help you, thank them for it! (See "Practice Gratitude," page 94, in Chapter 5.)

Saying No

Let's consider the flip side of the same coin: imagine that you are the one being asked to help out with some activity or task. Using communication skills that get at the specifics will avoid problems. It is important to understand any request fully before responding. It is probably best not to answer right away. Asking for more information or restating the request will often bring more clarity. "Before I answer . . ." will not only clarify the request but also prevent the person from assuming that you are going to say yes. If a request for help from someone leaves you feeling negative or unsure, trust your feelings. A good rule of thumb is don't answer until you know enough about the request to feel comfortable saying yes.

The moving example we just discussed is a good one. "Help me move" can mean anything from moving furniture up stairs to picking up pizza for the hungry troops. Or, if you are asked to help with a community fund-raising event, does it mean standing while serving coffee and sandwiches or sitting at a counter collecting donations?

If you are feeling overwhelmed and the request is unrealistic for you at this time, saying no is an important self-management tool. However, if you decide to say no, it is important to acknowledge the importance of the request. In this way, the person will see that you are rejecting the request rather than the person. Your turndown should not be a putdown. Instead, include a positive note in your refusal, such as, "That sounds like a worthwhile project you're doing, but it's beyond what I can do this week." Again, specifics are the key. Be clear about the conditions of your refusal: Will you always turn down this request, or is it just that today or this week or right now is a problem? You may wish to make a counteroffer, such as, "I won't be able to drive today, but I may be able to do it next week." But remember, you always have the legitimate right to decline a request, even if it is a reasonable one.

Listening

Good listening is probably the most important communication skill. Most of us are much better at talking than we are at listening. When others talk to us, we are often preparing a response instead of just listening. There are several steps to being a good listener:

1. **Listen to the words and tone of voice, and observe body language** (see page 177). There may be times when the words don't tell the whole story. Is the speaker's voice wavering? Is he or she struggling to find the right words? Do you notice body tension? Does he or she seem distracted? Do you hear sarcasm? What is the facial expression? If you pick up on some of these signs, the speaker probably has more on his or her mind.

2. **Let the person know you heard what he or she said.** This may be a simple "uh huh."

Sometimes when we are troubled, it is helpful just to talk to a sympathetic listener. Many times the only thing the speaker wants is acknowledgment or just someone who is willing to take the time to listen.

3. **Let the person know you heard both the content and the emotion behind what he or she said.** You can do this by restating the content. For example, "Sounds like you are planning a nice trip." Or you can respond by acknowledging the emotions: "That must be difficult" or "How sad you must feel." Responding to either the content or the emotion can help communication. It discourages the other person from simply repeating what has already been said. When you respond on an emotional level, the results are often startling. These responses tend to open the gates for more expression of feelings and thoughts. Don't try to talk people out of their feelings. They are real to them. Just listen and reflect.

4. **Respond by seeking more information** (see the Table 10.1 on page 172). This is especially important if you are not completely clear about what was said or what is wanted.

Getting More Information

Getting more information is a bit of an art. It can involve both simple and more complicated techniques.

The simplest way to get more information is to ask. "Tell me more" will probably get you more, as will "I don't understand; please explain," "I would like to know more about . . . " "Would you say that another way?" "How do you mean?"

"I'm not sure I got that," and "Could you expand on that?"

Another way to get more information is to paraphrase, or repeat what you heard in your own words. This is a good tool if you want to make sure you understand what the other person really meant. Paraphrasing can either help or hinder effective communication. It depends on the way the paraphrase is worded. It is important to paraphrase in the form of a question, not a statement. For example, someone says:

"I don't know. I'm really not feeling up to par. This party will be crowded and noisy, and I really don't know the hosts very well."

Provocative paraphrase:

"Obviously, you're telling me you don't want to go to the party."

This response might provoke an angry response such as, "No, I didn't say that! If you're going to be that way, I'll stay home for sure." Or the response might be no response—a total shutdown because of anger or despair ("he just doesn't understand"). People don't like to be told what they meant.

Here's a better paraphrase, expressed as a question:

"Are you saying that you'd rather stay home than go to the party?"

The response to this paraphrase might be:

"That's not what I meant. I'm feeling a little worried that my pain will act up. I'd appreciate it if you'd stay near me during the party and if I need to come home early, we can do that. I'd feel better about it, and I might be

able to relax and have a good time if I know it doesn't have to be a long night."

As you can see, the second paraphrase helps communication. The real reason for expressing doubt about the party has been discovered. As this example illustrates, you get more information when you paraphrase with questions.

Be specific. If you want specific information, you must ask specific questions. We often speak in generalities. For example:

Doctor: *"How have you been feeling?"*

Patient: *"Not so good."*

The doctor has not gotten much information. "Not so good" isn't very useful. Here's how the doctor gets more information:

Doctor: *"Are you still having those sharp pains in your right shoulder?"*

Patient: *"Yes. A lot."*

Doctor: *"How often?"*

Patient: *"A couple of times a day."*

Doctor: *"How long do they last?"*

Patient: *"A long time."*

Doctor: *"About how many minutes would you say?"*

. . . and so on.

Health care providers are trained to get specific information from patients, although they sometimes ask general questions. Most of us are not trained, but we can learn to ask specific questions. Asking for specifics is a good way to start: "Can you be more specific about . . . ?" "Are you thinking of something special?"

Avoid simply asking "Why?" This is far too general a question. "Why?" also forces a person to justify something and can put him or her on the defensive. A person may respond at an entirely different level than you had in mind. Rather than using *why*, begin your responses with *who, which, when,* or *where*. These words promote a specific response.

Sometimes you may not get the information you're seeking because you do not know what question to ask. For example, you may be seeking legal services from a senior center. You call and ask if there is a lawyer on staff and hang up when the answer is no. If instead you had asked where you might get low-cost legal advice, you might have gotten some referrals.

Body Language and Conversational Styles

Part of listening to what others are saying includes observing *how* they say it. Even when people say nothing, our bodies are talking. Sometimes they are even shouting. Research shows that more than half of what we communicate is done through our body language.

If you want to communicate really well, be aware of body language, facial expressions, and tone of voice. These should match what you say in words. If you do not do this, you are sending mixed messages and creating misunderstandings. For example, if you want to make a firm statement, look at the other person. Stand tall and confident, relax your legs and arms, and breathe. You may even lean forward to show your interest. Keep your expression friendly. Try not to sneer or bite your lip; this might indicate discomfort or doubt. Don't move away or slouch, as these communicate disinterest and uncertainty.

When you notice someone's body language does not match his or her words, gently point this out. Ask for clarification. For example, you might say, "Dear, I hear you saying that you would like to go with me to the family picnic, but you look tired and you're yawning as you speak. Would you rather stay home and rest while I go alone?"

In addition to reading people's body language, it is helpful to recognize and appreciate that we all express ourselves differently. Many things influence how we communicate—our culture, country of origin, education, occupation, and especially our gender.

For example, women tend to ask more personal questions than men do. These show interest and help form relationships. Men are more likely to offer opinions or suggestions and to state facts. They tend to discuss problems in an effort to find solutions, whereas women want to share their feelings and experiences. No one style is better or worse; they're just different. By acknowledging and accepting these differences, we can reduce some of the misunderstanding, frustration, and resentment we sometimes feel when we communicate with others.

Suggested Further Reading

To learn more about the topics discussed in this chapter, we suggest that you explore the following resources:

Beck, Aaron T. *Love Is Never Enough: How Couples Can Overcome Misunderstandings, Resolve Conflicts, and Solve Relationship Problems Through Cognitive Therapy.* New York: HarperCollins, 1989.

Caudill, Margaret A. *Managing Pain Before It Manages You.* New York: Guilford Press, 2009 (especially Chapter 8).

Davis, Martha, Kim Paleg, and Patrick Fanning. *The Messages Workbook: Powerful Strategies for Effective Communication at Work and Home.* Oakland, Calif.: New Harbinger, 2004.

Gottman, John M., and Joan DeClaire. *The Relationship Cure: A 5-Step Guide to Strengthening Your Marriage, Family, and Friendships.* New York: Three Rivers, 2001.

Gottman, John M., and Nan Silver. *The Seven Principles for Making Marriage Work: A Practical Guide from the Country's Foremost Relationship Expert.* New York: Three Rivers, 1999.

Hendrix, Harville. *Getting the Love You Want: A Guide for Couples.* New York: Henry Holt, 2007.

McKay, Matthew, Martha Davis, and Patrick Fanning. *Messages: The Communication Skills Book.* Oakland, Calif.: New Harbinger, 2009.

Tannen, Deborah. *You Just Don't Understand: Women and Men in Conversation.* New York: HarperCollins, 2001.

Turk, Dennis and Frits Winter. *The Pain Survival Guide: How to Reclaim Your Life.* Washington, D.C.: American Psychological Association, 2007 (Chapter 5).

CHAPTER 11

Communicating with Your Health Care Professionals

GOOD COMMUNICATION IS A NECESSITY when you have a long-term condition. It is the lifeblood of all relationships, and relationships are a lifeline to healthy coping when you are self-managing chronic pain. Your health care team in particular must understand you. And when you don't understand advice or recommendations from your doctors and other health professionals, serious problems can result.

One of the keys to getting good health care is to communicate well with your health care providers. This important self-management tool can be a challenge. You may be afraid to talk freely or feel there is not enough time during an appointment. Health professionals may use words you do not understand, or you may not want to share personal and possibly embarrassing information. These fears and feelings can hinder communication with your providers and harm your health.

Providers share the responsibility for poor communication. They sometimes feel too busy or important to take the time to talk with and know their patients. They may ignore or tune out questions. Their actions or inaction might offend you.

Although you do not have to become best friends with your providers, you should expect them to be attentive and caring. You also want them to be able to explain things clearly. But explanations aren't always easy with chronic pain conditions. Providers are often perplexed about this complex health problem. You may think that you can only get the best care by going to specialists. This may be true in some cases, but it can also greatly complicate the care you receive. You may be seeing several specialists. They may not get to really know you and may not be aware of what your other care providers are doing, thinking, or prescribing. These are good reasons to have a primary provider, or a medical "home." A relationship with a health care provider is much like a business partnership or even a marriage. Establishing and maintaining this long-term relationship may take some effort, but it can make a large difference to your health.

Many of us would like our healthcare providers to be like warmhearted computers— gigantic brains, stuffed with knowledge about the human body and mind (especially ours). We want our providers to analyze the situation, read our minds, make a perfect diagnosis, come up with a treatment plan, and tell us what to expect. At the same time, we want them to be warm and caring and to make us feel as though we are their most important patient.

Most providers wish they were just that sort of person. Unfortunately, no one provider can be all things to all patients. Providers are human. They have bad days, they get headaches, they get tired, and they get sore feet. They have families who demand their time and attention, and they may get frustrated by paperwork, electronic record keeping, and large bureaucracies.

Doctors and other health care professionals entered the health care system because they wanted to help people, and they took extensive training in order to be able to do so. They may be frustrated when they do not have all the answers about chronic pain. Many times they must take their satisfaction from improvements rather than cures, or even from slowing the decline of some conditions. Undoubtedly, you have been frustrated, angry, or depressed about your condition from time to time, but your doctor and other providers have probably felt similar emotions about their inability to cure your condition. In this, you are truly partners.

To keep the lines of communication open, be clear about what you want from your providers. You should feel comfortable expressing your fears, asking questions that you may think are "stupid," and negotiating a treatment plan to satisfy you both.

Doctors and other providers are typically on very tight schedules. This becomes painfully clear when you have to wait in the doctor's office because of an emergency or a late patient that has delayed your appointment. This sometimes causes both patients and doctors to feel rushed. Time is a threat to a good patient-provider relationship. Both you and your provider would probably greatly welcome more face-to-face time. When time is short, the resulting anxiety can bring about rushed communication. "You" messages and misunderstandings are common in these situations. (See Chapter 10, pages 170–172.)

One way to get the most from your visit is to take PART. This acronym stands for Prepare, Ask, Repeat, Take action. In this section of the chapter, we explain more about taking PART.

(See Chapter 10, pages 170–172.)

| **Take PART** |
| Prepare |
| Ask |
| Repeat |
| Take action |

Prepare

People with chronic pain are often referred to multiple health care providers. That's because no single provider has all the answers. This means that you have appointments with people who do not know your pain history. The importance of communicating clearly and directly with all these providers cannot be emphasized enough.

Pain is a personal experience. The pain you have is only felt by you. Your pain can't be compared to another person's, and only you can know how much pain you feel, when you feel it, and how it affects you physically, emotionally, and socially. While this may sound very basic, think about the frustration you feel when you try to describe your pain to your doctor. Not easy, is it? At the same time, your doctor and other providers can be frustrated because they are desperately trying to understand your pain problem better. Very often, there are no blood screens, X-rays, or other tests to help them sort out the problem. Doctors can use these tools to rule out other diseases but they cannot use them to assess your pain. They are relying on your communication to help them. No matter what kind of pain you have, it is important to describe it and any related symptoms precisely. This reduces everybody's frustration level. The following guidelines can help you gather detailed information about your pain that will make your visits with a healthcare provider more productive:

■ **Pain Profile:** When you go to a doctor or other provider's office, have a written "pain profile" with you so you are ready to answer questions about your pain. Whether you have had pain for six months or six years, it can be hard to remember details if you are not prepared. Before going to a new appointment, answer the questions in Figure 11.1 on page 182. By being as specific as possible, you can help your doctor better understand the nature of your pain. This is part of being a good self-manager, because you are helping to develop the best plan of care for you. Once your health provider knows your pain history, you usually will not need to review your entire pain profile except to report changes.

■ **Pain Language:** Although the word *pain* means many things to many people, specific kinds of words are commonly used for specific types of pain conditions. For example, *throbbing*, *pounding*, and *splitting* are words frequently used by people who have headaches. *Burning*, *tingling*, and *jumping* can describe pain that is associated with some

Figure 11.1 **Preparing Your Pain Profile**

1. When did the pain start? _____

   _____

   Was there a specific cause (e.g., a fall) or did it just seem to develop over time?

   _____

   _____

2. Has it gotten worse with time or has it remained the same?

3. Is it intermittent or constant?_____
   Does it come in waves and then subside?
   Yes ☐ No ☐

4. What does the pain feel like? (*Refer to Figure 11.2 on the next page*)

   _____

   _____

5. Is there a time of day when the pain is worse? _____

   _____

   Does it wake you from sleep? Yes ☐ No ☐
   Does it cause insomnia? Yes ☐ No ☐

6. Have you ever had this type of pain before? Yes ☐ No ☐
   When? _____

   _____

   Why?_____

   _____

7. What increases the pain? Sitting? _____
   Lying down? _____ Mild massage? _____
   Other? _____

   _____

8. Does the pain radiate to another part of your body such as your back, shoulder, or legs?_____

   _____

9. How severe is the pain? On a 0 to 10 scale, with 10 being the most severe, how does this pain rate?_____

   _____

10. Can you distract yourself from the pain either partially or completely? Or is the pain so intense that distraction is impossible? _____

    _____

11. How does it affect the quality of your life? Have you stopped visiting friends? Are you irritable, angry, depressed?

    _____

    _____

    _____

12. Is the pain accompanied by symptoms such as nausea, sweating, shortness of breath?_____

    _____

13. Which, if any, medications have you taken?_____

    _____

    _____

    Have they relieved the pain?
    Completely?   Yes ☐ No ☐
    Partially?   Yes ☐ No ☐
    Not at all?   Yes ☐ No ☐

14. Are you sensitive or allergic to any pain medication? _____

    _____

15. Miscellaneous comments

    _____

    _____

    _____

    _____

Figure 11.2 **Describing Your Pain**

Pain Intensity Scale

0 No Pain
1 Mild
2 Discomforting
3 Distressing
4 Horrible
5 Excruciating

___Flickering

___Quivering

___Pulsing

___Throbbing

___Beating

___Pounding

___Jumping

___Flashing

___Shooting

___Pricking

___Boring

___Drilling

___Stabbing

___Sharp

___Cutting

___Lacerating

___Pinching

___Pressing

___Gnawing

___Cramping

___Crushing

___Tugging

___Pulling

___Wrenching

___Hot

___Burning

___Scalding

___Searing

___Tingling

___Itching

___Smarting

___Stinging

___Dull

___Sore

___Hurting

___Aching

___Heavy

___Tender

___Taut

___Rasping

___Splitting

___Tiring

___Exhausting

___Sickening

___Suffocating

___Fearful

___Frightful

___Terrifying

___Punishing

___Gruelling

___Cruel

___Vicious

___Killing

___Wretched

___Blinding

___Annoying

___Troublesome

___Miserable

___Intense

___Unbearable

___Spreading

___Radiating

___Penetrating

___Piercing

___Tight

___Numb

___Drawing

___Squeezing

___Tearing

___Cool

___Cold

___Freezing

___Nagging

___Nauseating

___Agonizing

___Dreadful

___Torturing

_____

_____

_____

_____

These descriptions of pain were taken from the McGill Pain Questionnaire, © 1970 Ronald Melzack, PhD, and are used with permission of Dr. Melzack.

kinds of nerve involvement. People with arthritis sometimes use the words *achy*, *sore*, or *tiring*. The words you use to describe your pain can sometimes point to a type of pain problem, so a rich vocabulary can be very helpful. Figure 11.2 lists typical words to describe pain sensations and the emotions that pain can cause. Place a mark next to each one that describes your pain. If there are other words that you use to describe your pain, add

them to the list. Bring the list with you when you see your doctor or other providers.

■ **Pain Intensity:** Just as words describe the quality of your pain, numbers can help describe the intensity or strength of your pain. There are several ways to measure or monitor pain intensity with numbers. One is a 0 to 5 scale (Figure 11.2, top left). Another is to use a 0 to 10 scale, with 0 indicating no pain at all and 10 as the worst

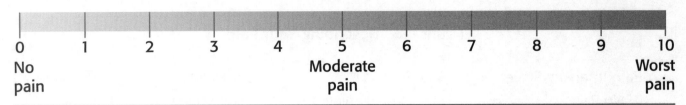

Figure 11.3

pain you have ever experienced (see Figure 11.3). When the doctor asks, "How bad is your pain now?" you can answer, "Well, on a scale from 0 to 10, I'd say it's a 5 or 6 right now." That is much more precise than saying, "Well, it's bad but not as bad as it gets." A numbering scale provides a point of comparison. It is also a good way for you to monitor your pain levels when you are trying to pace your activities (see Chapter 6, page 108). It's important to understand that your rating only applies to your pain, not anyone else's. Your rating of 6 might be very different from another person's rating of 6.

■ **Pain Effects:** In addition to the pain profile, think about how pain affects your everyday physical, mental, and social functioning. Does it affect your ability to walk, sit, do personal care, or get in and out of bed or a chair? Can you complete job responsibilities, prepare and enjoy meals, participate in leisure and family activities, and enjoy sexual intimacy? This is all important information for your health care provider. Come to your appointments prepared to talk about the specifics of how pain affects your activities and your life.

Make an appointment agenda

If you have a chronic pain condition, you will likely have regular appointments with your primary care doctor or other members of your pain team. Before each of these appointments, prepare an agenda. What are the reasons for the visit? What do you expect from your health care provider?

Before every appointment, write a list of your concerns or questions. After you walked out of the provider's office have you ever thought to yourself, "Why didn't I ask about . . . ?" or "I forgot to mention . . . " Making a list beforehand helps ensure that your main concerns get addressed. Be realistic. If you have 13 different problems, your provider probably cannot deal with all of them in one visit. Star or highlight the two or three most important items.

Give the list to your health care provider at the beginning of the visit and explain that you have starred your most important concerns. By calling attention to the starred items, you let the provider know which items are the most important to you. But by providing the complete list, you let the provider see everything in case there is something medically important that is not starred. If you wait until the end of your appointment to bring up concerns, there will not be time to discuss them.

Here is an example. Your doctor asks, "What brings you in today?" You might say something like, "I have a lot of things I want to discuss this visit" (glancing at his or her watch and thinking of the appointment schedule, the doctor immediately begins to feel anxious), "but I know that we have a limited amount of time. The things that most concern me are my shoulder pain, my dizziness, and the side effects from one of the medications I'm taking" (the doctor feels relieved because the concerns are focused and potentially manageable within the appointment time available).

List your medications and prepare your story

There are two other things you can do to prepare before your visit. List all your medications and their dosages and bring the list to all your appointments. If this is too difficult, put all your meds in a bag and bring them with you. Do not forget vitamins and over-the-counter medications and supplements.

The final thing to prepare is your story. Visit time is short. When the provider asks how you are feeling, some people will go on for several minutes about this and that symptom. It is better to be specific and succinct. Say, for example, "I think that overall my pain is about the same, but now I have more trouble sleeping and I'm feeling a bit depressed about things." Be prepared to describe your symptoms in detail, including:

- When they started
- How long they last
- Where they are located
- What makes them better or worse
- Whether you have had similar problems before
- Whether you have changed your diet, exercise, or medications in a way that might contribute to the symptoms
- What worries you most about the symptoms
- What you think might be causing the symptoms

If you were given a new medication or treatment during a previous visit, be ready to report how it went. If you are going to several providers, bring the results of all tests you have had in the past six months.

In telling your story, talk about trends: Are you getting better or worse, or are you the same? Also talk about frequency and degree: Are your symptoms more or less frequent or intense? For example, "In general, I am slowly getting better. I mostly feel the pain first thing in the morning and after I go grocery shopping. Last week, though, my pain did not get better over the course of the day, which is why I'm here."

Be as open as you can in sharing your thoughts, feelings, and fears. Remember, your provider is not a mind reader. If you are worried, explain why: "I'm worried that I may not be able to work," or "I'm worried I have cancer because no one can find the cause of my pain," or "My father had similar symptoms before he died." The more open you are, the more likely your provider can help. If you have a problem, don't wait for the provider to "discover" it. State your concern immediately. For example, "I'm worried about this mole on my chest."

The more specific you can be (without overdoing it with irrelevant details), the clearer a picture your health care provider will have of your problem, and the less time will be wasted for both of you.

Share your hunches or guesses about what might be causing your symptoms, as they often provide vital clues to an accurate diagnosis. Even if it turns out that your guesses are not correct, it gives your provider the opportunity to reassure you or address your hidden concerns.

Ask

In the doctor-patient partnership, your most powerful tool is the question. Your questions can help you to fill in important missing pieces of information and close critical gaps in communication. Asking questions is part of your active participation in the process of care, a critical ingredient to restoring your health. Accessing answers you understand is a cornerstone of self-management.

Be prepared to ask questions about the diagnosis, tests, treatments, and follow-up not just about your pain but about all your symptoms or other health concerns. Use the following guidelines to ask the right questions:

- **Diagnosis.** Ask what's wrong, whether there is a known cause, if it is contagious (for example, if you have an infection), what the future outlook (prognosis) is, and what can be done to prevent or manage the condition.

- **Tests.** If the doctor wants to perform tests, ask how the results are likely to affect treatment plans and what will happen if you are not tested. If you decide to undergo a test, find out how to prepare for it and what it will be like. Also ask how and when you will get the results.

- **Treatments.** Ask if there are any choices in treatments and the advantages and disadvantages of each. Ask what will happen if you are not treated (see Chapters 15 and 16).

- **Follow-up.** Find out if and when you should call or return for a follow-up visit. What symptoms should you watch for, and what should you do if they occur?

Repeat

To ensure you really understand everything, briefly repeat key points back to the doctor or other provider. For example, "You want me to do this set of exercises two times a day, in the morning and in the evening. Is that right?" Or "You want me to take this medicine three times a day." This gives the provider an opportunity to quickly correct any misunderstanding and miscommunication.

Sometimes it is hard to remember everything. You may want to take notes or bring another person to important visits. You can even tape-record the visit if the medical professional grants permission. If you don't understand or remember something the provider said, simply state that you need to go over it again. For example, "I'm pretty sure you told me some of this before, but I'm still confused about it." Don't be afraid to ask what you may consider a stupid question. Such questions are important and may prevent misunderstanding.

Take Action

At the end of a visit, you need to clearly understand what to do next. This includes making appointments for treatments, tests, and follow-up visits. You should also know any danger signs and what you should do if they occur. If necessary, ask your provider to write down instructions, recommend reading material, or indicate other places you can get help.

If for some reason you can't or don't intend to follow the provider's advice, let her or him know.

For example, "I don't want to take the aspirin. It gives me stomach problems," or "My insurance doesn't cover that much therapy. I can't afford it," or "I've tried to exercise, but I can't seem to keep it up." If your provider knows why you can't or won't follow advice, she or he may be able to make other suggestions. If you don't share the barriers to taking action, it's difficult for your provider to help.

Asking for a Second Opinion

Sometimes you may want to see another provider or have a second opinion. Asking for a second opinion can be hard, especially if you have had a long relationship with your provider. You may worry that asking for another opinion will anger your provider or that he or she will take your request in the wrong way.

Providers are seldom hurt by requests for a second opinion. If your condition is complicated or difficult, the doctor may have already consulted with a colleague or specialist (or more than one). This is often done informally. Asking for a second opinion is perfectly acceptable, and providers are taught to expect such requests. However, if you find yourself asking

for third, fourth, and fifth opinions, this may be unproductive.

Ask for a second opinion by using a non-threatening "I" message:

> *"I'm still feeling confused and uncomfortable about my pain treatment. I feel that another opinion might reassure me. Can you suggest someone I could see?"*

In this way, you have expressed your own feelings without suggesting that the provider is at fault. You have also confirmed your confidence in your provider by asking for his or her recommendation. (However, you are not bound by this suggestion; you may choose to see anyone you wish.)

Giving Feedback to Your Provider

Let your providers know how satisfied you are with your care. Everyone appreciates compliments and positive feedback, especially members of your health care team. Your praise can help nourish and console these busy, hardworking professionals. Letting them know that you appreciate their efforts is one of the best ways to improve your relationship with them—plus it makes them feel good!

Likewise, if you do not like the way you have been treated by any members of your health care team, let them know. Remember, they are not mind readers. They cannot improve the relationship if they don't know there's a problem.

Your Role in Medical Decisions

Many decisions in medical care are not clear-cut, and often there is more than one option. Except in life-threatening emergencies, the best decisions depend on your values and preferences and should not be left solely to your doctor or other health care provider. For example you might say, "I'm very conservative about taking strong medications. What's a reasonable period of time for me to try to address these symptoms with exercise, improving my diet, and relaxation, before I start taking this new medication?"

To make an informed choice about a proposed treatment, you need to know its cost and risks. This includes possible complications such as drug reactions, bleeding, infection, injury, or death. It also includes personal costs, such as absences from work, as well as financial considerations, such as how much of the proposed treatments your insurance will cover.

You also need to understand the likelihood that the proposed treatment will benefit you. Ask how it may or may not relieve your pain and other symptoms or improve your ability to function. Sometimes the best choice may be to delay a treatment decision in favor of "watchful waiting."

No one can tell you which choice is right for you. But to make an informed choice, you need information about your options. Informed choice, not merely informed consent, is essential to quality medical care. The best medical care for you combines your provider's medical expertise with your own knowledge, skills, and values.

Making decisions about treatments can be difficult. For some suggestions on how to make decisions, see page 21, and see Chapter 17 for help on how to evaluate new treatments.

Working with the Health Care System

Many health care providers these days work in larger systems such as clinics or hospitals. Appointments, billing, and telephone and e-mail protocol are often decided by someone other than your provider.

If you are unhappy with your health care system, don't just suffer in silence; do something about it. Find out who is running the organization and who makes decisions. Then share your feelings in a constructive way by letter, phone, or e-mail. Most health care organizations are concerned about their patients and therefore usually respond.

People who make the biggest decisions about health care tend to be removed from the people who seek treatment. It is easier to express our feelings to the receptionist, nurse, or doctor than it is to find an administrator. Unfortunately, the people we most frequently see during our appointments have little or no power in larger decisions about the way the system functions. However, these people can tell you whom to contact. If you can form a close partnership with your providers, together you will be better able to make the system more responsive.

If you decide to write or e-mail, keep your letter short and factual. Tell what actions you would find helpful. For example:

Dear Mr. Brown:

Yesterday I had a 10:00 A.M. appointment with Dr. Zim. She did not see me until 12:15 P.M., and my total time with the doctor was eight minutes. As I left, I was told to make another appointment so I could get my questions answered.

I know that sometimes there are emergencies. However, I would appreciate being called if my doctor is running late or told when to return. I would also like 15 or more minutes with my doctor.

I would appreciate a reply from you within two weeks.

Sincerely, Jane Healthcare Consumer

The following are some typical complaints about the health care system, as well as a few hints for addressing them. These problems and suggestions will not apply to all systems or countries, but they do apply to many.

- **"I hate the phone system."** Often when you call for an appointment or information, you reach an automated system. This can be frustrating but you cannot change this. However, keep in mind that phone systems do not change often. Once you memorize the numbers or keys to press, you can move more quickly through the system. Sometimes pressing the pound key (#) or 0 will get you to a real person. Once you do get through, ask if there is a way to do this faster next time.

- **"It takes too long to get an appointment."** Ask for the first available appointment. Take it. Then ask how you can learn about cancellations. Some systems are happy to call you when they have an empty spot. In others, you may have to call them once or twice a week to check on cancellations. Ask the person making the schedule what you can do to get an earlier appointment. Ask for a telephone number so you can reach the person making appointments directly. Some systems are now setting time aside each day for same-day appointments. If this is available, ask when you should call to schedule one. It is usually early in the morning. If your pain or other symptoms have changed and you believe you must see a doctor right away, tell the scheduler. If nothing is available, ask what you need to do to see someone sooner rather than later. No matter how frustrated you are, be nice. You want the person who schedules appointments to be on your side and you will feel better if you speak pleasantly and do not lose your temper.

- **"I have so many providers; I do not know whom to ask for what."** When you see any member of your pain team, ask who is in charge of coordinating your care. It will most likely be your primary care doctor or nurse practitioner. Call the provider to confirm that he or she is coordinating your care. Ask how you can help make coordination as efficient as possible. Let this coordinating provider know when someone else orders a test or new medication. Keeping your primary care provider informed is especially important when providers are not in the same system and do not share electronic medical records (EMRs).

- **"What is an electronic medical record (EMR) anyway?"** In much of the United States and in parts of Canada, most medical information is maintained on a secure computer system, so your records can be viewed by all providers in the same system. You should know what information is on the system. Sometimes the EMR has just test results; other times it has test results and medication information. Sometimes it has all the information the organization has collected about you.

  An electronic medical record is just like a paper record: it does no good if your providers don't read it. For example, when you have a test, the doctor ordering the test will know when the results are ready. However, your other doctors may not know anything

about the test unless you tell them to read the results. Learn about the medical records system so you can help all your providers use it more effectively.

In the United States, Canada, and many other countries, you have the right to a copy of almost any information in your medical record. Ask for copies of all your consultations, lab, and other test results so you can carry them with you from one provider to the next. In this way, you know that the information will not get lost.

- **"I can never talk to my doctor."** It can be difficult to get a provider on the phone, but many systems now have ways for doctors, nurse practitioners, and patients to communicate by text or e-mail. The next time you see your provider, ask if your healthcare system provides these options. In the United States, many health systems have a way to quickly process routine things like medication refills. It may mean calling a special number or talking to the nurse. Learn how to do this.

  A medical emergency is important. Do not waste time trying to contact your doctor. Rather, go to a hospital emergency department or call 911.

- **"I have to wait too long in the waiting room or the examination room."** Emergencies happen sometimes, and this can cause a wait. If your schedule is tight and a delayed appointment will cause problems for you, call before you head to the appointment and ask if the doctor is running late and if so, how long you will have to wait. If your doctor is running late, you can decide whether to bring a book to read or ask to reschedule. If you show up for your appointment and find there's a wait, don't get upset. Instead, let the receptionist know that you are going to step out to run a quick errand nearby or for a cup of coffee. Tell them you will return within a specified amount of time.

■ **"I don't have enough time with the provider."** This may be a systemic problem. Someone other than your provider often decides how many patients to schedule and for how long. The decision is sometimes based on what you tell the booking clerk or scheduler. If you say you need a blood pressure check, you will be given a short visit. If you say you are very depressed and cannot function, you may be given a longer appointment. When making the appointment, ask for the amount of time you want, especially if it is more than 10 or 15 minutes. Be prepared to make a case for more time. You can also ask for the last appointment in the day. You may have to wait a while, but at least the provider will not be pressured because there are more patients to see.

Once you are with a provider and you request more time than is allotted, you make other people wait. An extra five minutes may not seem like much. However, a doctor often sees 30 patients a day. If each one takes five extra minutes, this means that the doctor has to work an extra 2½ hours that day! Those little bits of extra time add up.

If you think that things should not be this way and it is not fair to place this burden on the patient, we wholeheartedly agree. Health care systems should change to be more responsive and patient-friendly. A few systems in the United States are already doing this. In both the United States and Canada, patient groups are advocating for more accessible services that are especially appropriate for people with chronic pain. In the meantime, we offer these suggestions to help you deal with a difficult situation:

■ If something in the health care system is not working for you, ask how you can help make it work better. If you learn how to navigate the system, you can often solve or at least partially solve your problems.

■ Be reasonable. If the system or your provider sees you as a difficult person, getting what you want out of the system may become more difficult for you.

Other Resources to Explore

American Chronic Pain Association: www.theacpa.org/Communication-Tools.

Medline Plus: www.nlm.nih.gov/medlineplus/talkingwithyourdoctor.html

Suggested Further Reading

To learn more about the topics discussed in this chapter, we suggest that you explore the following resources:

Caudill, Margaret A. *Managing Pain Before It Manages You*. New York: Guilford Press, 2009 (especially Chapter 8).

Feldman, William. *Take Control of Your Health: The Essential Roadmap to Making the Right Health Care Decisions*. Toronto; Key Porter Books, 2007.

Hadjistavropoulos, T., and Heather D. Hadjistavropoulos (eds). *Pain Management for Older Adults. A Self-Help Guide*. Seattle, Wash.: IASP Press, 2008 (see Chapter 9).

Jones, J. Alfred, Gary L. Kreps, and Gerald M. Phillips. *Communicating with Your Doctor: Getting the Most Out of Health Care*. Cresskill, N.J.: Hampton Press, 1995.

CHAPTER 12

Sex and Intimacy

*E*NJOYING A LOVING RELATIONSHIP WITH PHYSICAL INTIMACY and sexual pleasure is a basic human need. However, many individuals and couples with chronic pain problems find it challenging to maintain this important part of their lives. Fear of causing more pain or injury, worry about being unable to perform or of rejection by a partner, or just plain disinterest can interfere with healthy sexuality. Sex, after all, is supposed to be joyful and pleasurable, not a cause of worry, discomfort, and pain.

If you have these worries or feelings, you are not alone. About one-half to two-thirds of people with chronic pain report significant reduction or loss of sexual functioning because of pain or its treatment. Of course, sex is more than the act of sexual intercourse or achieving orgasm; it is also the sharing of our physical and emotional selves. We enjoy a special intimacy when we make love. Believe it or not, having a chronic pain problem may actually offer the opportunity to improve your sex life by encouraging you to experiment with new types of physical and emotional stimulation. This process of exploring sensuality with your partner can open communication and strengthen your relationship.

Furthermore, when we are sexually active, natural "feel-good" hormones, including endorphins, are released into our bloodstream. These help us achieve a deep sense of relaxation and a feeling of well-being. They may even provide pain relief, at least temporarily, by closing the pain gate.

Sex and Chronic Pain

For many people with chronic pain, intercourse is difficult because of the physical demands. It increases heart rate and breathing and can tax someone with reduced energy due to fatigue, poor sleep, and stress. Intercourse can also be physically uncomfortable by placing strain on muscles, tissues, and joints that may already be hurting or sensitive to touch. For these reasons, it may be more satisfying to spend more time on sensuality or foreplay and less on actual intercourse. By concentrating on ways to give pleasure to your partner in a relaxed, comfortable atmosphere, your intimate time together can last longer and be very satisfying. Many people enjoy climax without intercourse; others may wish to climax with intercourse. For some, climax may not be as important as sharing pleasure and time together. There are many ways to enhance sensuality. Because our minds and bodies are linked, we can increase sexual pleasure through both physical and mental stimulation.

Emotional concerns can also be a serious factor for people with chronic pain conditions. Someone with angina may be concerned that sexual activity will bring on another attack. People with migraine headaches may worry that climax may trigger an episode. People with neck, back, or joint pain may be anxious that sex will spike their pain if they happen to move the wrong way. Their partners may fear that sexual activity might cause these problems and that they would be responsible. Some conditions such as diabetes or just normal aging can make erections difficult or cause vaginal dryness. These worries can certainly hurt the relationship.

Loss of self-esteem and a changed self-image can be subtle and devastating sexual barriers. If pain has left you physically changed, unemployed, or not able to contribute to your home life the way you used to, you may think of yourself as unattractive or undesirable to your partner. Thinking this way can damage your sense of self, which could cause you to avoid sexual or intimate situations; you "try not to think about it." Ignoring the sexual part of your relationship or physically and emotionally distancing yourself from your partner can lead to isolation and depression, which in turn leads to lack of interest in sex and more depression—a vicious cycle. (For more on depression and how to help yourself overcome it, see Chapter 4. If self-management techniques are not enough, talk to your doctor or therapist.)

Even good sex can get better. Thankfully, there are ways you and your partner can explore sensuality and intimacy, as well as some ways to overcome fear during sex.

Misconceptions About Sex

Many of our sexual attitudes and beliefs are learned—they are not automatic or instinctual. We begin learning them when we are young. They come from friends, older children, parents, and other adults. We also learn them through jokes, magazines, TV, and movies. Much of what we learn about sex is distorted with inhibitions and misconceptions, as well as a good dose of "shoulds," "musts," "should nots," and "must nots."

To maximize your sexual enjoyment, you often have to break down your misconceptions so that you are free to discover and explore your own sexuality. For example, many people believe a number of things that simply aren't true such as:

- Older people can't enjoy sex.
- Sex is for people with beautiful bodies.
- A "real man" is always ready for sex.
- A "real woman" should be sexually available whenever her partner is interested.
- Sex must lead to orgasm.
- Lovemaking has to involve sexual intercourse.
- Orgasm should occur simultaneously in both partners.
- Kissing and touching should only be done when they lead to sexual intercourse.

Overcoming Fear During Sex

With a condition like chronic pain, you probably worry that your pain will get worse and spin out of control. Fear and anxiety can really get in the way of the activities that you want and need to do. When sex is one of those activities, you face a difficult problem. Not only are you denying yourself an important, pleasurable part of life, but you probably also feel guilty about disappointing your partner. On the other hand, your partner may feel more fearful and guilty than you do. Your partner may be afraid he or she might hurt you during sex, or feel guilty for feeling resentful due to lack of sex. This dynamic can cause serious relationship problems. The resulting stress and depression can produce even more symptoms. You don't have to allow this to happen!

For successful sexual relationships, the most important thing is communication. The most effective way to address the fears of both partners is to talk about your concerns openly and find ways to alleviate them through good communication and problem solving. Effective communication will not only help you and your partner explore your fears and desires about sexuality, it will lead you to new ways of expressing intimacy. This is particularly important for people who worry about how their pain and other health problems may make them look physically to others. Often they find that their partner is far less concerned about their looks than they are.

When you and your partner are comfortable with talking about sex, you can go about finding solutions to your concerns. Start by sharing what kinds of physical stimulation you prefer and which positions you find most comfortable. Then you can share the fantasies you find most arousing. It's difficult to dwell on fears and worries when your mind is occupied with a fantasy.

Get started by reviewing the communication skills in Chapter 10 and the problem-solving techniques in Chapter 2. It takes really good communication and problem-solving skills to discuss sexuality openly and sort out your different needs. Remember, if these techniques are new, give them time and practice. As with any new skill, it takes patience to learn to do them well.

Sensual Sex

In our society sexual attraction has become almost solely dependent on the visual experience. This leads to an emphasis on our physical image. Sight, however, is only one of our five senses. Therefore, when we think about being sensual, we must also consider the seductive qualities of our partner's voice, scent, taste, and touch. Sensual sex is about connecting with our partner through all the senses, making love not only with the eyes but with our ears, nose, mouth, and hands as well.

Sensual touch is particularly important because the largest sensual organ of our bodies is the skin. The right touch on almost any area of our skin can be very erotic. Fortunately, sexual stimulation through touch can be done in just about any position and can be enhanced with the use of oils, flavored lotions, scents, feathers, fur gloves—whatever the imagination desires. Just about any part of the body is an erogenous zone. The most popular are the mouth, ear lobes, neck, breasts and nipples (for both genders), navel area, hands (fingertips if you are giving pleasure, palms if you are receiving pleasure), wrists, small of the back, buttocks, toes, and insides of the thighs and arms. Experiment with different types of touch—some people find a light touch arousing; others prefer a firm touch. Many people also become very aroused when they are touched with the nose, lips, and tongue. Even sex toys can play a part.

Some chronic pain conditions can cause hypersensitivity to even light touch. It is especially important that you determine what type of touch is pleasurable for you and what is not. Then talk to your partner about this. By working together you should be able to find ways to increase sensual pleasure and decrease your fear and anxiety about being touched in the wrong places or in the wrong ways.

If you decide that you wish to abstain from sexual activity because it is not an important part of your life, that's okay—but it is important that you discuss this decision with your partner. Good communication skills are essential in this situation, and you may even benefit from discussing it with a professional therapist present. Someone trained to deal with important interpersonal situations can help facilitate the discussion.

Sensuality with Fantasy

What goes on in our mind can be extremely arousing. If it weren't, there would be no romance novels, pornography, or strip clubs. Most people engage in sexual fantasy at some time or another. There are probably as many sexual fantasies as there are people. It is okay to mentally indulge in fantasy. If you discover a fantasy that you and your partner share, you can play it out in bed, even if it is as simple as a particular phrase you or your partner like to hear during sex.

Engaging the mind during sexual activity can be every bit as arousing as the physical stimulation. It is also useful when pain or symptoms during sex interfere with your enjoyment. But you want to be careful—sometimes fantasy leads to unrealistic expectations. Your real partner might not compare favorably to your dream lover. Your sexual satisfaction could suffer if you regularly fire up your imagination with explicit photos or videos of young, hard bodies.

Overcoming Symptoms During Sex

Sometimes people are unable to find a sexual position that is completely comfortable. Other times, pain, fatigue, stress, or even negative thoughts (self-talk) during sex are so distracting that they interfere with your enjoyment of sex or your ability to have an orgasm. This can pose some special problems. If you are unable to climax, you may feel resentful of your partner. If he or she is unable to climax, you may feel guilty about it. If you avoid sex because you are frustrated, your partner may become resentful and you may feel guilty. Your self-esteem may suffer. Your relationship with your partner may suffer. Everything suffers.

One thing you can do to help deal with this situation is to review your medications. It may be important to take a pain medication for example so it is at peak effectiveness when you are ready to have sex. Of course, this involves planning ahead. The type of medication may be important too. Such medications as narcotic-type pain relievers and some antidepressants can reduce interest in sex or inhibit sexual functioning. Your doctor may be able to reduce the dosages of these drugs or prescribe other medications that are effective for treating pain and other symptoms but have less effect on sexuality. Drugs such as muscle relaxants may also muddle your thinking, making it more difficult to focus. Alcohol and marijuana (cannabis), which are used by some people to reduce pain, can also impact sexual functioning. Some medications can make it difficult for a man to achieve an erection; others can help with an erection. Likewise, there are water-based lubricants that can help with vaginal dryness. Ask your doctor, nurse practitioner, or pharmacist about timing of your medications, and alternative medications, as well as medications to help with other concerns such as erection or dryness.

Another way to deal with uncomfortable symptoms is to become an expert at fantasy. To be really good at something, you have to train for it, and this is no exception. The idea here is to develop one or more sexual fantasies that you can indulge in when needed, making it vivid in your mind. Then, during sex, you can call up your fantasy and concentrate on it. By concentrating on the fantasy or picturing you and your partner making love while you actually are, you are keeping your mind consumed with erotic thoughts rather than your symptoms or negative thoughts.

If you have not had experience with visualization and imagery techniques, you will need to practice several times a week to learn them well. All of this practice does not need to be devoted to your chosen sexual fantasy, however. You can start with any guided imagery tape or script such as the ones in Chapter 5, working to make it more vivid each time you practice.

Start with just picturing the images. When you get good at that, add and dwell on colors. Then listen to the sounds around you. Then concentrate on the smells and tastes in the image, and feel your skin being touched by a breeze or mist. Finally, feel yourself touch things in the image. Work on one of the senses at a time. Become good at one scene before going on to another. Once you are proficient at imagery, you can invent your own sexual fantasy and picture it, hear it, smell it, and feel it. You can even begin your fantasy by picturing yourself setting your symptoms aside. The possibilities are limited only by your imagination.

Learning to call on this level of concentration can also help you focus on the moment. Really focusing on your physical and emotional sensations during sex can be powerfully erotic. If your mind wanders (which is normal), gently bring it back to the here and now.

> *Important:* Do not try to overcome chest pain or sudden weakness on one side of the body with imagery. These symptoms should not be ignored. If you experience them, consult a physician right away.

Sexual Positions

A comfortable sexual position can minimize pain and fear of injury during sex for both partners. Experimentation may be the best way to find the right positions for you and your partner. Everybody is different; no one position is good for everyone. Experiment with different positions that lessen strain, such as lying side by side or sitting on a chair. Experiment with placement of pillows under different parts of your body to make you more comfortable. You might want to try these new positions before you and your partner are too aroused. Experimentation itself can be erotic.

No matter which position you try, it is often helpful to do some warm-up exercises before sex. Look at some of the exercises in the Moving Easy Program in Chapter 8. Exercise can help your sex life in other ways as well as increasing your general fitness. Becoming more fit is an excellent way to increase your comfort and endurance during sex. Walking, swimming, bicycling, and other activities can benefit you in bed by reducing shortness of breath, fatigue, and pain. They also help you learn your limits and how to pace yourself during sexual activity, just as in any other physical activity.

During sexual activity, it may be advisable to change positions once in a while. This is especially true if your symptoms come on or increase when you stay in one position too long. This can be done in a playful fashion, whereby it becomes fun for both of you. As with any exercise, pacing activity and stopping to rest is okay.

Sex and Other Health Conditions

Of course other health conditions, not just chronic pain, can cause concerns about sex and intimacy. For example, people who are recovering from a heart attack or stroke are often afraid to resume sexual relations. They fear they will be unable to perform, or sex will bring on another attack or even death. This fear is even more common for their partners. Fortunately, there is no basis for this fear, and sexual relations can be resumed as soon as you feel ready to do so. Studies show that the risk of sexual activity contributing to a heart attack is less than 1 percent. This risk is even lower in individuals who do regular physical exercise. After a stroke, any remaining paralysis or weakness may require that you pay a little more attention to finding the best positions for support and comfort and the most sensitive areas of the body to caress. There may also be concerns about bowel and bladder control. The American Heart Association (www.heart.org) has some excellent guides about sex after a heart attack or stroke.

People with diabetes sometimes report problems with sexual function. Men may have difficulty achieving or maintaining an erection.

These difficulties can be caused by medication side effects or other medical conditions associated with diabetes. Women and men may also have reduced feeling in the genital area. The most common complaint from women with diabetes is not enough vaginal lubrication.

If you have diabetes, the most effective ways to prevent or lessen these problems are to maintain tight management of blood sugar, exercise, keep a positive outlook, and generally take care of yourself. Lubricants can help with sensitivity for both men and women. If you are using condoms, be sure to use a water-based lubricant; petroleum-based lubricants destroy latex. A vibrator can be very helpful for individuals with neuropathy, and concentrating on the most sensual parts of the body for stimulation can help make sex pleasurable. There are new therapies for men with erectile problems. The American Diabetes Association (www.diabetes.org) has more detailed information about sex and diabetes.

People who are missing a breast, testicle, or another part of their body as a result of their treatment for cancer or other medical condition may also have fears about sex and intimacy.

The same is true of people with surgical scars or swollen or disfigured joints from arthritis. In these cases, people may worry about what their partner will think. Will their partner or potential partner find them undesirable? Although this may happen sometimes, it actually occurs less often than you think. Usually when we fall in love with someone, we fall in love with who the person is, not that person's breast, testicle, or other body part. Here again, good communication and sharing your concerns and fears with your partner can help. If this is difficult, talking with a couples counselor may help you. Often what you imagine will be a problem really is not.

Fatigue is another symptom that can kill sexual desire. In Chapter 4 we discuss dealing with fatigue. Here we will add one more hint: plan your sexual activities around your fatigue. That is, try to engage in sex during the times you are less tired. This might mean that mornings are better than evenings.

Many mental health conditions and the medications used to treat their symptoms can also interfere with sexual function and desire. It is important to talk with your doctor or nurse practitioner about these side effects so that together you can find alternatives. Sometimes the provider may find another medication, change the dosage and timing of the medication, or refer you to a therapist who may help you and your partner learn alternative coping strategies to decrease or eliminate symptoms. Individual or couples therapy can also help in dealing with personal relationship, intimacy, and sexual problems unrelated to your medications.

Your doctor or nurse practitioner should be your first consultant on sexual problems related to your condition. It's unlikely that your problem is unique. Your doctor has probably heard about it many times before and may have some solutions. Remember, this is just another problem associated with your chronic condition, just like pain, fatigue, and physical limitations, and it is a problem that can be addressed. Chronic health problems need not end sex. Through good communication and planning, satisfying sex can prevail. By being creative and willing to experiment, both the sex and the relationship can actually be better.

Other Resources to Explore

American Diabetes Association: www.diabetes.org

American Heart Association: www.heart.org

Arthritis Foundation: www.arthritis.org

Cleveland Clinic: www.my.clevelandclinic.org

Mayo Clinic: www.mayoclinic.org/

Pain Concern: www.painconcern.org.uk

WebMD: www.webmd.com

Suggested Further Reading

To learn more about the topics discussed in this chapter, we suggest that you explore the following resources:

Agravat, Pravin. *A Guide to Sexual and Erectile Dysfunction in Men*. Leicester, England: Troubador, 2010.

American Heart Association. *Sex and Heart Disease*. Dallas, Tex.: American Heart Association, 2008.

American Heart Association and American Stroke Association. *Sex After Stroke: Our Guide to Intimacy After Stroke*. Dallas, Tex.: American Heart Association and American Stroke Association, 2011.

Ford, Vicki. *Overcoming Sexual Problems*. London: Constable & Robinson, 2010.

Garrison, Eric Marlowe. *Mastering Multiple-Position Sex: Mind-Blowing Lovemaking Techniques That Create Unforgettable Orgasms*. Beverly, Mass.: Quiver Books, 2009.

Hall, Kathryn. *Reclaiming Your Sexual Self: How You Can Bring Desire Back into Your Life*. Hoboken, N.J.: Wiley, 2004.

Kaufman, Miriam, Cory Silverberg, and Fran Odette. *The Ultimate Guide to Sex and Disability: For All of Us Who Live with Disabilities, Chronic Pain, and Illness*. Berkeley, Calif.: Cleis Press, 2007.

Klein, Marty. *Beyond Orgasm: Dare to Be Honest About the Sex You Really Want*. Berkeley, Calif.: Celestial Arts, 2002.

McCarthy, Barry W., and Michael E. Metz. *Men's Sexual Health: Fitness for Satisfying Sex*. New York: Routledge, 2008.

Schnarch, David. *Intimacy and Desire: Awaken the Passion in Your Relationship*. New York: Beaufort Books, 2009.

Schnarch, David. *Resurrecting Sex: Solving Sexual Problems and Revolutionizing Your Relationship*. New York: HarperCollins, 2002.

Let food be thy medicine.
—Hippocrates, father of medicine, 431 B.C.E.

CHAPTER 13

Healthy Eating

HEALTHY EATING IS ONE OF *THE* WISEST personal investments you can make. The food you consume is a central player that influences your health.

Eating healthy simply means that most of the time you make good and healthful food choices. It does not mean being rigid or perfect. No matter what the media or your friends say, there is no one best way of eating that fits everyone; there is no perfect food. Eating healthy can mean finding new or different ways to prepare your meals to make them tasty and appealing. If you have certain health conditions, it may mean that you have to be choosier. Eating well does not usually mean you can never have the foods you like most.

Thanks to the Internet, books, other media, friends, and relatives, we can get overloaded with information about what we should and should not eat. The whole eating thing gets very confusing. In this chapter we give you basic science-based nutrition

Special thanks to Bonnie Bruce, DrPH, RD, and Yvonne Mullan, MSc, RD, for their help with this chapter.

and dietary information. We do not tell you what to eat or how to eat. That is your decision. We do tell you what is known about nutrition for adults, some new information about nutrition and chronic pain, and some ways to help you fit that information to your specific likes and needs. We hope this chapter will put you on the path to healthier eating.

Please note that most of the nutrition information presented in this chapter is from the United States Department of Agriculture (USDA) Dietary Guidelines for Americans published in 2010 and the USDA MyPlate program launched in 2011. Health Canada also has dietary recommendations called *Eating Well with Canada's Food Guide*, first published in 2007. Most of the Canadian recommendations are similar to the American ones, but there are some differences. Food amounts in this chapter are listed in both imperial and metric measure. See the Health Canada website listed under Other Resources at the end of the chapter for more Canadian-specific information.

Why Is Healthy Eating So Important?

The human body is a complex and marvelous machine, much like an automobile. Autos need the proper mix of fuel to run right. Without it, they may run rough and may even stop working. The human body is similar. It needs the proper mix of good food (fuel) to keep it running well. It does not run right on the wrong fuel or on empty.

Healthy eating cuts across every part of your life. It is linked to your body and your mind's well-being, including how your body responds to some illnesses and conditions.

When you give your body the right fuel and nourishment, here's what happens:

- You have more energy and feel less tired.

- You increase your chances of preventing or lessening health conditions such as heart disease, diabetes, cancer, and some chronic pain conditions.

- You feed your central nervous system and brain, which can help you handle life's challenges as well as its emotional ups and downs.

What Is Healthy Eating?

At the heart of healthy eating are the choices we make over the long run. Healthy eating is being flexible and allowing yourself to occasionally enjoy small amounts of foods that may not be so healthy. There is no such thing as a perfect eating style. Being too strict or rigid and not allowing yourself to ever have treats will likely cause your best efforts to fail.

If you have chronic pain or other conditions, healthy eating means having to be somewhat choosy about the foods you eat. For example, some people with migraines need to avoid certain foods that might trigger a headache. People with diabetes need to watch their carbohydrate intake to manage their blood sugar levels. They do best by deciding which carbohydrate foods (fruit, breads, cereals, rice, etc.) they will eat each day. People who have or are at risk for heart disease control their blood cholesterol levels by watching the amount and kinds of fat they eat. Consuming the right amount and types of fat can also reduce inflammation for some kinds of chronic pain conditions. Those with high blood pressure can help lower it by eating lots of fruits, vegetables, and low-fat dairy foods. For some, cutting back on salt also lowers high blood pressure. And, to maintain, lose, or gain weight, everyone needs to pay attention to how many calories we eat.

We have come a long way since meat and potatoes were considered the backbone of a great diet. Today, vegetables, fruits, whole grains, low-fat milk and milk products, lean meats, poultry, and fish are at the core of a healthy diet. There is still a place for meat and potatoes; it is just not the most important place.

The real issue for most of us is not the healthy foods we consume but the less healthy ones. One-third of most North American diets is made up of foods that are high in added sugars, solid fats (butter, beef fat, pork fat, chicken fat, stick margarine, shortening), and salt. We also eat a lot of food that is made from white flour and other refined grains. These added sugars, fats, and salt contribute to high blood pressure, diabetes, and obesity. There is some evidence that unhealthy diets may be associated with chronic pain as well.

Trade-offs are a big part of healthy eating. This means learning how food affects you and then deciding when you can treat yourself and when you should pass. For instance, it may be important for you to have a special meal on your birthday. If so, then you can make healthier choices when you are out for casual lunches on days that are not special occasions. Trading off like this can help you stay on the path of healthy eating. It gets easier with practice, and it even becomes part of your everyday life.

A good starting place is to move toward eating more plant foods: fruits, vegetables, whole grains, legumes, nuts, and seeds. This does not mean giving up meats and foods that may be high in sugar, fat, or salt but rather eating them in smaller amounts or less often. The goal is to maintain a healthy balance in the kinds of foods you eat and how much you eat. (We'll have more to say about this a little later in this chapter.)

This all sounds simple, but every day we are faced with hundreds of food choices. It is often easier and quicker to grab something less healthy than to think about what we will eat. So how do we put together meals that are tasty and enjoyable yet healthful? In this chapter, we try to make it as simple as possible.

Key Principles of Healthy Eating

■ **Choose foods as nature originally made them.** This means the less processed the better. By *processed* we mean foods that have been changed from their original state by having ingredients added (often sugar, salt, or fat) or removed (often fiber or nutrients) to make them tastier. Examples include whole grains made into white flour for bakery products or animal foods made into deli meats. Choosing the least-processed option isn't difficult.

Go for a grilled chicken breast instead of fried breaded chicken nuggets, a baked potato (with skin) rather than French fries, and whole-grain bread and brown rice instead of white bread and white rice.

- **Get your nutrients from food, not supplements.** For most people, vitamin, mineral, and other dietary supplements cannot completely take the place of food. Unprocessed foods contain nutrients and other healthy compounds (such as fiber) in the right combinations and amounts. When manufacturers remove nutrients from their natural state in food, the foods may not fuel your body the way they should.

For instance, take beta-carotene, an important source of vitamin A, found in plant foods such as carrots and winter squash. It helps our vision and enhances our immune system. However, artificial beta-carotene supplements have been shown in some people to increase some cancer risks. This same risk is not present when beta-carotene is eaten as it is naturally found in food. Another reason to get your nutrition from foods as close as possible to how nature made them is that these choices could contain as yet unknown healthy compounds. When you take a supplement such as a vitamin pill, you could be missing out on many other helpful substances that are naturally packaged with the food from which the vitamin was removed.

In many countries, including the United States, there are no government-imposed quality controls for diet and nutrition supplements. Unlike over-the-counter medications, with supplements there is no guar-antee you are getting what you pay for or that you are not getting harmful substances. In Canada, many vitamin and mineral supplements and "natural" health products are licensed by Health Canada. Health Canada assesses these products to be sure they are safe, effective, and of high quality. You can check if a product is licensed in Canada by going to the Licensed Natural Health Products Database of Health Canada. The web address is listed under Other Resources at the end of this chapter.

Can dietary supplements ever play a role in healthy eating? Yes—sometimes we cannot get enough of one or more of the nutrients we need. Vitamin D is an example. People who live in more northern climates can have low levels of vitamin D. In Canada, Health Canada advises everyone over the age of 50 to take a daily supplement of at least 400 IU of vitamin D. Another example is calcium. Older men and women need a large amount of calcium to help prevent or slow osteoporosis. Although you should aim to get enough calcium from milk and milk products such as yogurt or cheese, it may be difficult to get the necessary amount. If you are thinking of taking supplements, it is important to talk to your health care professional or a registered dietitian first.

- **Eat a wide variety of colorful minimally processed foods.** Your goal is to get more variety, more colors, and fewer processed foods on your plate. These three simple rules will give your body all the good things it needs. Choose minimally processed meat, fish, or poultry and a lot of colorful fruits and vegetables. Think blue and purple for grapes and blueberries; yellow and orange for pineapple, oranges, and carrots; red for tomatoes, strawberries, and watermelon; and green for spinach, kale, and green beans. Don't forget the white and warm brown tones from mushrooms, onions, and cauliflower and whole grains such as brown rice.

■ **Eat foods high in phytochemicals.** Phytochemicals are compounds that are found only in plant foods—fruits, vegetables, whole grains, nuts, and seeds (*phyto* means "plant"). There are hundreds of health-promoting and disease-fighting phytochemicals. These include compounds that give fruits and vegetables their bright colors. Whenever a food is refined or processed, as when whole wheat is made into white flour, phytochemicals are lost. The more often you choose foods that are not refined, and as close as possible to how nature made them, the better.

■ **Eat regularly.** A gas-fueled vehicle will not run without the gas, and a fire eventually burns out without more wood. Your body is much the same. It needs refueling regularly to work at its best. Eating something, even a little bit, at regular intervals helps keep your "fire" burning.

Eat at regular times during the day, preferably at evenly spaced intervals during the day. This helps maintain and balance your blood sugar level. Blood sugar is a key player in supplying the body, especially the brain, with energy. If you do not eat regularly, your blood sugar drops. If it becomes too low, it can cause weakness, sweating, shaking, mood changes (irritability, anxiety, or anger, for example), nausea, headaches, or poor coordination. This can be dangerous for many people.

Eating regularly helps you get the nutrients you need and helps your body process those nutrients. Not skipping meals or not letting too many hours go between meals also helps keep you from getting overly hungry. Being overly hungry often leads to overeating. This can in turn lead to such problems as indigestion, heartburn, and weight gain. You may find that sometimes several small meals throughout the day works well while at other times fewer, bigger meals work best. So eating regularly does not mean you must stick to the same routine every day. Nor does it mean you must follow the "normal" pattern of eating three meals a day. Allow yourself room for give and take.

■ **Eat what your body needs** (not more or less). This is easy to say but more difficult to put into action. How much you should eat depends on things like the following:

♦ Your age (we need fewer calories as we get older)

♦ If you are a man or woman (men usually need more calories than women)

♦ Your body size and shape (in general, if you are taller or have more muscle, you can eat more calories)

♦ Your health needs (some conditions affect how your body uses calories)

♦ Your activity level (the more you move or exercise, the more calories you can eat)

A Note About Breakfast

Breakfast is just that: "breaking the fast." It refuels your body after going without eating for many hours and helps you resist the urge to eat extra snacks or overeat the rest of the day.

You may not want to eat breakfast, because you don't have the time or aren't hungry or maybe because you do not like the usual breakfast foods. But there are no set rules about what you should eat in the morning. Breakfast can be anything—fruit, beans, rice, bread, broccoli, even leftovers. The important thing is to kick-start your body each day by refueling it with a healthy breakfast.

Tips to Help You Manage How Much You Eat

- **Stop eating when you first feel full.** This helps you control the amount you eat so you don't overeat. Pay attention to your body so you can learn what fullness feels like. Like all new skills, it takes some practice. If it is hard to stop eating when you begin to feel full, remove your plate or get up from the table if you can.

- **Eat slowly.** Eating slowly gives you more enjoyment and helps prevent overeating. Make your meals last at least 15 to 20 minutes. It takes that long for the brain to catch up and tell your stomach that it is getting full. Put down your utensils between bites. If you finish quickly, wait at least 15 minutes before getting more food. If this is difficult for you, see the additional tips on pages 222–225.

- **Be mindful of what you eat.** If you are not paying attention to what you are doing, it is easy to eat an entire bag of chips or cookies or eat too much of any bite-sized pieces of food without even knowing it. This can happen easily when we are with friends,

using the computer, or watching television. In these situations, try portioning out what you want to eat before you begin eating, or keep food out of reach or out of sight. Don't eat right out of the package—place food in an appropriate serving-sized container. Take time to enjoy what you are eating.

- **Know a serving size when you see one.** To do this, you need to know what a serving size or portion looks like. A 1/2-cup (125 mL) portion is about the size of a tennis ball or a closed fist. A 3-ounce (84 g) portion of cooked meat, fish, or poultry is about the size of a deck of playing cards or the palm of your hand. The end of your thumb to the first joint is about one teaspoon (5 mL); three times that is a tablespoon (15 mL). (*Tip:* Use a measuring spoon or cup to see what a serving size looks like.)

- **Watch out for supersizing and portion inflation.** In recent years, serving sizes at restaurants and in packaged foods have literally "beefed up." The typical adult cheeseburger used to have about 330 calories; now it has a whopping 590 calories. Twenty years ago, an average cookie was about 1½ inches (3.8 cm) wide and had 55 calories; now it is 3½ inches (8.9 cm) wide and has 275 calories—*five times* the calories! Soda typically came in 6½-ounce (195 mL) bottles with 85 calories; today a typical bottle of soda is 20 ounces (600 mL) and 250 calories.

If we consume 3,500 calories more than we need, we gain a pound of body fat. Over a single year, consuming just an extra 100 calories a day will cause you to put on 10 pounds (4 kg). That is equal to eating only an extra third of a bagel each day! There are many published ranges of recommended serving sizes for different foods. In the food guide on pages 226–233, we list some common serving sizes for a variety of foods.

- **When practical, select single-size portions.** Foods that are prepackaged as single servings can help you see what a suggested serving should look like.

- **Make your food attractive.** We really do eat with our eyes! Compare the appeal of a plate of white rice, white cauliflower, and white fish with one of baked sweet potato, bright green spinach, and grilled white fish with salsa. Which of these two meals seems more appetizing?

An Easy Map for Healthy Eating

The U.S. Department of Agriculture's MyPlate Map for Healthy Eating in Figure 13.1 shows what a healthy meal should look like. Put your meal together so that one-fourth of the plate is covered with colorful fruit, one-fourth with vegetables, one-fourth with a protein source (lean meat, fish, or poultry, or better yet, plant foods such as tofu, cooked dry beans, or lentils), and the remaining one-fourth with grains (preferably at least half from whole grains) or other starches such as potatoes, rice, yams, or winter squash. Finish off your plate with calcium-rich foods. These could be milk or foods made from milk (preferably fat-free or low-fat), such as cheese, yogurt, frozen yogurt, puddings, or calcium-fortified soy foods such as soy milk. Of course, your food choices and amounts will depend on what you like and need. If you would like more information about this way of eating, check out the USDA's MyPlate website at www.choosemyplate.gov.

Even with this map as a guide, calories and portion sizes are important. Plate sizes are now

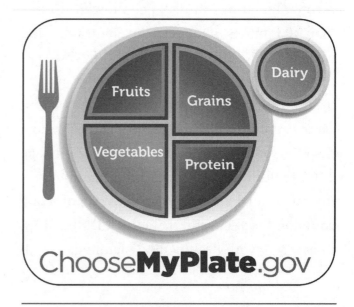

Figure 13.1 **MyPlate: A Map for Healthy Eating**

larger, making it easier to get more calories than you need. Table 13.1 on page 214 can help you as you plan. It gives you examples of recommended daily portions from different food groups. Note that these amounts are general recommendations and may be different if you have special dietary needs. If you have questions, check with your doctor or a registered dietitian.

Note, too, that when you go to the Internet for information and recommendations, you will find many people who say they are nutrition experts. They may not be. If you want a real expert, look for a registered dietitian (RD). These health professionals are specially trained and are the best sources for diet and nutrition advice and information.

Nutrients: What the Body Needs

Earlier we talked about the benefit of getting nutrients from food not from supplements. In the following sections, we talk about carbohydrates, fats, protein, a few vitamins and minerals, and plain old water. Although it is technically not a nutrient, we also talk about fiber.

First, take a look at Table 13.1 on page 214, Daily Recommended Servings, with Examples for Healthy Meal Planning. It lists the number of recommended servings for adult women and men along with examples of serving sizes. These recommendations are for people who do less than 30 minutes of moderate exercise a day and eat 1,000 to 3,000 calories. If you have a special health problem or condition, such as diabetes, you may need to change how much you eat of certain foods. Even so, you can still follow the Map for Healthy Eating. Table 13.2 on page 226 provides more detailed information about the nutritional values per serving size of many common foods. Use both Tables 13.1 and 13.2 to help you with healthy meal planning.

Carbohydrates: Your Body's Chief Energy Source

With few exceptions, carbohydrates are your body's go-to fuel for the brain, central nervous system, and red blood cells. Carbohydrates largely determine your blood sugar level—more so than protein or fat. And carbohydrates do a great deal more. They provide the basic materials for the vital components in your body. The construction of nearly every part of your body, from your toenails to the top of your head, involves carbohydrates. These include hormones, fats, cholesterol, and even some vitamins and proteins.

Carbohydrates are found mostly in plant foods such as grains, starchy vegetables, and fruits. Milk and yogurt are about the only animal foods that have more than a very small amount of carbohydrate. Sugary carbohydrates are found in fruit and juice, milk, yogurt, table sugar, honey, jellies, syrups, and sugar-sweetened drinks. Starchy carbohydrates are found in vegetables such as corn, green peas, potatoes, winter squash, dried beans and peas, lentils, and grains such as rice. Pasta, tortillas,

Tips for Choosing Healthier Carbohydrates and Increasing Fiber

- Fill at least half of your plate with a variety of vegetables and whole fruits.

- At least half of the grains you eat should be whole grains (brown rice, whole-grain breads and rolls, whole-grain pasta, and tortillas).

- Choose foods with whole wheat or a whole grain (such as oats) listed first on the food label ingredients list.

- Choose dried beans and peas, lentils, or whole-grain pasta instead of meat or as a side dish at least a few times a week.

- Choose whole fruit rather than fruit juice. Whole fruit contains fiber, takes longer to eat, fills you up better than juice, and can help keep you from overeating.

- Choose higher-fiber breakfast cereals such as shredded wheat, Grape-Nuts, All-Bran, or raisin bran.

- Eat higher-fiber crackers, such as whole-rye or multigrain crackers and whole-grain flatbread.

- Snack mostly on whole-grain crackers or breads, whole fruit, or nonfat yogurt rather than sweets, pastries, or ice cream.

- When you add fiber to your diet, do it gradually over a period of a few weeks. Drink plenty of water to process the fiber.

and bread are high in starchy carbohydrates. The amount of carbohydrate in whole grains, brown rice, and whole-wheat bread is similar to that in refined grains, such as white bread and white rice. The big difference between whole grain foods and refined foods is that the refined grains have lost nutrients, phytochemicals, and fiber, and other important compounds during processing.

Fiber is found naturally in whole and minimally processed plant foods with "skins, seeds, and strings." For example, whole grains, dried beans, peas, lentils, fruits, vegetables, nuts, and seeds all have some fiber. Some foods have added fiber (as when pulp is added to juice). Animal foods and refined and processed foods (white flour, bread, many baked and snack foods) have little or no fiber unless it was added by the manufacturer.

Fiber helps you in important ways. The fiber in wheat bran, some fruits and vegetables, and whole grains keeps your digestive system moving and helps prevent constipation. The fiber in oat bran, barley, nuts, seeds, beans, apples, citrus fruits, and carrots can help manage your blood sugar because it slows the amount of time it takes for sugar to get into the bloodstream. It can also help lower blood cholesterol. High-fiber diets are also thought to help reduce the risk of rectal and colon cancers.

Oils and Solid Fats: The Good, the Bad, and the Deadly

Not all fat is bad for you. You need some fat for survival and for your body to work properly. Your body needs about one tablespoon (15 mL) of fat a day to work properly.

Although all fats have the same number of calories per portion, some fats are more healthful than others, and some can be harmful when we eat too much.

Good fats (also called unsaturated fats) are oils that are usually liquid at room temperature. They help keep your cells healthy, and some can help reduce blood cholesterol. Good fats include soybean, safflower, corn, peanut, sunflower, canola, and olive oils. Nuts, seeds, and olives (and their oils), as well as avocados, are also rich in good fats.

Omega-3s are another group of good fats that can reduce the risk of heart disease and may help with some types of chronic pain symptoms. (They may, for example, reduce inflammation.) These fats are found in fatty fish such as salmon, mackerel, sardines, arctic char, trout, and tuna. Other sources of omega-3s include wheat germ, flaxseed, and walnuts, although the body may not use omega-3s from plants as well as it does the omega-3s from fish.

The bad fats (also called saturated fats) are usually solid at room temperature (think shortening, butter, lard, and bacon grease). They can increase blood cholesterol and the risk of heart disease. Most bad fats are found in animal products such as butter, beef fat, chicken fat, and pork fat (lard).

Tips for Choosing Healthier Fats

The following tips will help you eat less bad fat and more good fat. If you decide to choose more good fats, be sure you are eating less bad fat. You do not want to increase the total amount of fat you eat.

When Choosing Foods

- Eat cooked portions of meat, fish, and poultry that are 2 to 3 ounces (56 to 84 g). This is about the size of a deck of cards or the palm of your hand.
- Eat more fish rich in omega-3s (salmon, tuna, mackerel, sardines).
- Choose leaner cuts of meat (round, sirloin, flank).
- Choose low-fat or fat-free milk and dairy foods (cheese, sour cream, cottage cheese, yogurt, ice cream).

When Preparing and Eating Foods

- Use a nonstick pan or a small amount of cooking oil spray.
- When cooking and baking, use oil (such as olive or canola oil) and soft (tub) margarines instead of shortening, lard, butter, or stick margarine.
- Broil, barbecue, or grill meats.
- Avoid frying or deep-frying foods.
- Trim off all the fat you can see from meat before cooking it.
- Skim the fat from stews and soups during cooking. (If you refrigerate them overnight, the solid fat lifts off easily.)
- Do not eat the skin on poultry.
- Use less butter, margarine, gravies, meat-based and cream sauces, spreads.

Other foods high in bad fats include stick margarines, red meat, regular ground meat, processed meats (sausage, bacon, deli meats), poultry skin, whole- and low-fat milk, sour cream, and cheese (including cream cheese). Palm kernel oil, coconut oil, and cocoa butter are also considered bad fats because they are high in saturated fat. However, research is being done on some possible health benefits of coconut oil.

The fats classed as "deadly" are the trans fats. They can increase blood cholesterol and risk of heart disease even more than the bad fats. Trans fats are in many processed foods, including pastries, cakes, cookies, crackers, icing, margarine, and most microwave popcorn. The best strategy is to eat as little trans fats as possible. They are listed on food labels as "partially hydrogenated" or "hydrogenated" oils. Be warned! Food companies can legally claim "no" or "0" trans fats on the label even when the food has up to half a gram (0.5 g) per serving. There are no specific daily recommendations for how much fat you should eat. Most people get more than enough in their diet. The best recommendation is to eat very little bad and deadly fats. Replace bad and deadly fats with good fats, but do not increase the total amount of fat you eat.

There is one more thing you should know about fat. All fats contain twice the calories per teaspoon as protein or carbohydrates. Calories from fat add up quickly. For instance, one teaspoon (5 mL) of sugar has about 20 calories, but the same amount of oil or solid fat has about 35 calories. When we eat more calories than we need—no matter where they come from—the extra calories get stored as body fat, which leads to weight gain.

Protein: Muscle Builder and More

Protein is vital for hundreds of biological processes that keep you alive and healthy. Protein is part of your muscles, red blood cells, and the enzymes and hormones that help regulate the body. Protein helps your immune system fight infection and builds and repairs damaged tissues. It can also give you some energy. But like fat, protein is not as good a source of energy for the body as carbohydrates.

There are two types of proteins: complete and incomplete. Complete proteins have all the right parts in the right amounts. Your body uses them just as they are. Complete proteins are found in animal foods—meat, fish, poultry, eggs, milk, and other dairy products—as well as in soy foods such as soybeans, tofu, and tempeh. Incomplete proteins are low in one or more parts. They are found in plant foods such as grains, dried beans and peas, lentils, nuts, and seeds. Most fruits and vegetables contain little, if any, protein. For your body to be able to use incomplete proteins best, eat them with at least one other incomplete protein or along with a complete protein. Two of the most commonly eaten incomplete protein pairs are beans and rice and peanut butter and bread.

Nearly all plant proteins are incomplete proteins, yet they are at the heart of eating healthy. By eating a small amount of an animal protein such as chicken with a plant food such as lentils or black beans, you get all the benefits of a complete protein. In addition, some plant foods, such as nuts and seeds, are sources of the good fats, and many plant foods are good sources of fiber. Plant foods have no cholesterol and little to no trans fats.

Table 13.1 **Daily Recommended Amounts, with Examples for Healthy Meal Planning**

These recommendations are for average adults (19 years and older) who exercise less than 30 minutes daily and eat 1,000 to 3,000 calories. They are based on the United States Dietary Guidelines. (For Canada's guidelines, please see www.healthcanada.gc.ca/foodguide.)

If you have a special condition, you may need to modify portion sizes of certain foods but should still aim for an overall balance.

Household Measure Equivalencies

Imperial (United States)	Metric (Canada)
1 teaspoon (tsp)	5 milliliters (mL)
1 tablespoon (Tbsp)	15 mL
1/4 cup	60 mL
1/3 cup	75 mL
1/2 cup	125 mL
2/3 cup	150 mL
3/4 cup	175 mL
1 cup	250 mL
1 ounce (oz)	28 grams (g)
1 fluid ounce (oz)	30 mL
1 inch	2.54 centimeters (cm)

Recommended Daily Amount			
Protein-Rich Foods	**Women**	**Men**	**Examples**
Animal (meat, fish, poultry) and plant sources (beans, nuts, seeds)	5–5 1/2 ounces (140–154 g)	5 1/2–6 1/2 ounces (154–182 g)	**What counts as a 1-ounce (28 g) serving:** _Contains Little to No Carbohydrate_ 1 ounce (28 g) cooked lean meat, poultry, or fish 1 egg 1 tablespoon (15 mL) nut butter (peanut, almond, soy, etc.) About 2 tablespoons (1 ounce, 30 mL, or 30 g) nuts (12 almonds, 7 walnut halves) _Contains Carbohydrates_ 1/2 cup (125 mL) cooked dry beans, peas, or lentils 1/2 cup (125 mL) baked or refried beans 1 ounce (28 g) cooked tempeh 2 tablespoons (30 mL) hummus 1/2 cup (125 mL) roasted soybeans 4-ounce (112 g) falafel patty

Recommended Daily Amount			
Protein-Rich Foods	**Women**	**Men**	**Examples**
Milk, cheese (except cream cheese), yogurt, milk-based desserts (Choose fat-free or low-fat most of the time)	3 cups (750 mL)	3 cups (750 mL)	**What counts as a 1-cup (250 mL) serving:** *Contains Little to No Carbohydrate* 1½ ounces (42 g) cheese 1/3 cup (75 mL) shredded cheese 2 cups (500 mL) cottage cheese *Contains Carbohydrates* 1 cup (250 mL) milk, yogurt, or kefir 1 cup (250 mL) pudding or frozen yogurt 1½ ounces (42 g) ice cream 2 ounces (56 g) processed cheese or cottage cheese
Grains (At least half should be whole grains)	5–6 ounces (140–168 g)	6–8 ounces (168–224 g)	**What counts as a 1-ounce (28 g) serving:** 1-ounce (28 g) slice of bread 1/2 English muffin 1 cup (250 mL) ready-to-eat flaked cereal 1/2 cup (125 mL) cooked rice, cooked pasta, or cooked cereal 6-inch flour or corn tortilla
Vegetables	2–2½ cups (500–625 mL)	2½–3 cups (625–750 mL)	**What counts as a 1-cup (250 mL) serving:** *Low in Starch* 1 cup (250 mL) cooked vegetables (greens, broccoli family, green beans) or vegetable juice 2 cups (500 mL) raw leafy greens 12 medium baby carrots *High in Starch* 1 cup (250 mL) cooked sweet potato, white potato, or winter squash 1 cup (250 mL) cooked dry beans, peas, or lentils 1 cup (8 ounces) (250 mL or 224 g) tofu 1 cup (250 mL) corn or green peas
Fruit	1½–2 cups (375–500 mL)	2 cups (500 mL)	**What counts as a 1-cup (250 mL) serving:** 1 cup (250 mL) fruit 1 cup (250 mL) 100% juice 1/2 cup (125 mL) dried fruit 1 banana (8–9 inches) (20–23 cms) 8 large strawberries
Oils and Solid Fats	5–6 teaspoons (25–30 mL)	6–7 teaspoons (30–35 mL)	**What counts as a 1-teaspoon (5 mL) serving:** About 1 teaspoon (5 mL) salad or cooking oil, margarine, mayonnaise, or salad dressing 1 teaspoon (5 mL) butter or margarine

The good news is that most people already eat more than enough protein. Unless you have a special medical condition, there is no need to be concerned about not getting enough from your normal diet. Unfortunately, many people get most of their protein from meat, which tends to be high in the bad fats. The best way to get protein is mainly from plant foods, along with small amounts of lean meat, poultry, or fish.

Vitamins and Minerals

Vitamins help regulate the body's inner workings. Minerals are part of many cells and cause important reactions to happen in the body. All vitamins and minerals are essential for survival and good health. Most of us can get the vitamins and minerals we need from healthy eating. But the minerals sodium, potassium, and calcium stand out because many of us eat either too much or too little of these nutrients.

Sodium

For some people, too much sodium (salt) can raise blood pressure. This can lead to heart disease, stroke, and kidney failure. Cutting back on sodium may help lower blood pressure and help prevent high blood pressure.

It is easy to get enough sodium to meet your bodies' needs. In fact, most of us get way too much. We need only about 500 mg a day (in terms of table salt, this is less than a fifth of a teaspoon, or 1 mL). Yet the majority of people eat 8 to 12 times that much. Adults should limit sodium intake to 2,300 mg a day, which is about the amount in 1 teaspoon (5 mL) of table salt. People who have high blood pressure, kidney disease, or diabetes, are African American, or who are middle-aged or older should not consume more than 1,500 mg of sodium a day.

There is sodium in most foods we eat—from trace amounts in some plant foods to higher amounts in some animal foods. But the real culprits are processed foods, which typically contain a lot of added sodium.

Eating less sodium takes some getting used to, but over time you will learn to enjoy the natural flavors of food. The following are some tips to help you keep your sodium intake in check:

- Always taste your food before salting it. Many times, it is good as is.

- Don't add salt to food when cooking. Season with spices, herbs, pepper, garlic, onion, or lemon.

- Use fresh or frozen, minimally processed poultry, fish, and lean meat instead of canned, breaded, or prepared packaged food.

- Choose foods labeled "low sodium" or those with 140 mg or less per serving. (Check out the Nutrition Facts label for this information.)

- Save high-sodium food for special occasions. Serve bacon, deli meats, frozen dinners, packaged mixes, salted nuts, salad dressings, and high-sodium canned soups as part of celebrations, not as everyday fare.

- In restaurants, ask that your food not be salted during preparation.

Potassium

Potassium is a mineral that helps your heart beat regularly, helps maintain normal blood pressure, and allows your muscles and nerves to work together. It may also reduce your risk of kidney stones and bone loss as you age. Most people do not get enough potassium. But when you follow the MyPlate Map for Healthy Eating (see Figure 13.1), it's easy to get enough of this important mineral. Lots of healthy foods are good sources. These include tomatoes, potatoes, sweet potatoes, and winter squash; fruits, including oranges, cantaloupe, bananas, kiwifruit, prunes, and apricots; and nuts. Dairy products like milk, buttermilk, and yogurt also contain some potassium.

Calcium

You probably know that calcium helps build bones, but did you know it is also needed for blood clotting and helps with blood pressure? It may also help protect against colon cancer, kidney stones, and breast cancer.

Unfortunately, most people, especially women and young children, do not get enough calcium. Most women under 60 should get the amount of calcium found in 3 cups (750 mL) of milk every day. Other good sources of calcium are yogurt and kefir (a beverage similar to yogurt); calcium-fortified soy, rice, and almond milks and calcium-fortified orange juice; and seaweed. It is also found in smaller amounts in such leafy greens as kale, Brussels sprouts, broccoli, kohlrabi, collards, and bok choy. Most fruits are low in calcium, except for dried figs (there's not much in fig cookies, though) and the tropical cherimoya (custard apple).

Water

Water is your most important nutrient. Like the air you breathe, you cannot live without it. More than half of your body is made up of water, and each of your cells is bathed in it. Water helps keep your kidneys working, helps prevent constipation, and helps you eat less by making you feel full. It also helps prevent some medication side effects.

Although people can survive for weeks without food, you cannot typically live longer than a week or so without water. Most adults lose about 10 cups (2500 mL) of water a day. Fortunately, people usually have no problem getting the six to eight glasses each day many experts recommend. This is especially true because you get water from the food you eat as well as from what you drink. Most foods, even the driest cracker, contain some water.

To see if you are drinking enough, check your urine. If it is light-colored, you are fine. When you feel thirsty, you need more water. Milk, juice, and many fruits and vegetables are good sources of water. Beware, though: coffee, tea, and other drinks with caffeine or alcohol, can cause you to lose water. Do not depend on these drinks for your water.

If you take certain kinds of medication or have other health conditions such as kidney disease or congestive heart failure, your needs for water may be different. Talk to a registered dietitian or your health care provider.

Healthy Eating and Chronic Pain

The relationship between nutrition and pain is at a relatively early stage of research. However, everyone agrees that the best eating plan for someone with chronic pain is a balanced and varied diet. It should include lots of fruits and vegetables; legumes and nuts; protein sources like fish, poultry, or alternative plant sources; and whole grains. It's also important to get adequate amounts of liquids in order to stay hydrated. Such a diet appears to reduce inflammation, decrease stress, and improve mood and depression. If you are living with chronic pain, follow the healthy diets in the USDA MyPlate and Eating Well with Canada's Food Guide programs. Remember to eat regularly and not to skip meals.

Self-management of your food choices does not end with eating a healthy diet. Some substances in foods may be helpful or harmful for chronic pain. Here are some of them.

- Omega-3 fatty acids are "good fats" that need to be in balance with other fats in our diet. Increasing the intake of foods rich in omega-3 may improve pain due to headaches, migraines, rheumatoid arthritis, and other types of inflammatory pain such as fibromyalgia. Foods that are high in omega-3s include fatty fish (such as salmon, mackerel, sardines, arctic char, anchovies, and trout), flaxseeds and flaxseed oil, canola oil, soybean oil, soy products like tofu, and walnuts. To increase the amount of omega-3 in your diet, try the following: eat fish twice a week; use canola or soybean oil for cooking and in recipes; use flaxseed oil for making salad dressings or uncooked dips; use 1/4 cup (60 mL) of walnuts or tofu in salads; and replace regular eggs with omega-3 eggs. (The websites listed under Other Resources at the end of the chapter contain more information on omega-3 food sources.) There is no need to purchase supplements. In fact, it is much better if you get your omega-3s from food sources.

- Vitamin D is thought to be a factor in pain regulation. It is estimated that as many as 50 percent of people with chronic pain have low levels of vitamin D. Scientists do not know for certain if vitamin D helps people with chronic pain but they think it might. There are other reasons to increase vitamin D. It can help you absorb calcium for your bones and teeth, and it may help prevent diabetes, multiple sclerosis, and some cancers. Vitamin D can be obtained from sunlight; therefore it is important to get outdoors every day when possible. It can also be obtained through some foods, including milk; fortified yogurt, orange juice, and soy beverages; margarine; fish (many of the same varieties high in omega-3s); and cod liver oil. It can also be taken as a supplement. Health Canada suggests that Canadians over the age of 50 take at least 400 IU a day. (Low levels of vitamin D are a common problem for people who live in more northern countries.) Safe tolerable levels are up to 4000 IU a day. Talk to your doctor about whether you should take vitamin D supplements and at what dose.

- Magnesium may reduce migraine headache, fibromyalgia, and some neuropathic pain. Magnesium-rich foods include flaxseed, sesame seeds, pumpkin seeds, Brazil nuts, almonds, pine nuts, fatty fish (salmon, halibut, mackerel), beans (black, lima, navy), black-eyed peas, green vegetables (cooked spinach and swiss chard), and wheat germ. Consult your doctor before you take a magnesium supplement, as too much may cause diarrhea.

■ Caffeine should be limited to about 400 mg, which is the equivalent of two to three 8-ounce cups of coffee a day. Caffeine isn't only found in coffee; it is also in tea, colas, cocoa, and some energy drinks. Cold remedies and some mild analgesics that you might take for pain may contain caffeine. Always read the label. Excess amounts of caffeine can increase feelings of anxiety, restlessness, irritability, chest palpitations, and stomach complaints and can interfere with sleep. These symptoms can further intensify your pain.

If you consume a lot of caffeine, it's important to gradually reduce your caffeine intake over two to three weeks. You may develop symptoms of withdrawal if you reduce it too quickly. These symptoms include headache, fatigue, irritability, and mood swings. If you reduce gradually, you should have no ill effects. Try to decrease your intake by substituting decaffeinated coffee, teas, and caffeine-free drinks. Brewed decaf coffee, for example, has 2 mg of caffeine per 6-ounce cup compared to 103 mg of caffeine in regular brewed coffee.

Other Eating Choices that Can Affect Chronic Pain

In addition to eating healthy foods, you can make other choices that may help you self-manage your chronic pain such as the following:

■ Stay hydrated. There may be a link between chronic dehydration and muscle soreness. (See p. 217 for more details on the recommended amount of liquid to consume.)

■ People with chronic migraines often report that certain foods may trigger their headaches. Some of these common triggers include alcohol, sulphites (found in dried fruits and some alcohol), tannins (wine, strong tea), various cheeses (especially aged or fermented), food additives like nitrates and nitrites found in processed meats, monosodium glutamate (MSG, a flavor enhancer in Asian and processed foods), aspartame and other artificial sweeteners, and fatty foods. Other reported triggers include fasting or missing a meal and becoming dehydrated. The exact cause of migraines is still not known, so it may be useful to experiment by avoiding foods you might suspect are triggers for you. As long as entire food groups are not eliminated, avoiding certain foods won't harm you.

Food Sensitivities

Other kinds of chronic pain, not just migraine, can be triggered by certain foods. To determine if you have sensitivities to certain foods, keep a food journal. (See, for example, the Lifestyle Tracking Diary in the next chapter.) Write down all the foods and beverages you consume in two weeks. Also, note if you have missed a meal. Then note whether your symptoms—your pain, mood, and emotions—are worse, better, or not affected. Then look for patterns to see if certain foods make your symptoms better or worse. You may not have realized that some common foods may be causing you problems. If you suspect some foods are a problem, eliminate them one at a time to test your idea. Again, it is important not to eliminate entire food groups. Always eat a balanced diet of fruits, vegetables, grains, proteins, and healthy dairy choices. And don't forget to hydrate!

The Nutrition Facts Label: "What's in That Package of Food?"

Food labels inform you about what is in the packaged foods you eat. The Nutrition Facts panel and the ingredients list are two important sources of information. Together they tell you what a food contains, which can help you make better choices. Reading and understanding the information on food labels isn't as daunting as it may seem. The following guidelines focus on the serving size, calories, total fat, trans fat, cholesterol, sodium, and total carbohydrates.

Serving Size

Look at the serving size information first. All the other information on the label is based on the serving size. If you will be having a single serving, then interpreting the Nutrition Facts panel is a straightforward process. But the serving size on the package may not be the amount you usually eat. If you would usually have less or more than the stated serving size, you need to adjust all the amounts listed in the Nutrition Facts. For example, if a serving size is one half a cup of cooked rice and you eat one cup, which is two servings, you need to double all the values. Most serving sizes are stated in cups, ounces, or pieces of the food. Beware: many packages that appear to be a single serving size contain more than one serving.

Calories

Total calories are given for the stated serving size, so if you eat more or less than one serving, you again will have to do a little arithmetic. There is also a listing for the number for calories from fat, although it doesn't tell you the kind of fat. From this number, you can figure out the percentage of calories you will get from fat. This is important if you are interested in how much fat you are eating. Divide the calories from fat by the calories in the serving size and then multiply

Nutrition Facts		
Serving Size 1 package (28 g/1 oz.)		
Servings Per Container		1

Amount Per Serving

Calories 280 Calories from Fat 45

		% Daily Value*
Total Fat 5 g		7%
Saturated Fat 2 g		10%
Trans Fat 0 g		
Polyunsaturated Fat 1 g		
Monounsaturated Fat 2 g		
Cholesterol 20 mg		7%
Sodium 540 mg		22%
Total Carbohydrate 12 g		16%
Dietary Fiber 3 g		12%
Sugars 7 g		
Protein 10 g		
Vitamin A 4%		Vitamin C 4%
Calcium 15%		Iron 4%

*Percent Daily Values are based on a 2,000 calorie diet. Your daily values may be higher or lower depending on your calorie needs.

	Calories:	2000	2500
Total fat	Less than	65 g	80 g
Sat fat	Less than	20 g	25 g
Cholesterol	Less than	300 mg	300 mg
Sodium	Less than	2,400 mg	2,400 mg
Potassium	Less than	3,500 mg	3,500 mg
Total Carbohydrate		300 g	375 g
Fiber		25 g	30 g

Figure 13.2

by 100. For the label in Figure 13.2, divide the 45 fat calories by the 280 in the serving and you get 0.16. Then multiply by 100 to get 16 percent.

Total Fat, Cholesterol, and Sodium

The total fat number includes good fat (polyunsaturated and monounsaturated), bad fat (saturated), and trans fat in grams (a unit of weight). If you are more comfortable thinking in terms of calories, you can change grams to calories by multiplying by 9. For the label in Figure 13.2 multiply the 5 g (total fat) by 9 to get 45 calories. This is the same number of calories shown in the calories from fat line. The amount of calories in all the fats should add up (or at least be close) to the calories for total fat.

Remember our warning about deadly trans fats! Due to the way food companies are allowed to do the arithmetic, any food with up to 1/2 (0.5) g per serving of trans fat can be listed as having no trans fat, but you still may be getting some. If the ingredients list has the words *partially hydrogenated* or *hydrogenated*, the product contains trans fat (even if the amount of trans fats per serving is 0 g).

So when you eat anything that lists *partially hydrogenated* or *hydrogenated* fat on the ingredients label, trans fats could add up, especially if you have more than one serving.

The cholesterol line tells you the amount of cholesterol by serving size. Because cholesterol is found only in animal foods, this line may be missing or show 0 g for foods not made with animal products. If you are watching the amount of cholesterol you eat, you need to be especially careful because even if a food does not have any cholesterol, it may contain bad or trans fat, particularly if it is a processed food. Trans fats can raise your blood cholesterol level more than the cholesterol from food.

To tell if the fat, cholesterol, or sodium is high or low, look at the "% Daily Value" or "% DV" column. Any value of 20 percent or more is high. If you want to eat less fat, cholesterol, or salt, or you plan to eat more than one serving, look for values of 5 percent or less. You can see in this example that the values for total fat, saturated fat, and cholesterol are low but sodium is high. Note that percent values are not available for trans fats and protein, as there are no recommended Daily Values for them. If you want to learn more about these recommended Daily Values, go to the MyPlate website (www.choosemyplate.gov).

Total Carbohydrate, Dietary Fiber, and Sugars

This section breaks out values for dietary fiber and sugars. It is important for people who want to monitor their carbohydrates or get more fiber in their diet. (Most of us should be eating more fiber.) Note that there is no Daily Value percent for sugar. However, for many people with diabetes, it's the total amount of carbohydrate that matters, not the specific kind. A general guideline is to keep this amount between 45 to 60 g per meal, assuming three meals a day.

Ingredients List

Always check a package's ingredients list. It will show you what is in the food you will be eating. Ingredients are listed in order *by weight*. If you see sugar listed first, then the food contains more sugar than anything else. And remember: when you see the words *partially hydrogenated* or *hydrogenated*, the product contains trans fats (even if the amount for trans fats is 0 g).

To learn more about Canada's Nutrition Facts label, please see: *www.healthcanada.gc.ca/foodguide*

Eating and Your Mood

Do you eat when you're bored, sad, or feeling lonely? Many people find comfort in food. They eat when they need to take their minds off something or have nothing else to do. Some people eat when they are feeling angry, anxious, or depressed. At these times, it is easy to lose track of how much you eat. It is also easy to make unhealthy choices—when you're feeling this way, celery sticks, apples, or popcorn just won't do! Here are some ways to help control these urges:

- Keep a "food mood" journal. Every day, list what, how much, and when you eat. Note how you are feeling when you have the urge to eat. Try to spot patterns so you can anticipate when you will want to eat without really being hungry.

- If you catch yourself feeling bored and thinking about eating, ask yourself, "Am I really hungry?" If the answer is no, make yourself do something else for two to three minutes. Go for a short walk in the house or around the block, work on a jigsaw puzzle, brush your teeth, or play a computer game.

- Keep your mind and hands busy. Getting your hands dirty is helpful (as with gardening).

- Write down action plans (see Chapter 2) to have on hand for when these situations arise. Sometimes it is easier to refer to the written word than to remember what you said you would do.

Common Challenges to Making Healthier Food Choices

"Healthy food doesn't taste the same as food I am used to. When I eat, I want something with substance, like meat and potatoes or a piece of apple pie! The healthy stuff just doesn't fill me up!"

Making healthier food choices does not mean you cannot have something you want or crave. It just means trading off some foods for others. You can still fit in favorites on special occasions while making healthier choices most of the time. Some tips about making good choices are discussed in Chapter 14, and sources for more information are listed at the end of this chapter. There are also many excellent cookbooks and websites with good, healthful recipe ideas. The following tips will help you overcome common excuses people use to justify poor eating choices:

"But I love to cook!"

If you love to cook, you are in luck. Take a cooking class, or watch a cooking show on TV that focuses on healthy foods. Buy a new cookbook on healthy cooking, or find a website with healthy recipes. If you have odds and ends, even leftovers, in your kitchen, do a computer search to see what recipes you can find. Play around with ways to modify your favorite recipes, making them lower in fat, sugar, and salt.

"I'm living alone now, and I'm not used to cooking for one. I find myself overeating so that food isn't wasted."

This can be a problem, particularly when the situation is new. But it might not have anything to do with wasting food. You may be overeating to fill time. Many people simply eat for as long as food is in front of you. Whatever the reason, there are some ways you can deal with the extra food.

- Don't eat "family style" by putting serving dishes on the table. Put as much as you feel you can comfortably eat on a plate, and bring only that plate to the table. Another strategy is to use a smaller plate.

- As soon as you have finished eating, or even right after you have served your portion, immediately put any remaining food in the refrigerator or freezer. You can enjoy leftovers the next day or whenever you don't feel like fixing a meal.

- Have guests over for dinner once in a while so you can share food and other people's company. Plan a potluck supper with neighbors, relatives, or members of your house of worship, clubs, or other groups.

"Food doesn't taste as good as before."

Many things can affect how food tastes. Surgery, certain medications, and even the common cold can make food taste off, bad, or funny. When this happens, you tend to eat less. Many people automatically add extra salt to their food to try to make it taste better. Unfortunately, this can cause you to retain water or feel bloated, which can increase blood pressure.

Here's how you can make foods taste better:

- Use herbs (basil, oregano, tarragon) and spices (cinnamon, cumin, curry, ginger, nutmeg) in cooking or sprinkle them on top of food when you are ready to serve.

- Squirt fresh lemon juice on foods.

- Use a small amount of vinegar in or on top of hot or cold foods. There are dozens of choices, from balsamic to berry- and fruit-flavored varieties. Experiment with new flavors.

- Add healthy ingredients to the foods you usually eat (add carrots or barley to soup, for example, or dried fruits and nuts to salads) to give them more texture and make them tastier.

- Chew your food slowly and well. This will allow the food to remain in your mouth longer and release more flavor.

If the lack of taste is keeping you from eating enough, you may need to add more calories to your meals or snacks. Tips for doing this are given in Chapter 14.

"It takes so long to prepare meals. By the time I'm done, I'm too tired to eat."

This is a common issue, especially for people who do not have much energy. Here are some hints to help:

- When you do have energy, cook enough for two, three, or even more servings or meals, especially if it is something you really like. Freeze the leftovers in single-serving sizes.

- Do a meal exchange with friends or family, and freeze what you get in single-serving sizes. When you are tired, choose one of these precooked meals, thaw it, reheat, and enjoy.

- Break your food preparation into steps, resting in between.

- Ask for help, especially for big holiday meals or family gatherings.

"Sometimes eating causes discomfort."

"I really have no appetite."

People who find it physically uncomfortable to eat meals tend to eat less. For some, eating a large meal causes stomach problems such as indigestion, discomfort, or nausea. Chronic pain symptoms can also suppress appetite.

If you face these challenges sometimes, try the following:

- Eat four to six small meals a day rather than the usual three large meals. You will be using less energy for each meal.

- Avoid foods that produce gas or make you feel bloated. Among the more common foods that can cause discomfort are cabbage, broccoli, Brussels sprouts, onions, beans, and certain fruits, including bananas, apples, melons, and avocados.

- Eat slowly, take small bites, and chew your food well. Pause occasionally during a meal. Slowing down and breathing evenly reduces the amount of air you swallow while eating.

- Do a relaxation exercise about half an hour before mealtime, or take time out for a few deep breaths during the meal.

- Choose food that is easy to eat, such as yogurt or pudding, or to drink, such as a protein shake or fruit smoothie.

"I love to eat out and can't resist all the tasty foods on the menu!"

If you don't have time, you hate to cook, or you just don't have the energy to shop for groceries or fix meals, eating out may suit your needs. This is not necessarily bad if you know how to make the best choices possible. Here are some tips for eating out:

- Select restaurants that have a variety of menu items prepared in healthy ways (for example, grilled or steamed dishes in addition to or instead of fried foods).

- Ask what is in the dishes you are considering and how they are prepared, especially if you are eating in an unfamiliar restaurant.

- Before you go out, decide what type of food you will eat and how much. Many restaurants post their menus on the Internet or at the front of the restaurant.

- Order small plates or appetizers instead of main courses.

- When you are with a group, order first so you aren't tempted to change your mind after hearing what others have selected.

- See if you can split an entrée with a dining companion, or order a half portion. You could also eat only half of what you are served and take the rest home for another meal. Ask to have the take-home container brought to you with your food, and box up half of your meal before you start eating.

- Choose menu items that are low in fat, salt, and sugar, or ask if they can be prepared that way.

- Whenever possible, order broiled, barbecued, baked, grilled, or steamed dishes rather than foods that are breaded, fried, sautéed, creamed, or covered in cheese.

- Ask for vegetables to be steamed or served raw without butter, sauces, or dips.

- Eat bread without butter. If you can't resist the temptation, ask the waitstaff to remove butter or dipping oil from the table.

- Request salad with dressing on the side, and dip your fork into the dressing before spearing each mouthful.

- For dessert, select fruit, nonfat yogurt, sorbet, or sherbet.

- Share a dessert with at least one other person.

  "I snack while I am doing other things—watching TV, working on the computer, or reading."

If this is a problem for you, keep healthier snacks in your fridge and cupboard. Here are some examples:

- Rather than snacking on crackers, chips, and cookies, munch on fresh fruit, raw vegetables, or fat-free or plain popcorn.

- Measure out your snack in a single-portion size so you won't be tempted to eat more.

- Designate specific places at home and the workplace "eating areas," and don't eat anywhere else.

Healthy eating is about the food choices you make most of the time. It is not about never being able to eat certain foods. There is no such thing as a perfect food. Healthy eating means enjoying a moderate amount of a wide variety of minimally processed foods in the proper amounts while allowing for occasional treats. Eating this way can help you maintain your health, prevent future health problems, and manage your pain condition symptoms as best as possible.

Eating healthy may mean making some changes to what you are now doing. These could include choosing more foods that are higher in good fats and fiber and fewer foods that are high in bad fats, sugar, and salt. Think of it as doing something positive and wonderful for yourself, not as punishment. As a self-manager, it's up to you to find the changes that are best for you. If you experience setbacks, identify the problems and work at resolving them. You can do it!

Table 13.2 **Food Guide for Healthy Meal Planning**

Nutritional values are based on data from the U.S. Department of Agriculture and the American Diabetes Association.

Abbreviations:

g = grams, mg = milligrams, oz = ounce, c = cup, Tbsp = tablespoon, tsp = teaspoon mL = milliliters, cm = centimeters

---

PROTEIN FOODS

Protein Sources with Little or No Carbohydrate

Beef, Pork, Lamb, Veal, Poultry, and Fish

Serving Size: 3–4 oz (84–112 g), cooked, NOT breaded, fried, or cooked with added fat unless noted. This portion is the size of the palm of your hand and 1/2 to 1 inch (1.0–2.5 cm) thick.
Per Serving: approx. 21–28 g protein; fat and calories vary

Lean *(up to 9 g fat, 135–180 calories per serving)*	Beef (fat trimmed) from the round, sirloin, and flank, tenderloin sirloin, ground round
	Pork, fresh, cured, boiled ham, Canadian bacon, tenderloin, center loin chop
	Lamb and veal, rib roast, chop, leg
	Chicken and turkey, white or dark meat, no skin
	Duck and goose, drained of fat, no skin
	Game, buffalo, ostrich, rabbit, venison
	Fish (fresh or frozen), catfish, cod, flounder, haddock, halibut, orange roughy, salmon, tilapia
	Fish (canned), tuna, in water or oil, drained; herring, uncreamed or smoked, 6–8 sardines
	Shellfish, clams, crab, lobster, scallops, shrimp, imitation shellfish
	Oysters (fresh or frozen), 18 medium
	Processed meats (luncheon meat, deli meat), turkey ham, kielbasa, pastrami, chipped beef, shaved meats
Medium-fat *(12–21 g fat, 150–300 calories per serving)*	Ground beef, meatloaf, corned beef, short ribs, prime rib, tongue
	Pork, shoulder roast, Boston butt (picnic), cutlets
	Lamb, rib roast and chops, roasts, ground
	Veal, cutlet
	Chicken, turkey, with skin, fried, ground
	Pheasant, dove, wild duck, wild goose
	Fish, all fried
High-fat *(24 g or more fat, 300–400 calories per serving)*	Pork, spareribs, ground
	Sausage, pork, bratwurst, chorizo, Italian, Polish, smoked, summer
	Processed meats, luncheon meat and deli meats, bologna, salami
	Bacon, 6 slices

Protein Sources with Little or No Carbohydrate (*continued*)

Organ Meats *Serving Size: 2–3 oz (56–84 g)* *Per Serving: 14–21 g protein; fat and calories vary; high in cholesterol*	Kidney (1–3 g fat, 70–105 calories) Liver, heart (6–9 g fat, 55–100 calories)
Eggs *Per Serving: 7 g protein*	Whole egg, 1 large, cooked (5 g fat, 75 calories) Egg whites, 2 large, cooked (0–1 g fat, 35 calories) Egg substitute, plain, 1/4 c (60 mL) (1 g fat, about 50 calories)
Cheese *Per Serving: 7 g protein; fat and calories vary*	
Fat-free and low-fat *(0–1 g fat, 35 calories)*	Fresh (Mexican) and nonfat cheese, 1 oz (28 g) Cottage cheese, fat-free, 1/4 c (2 oz) (60 mL or 56 g)
Medium-fat *(4–7 g fat, 75 calories)*	Feta, skim-milk mozzarella, string cheese, reduced-fat and processed cheese spreads, 1–2 oz (28–56 g) Ricotta, 1/4 c (2 oz) (60 mL or 56 g) Grated parmesan, 2 Tbsp (1 oz or 30 mL)
High-fat *(8 g fat, 100+ calories)*	All regular full-fat cheese: American, blue, Brie, Swiss, cheddar, Monterey jack, Swiss, provolone, whole-milk mozzarella, goat, queso, 1–2 oz (28–56 g)
Nuts and Seeds* *Per Serving: Little to no carbohydrate; fat and calories vary* **(These foods contain good fats—see page 212.)*	Almonds, cashews, mixed nuts, 6 nuts Peanuts, 10 nuts Pecans, walnuts, 4 halves Tahini (sesame paste), 1 Tbsp (15 mL) Pumpkin seeds (pepitas), sunflower seeds, 1 Tbsp (15 mL) Nut butters (peanut, almond, etc.), 2 Tbsp (30 mL) (8 g fat)

PROTEIN FOODS (*CONTINUED*)

Protein Foods with Carbohydrate

Milk *Serving Size: 1 c (250 mL)* *Per Serving: 8 g protein,* *12 g carbohydrate; fat and* *calories vary*	Nonfat, fresh or evaporated 1%, nonfat or low-fat buttermilk (0–3 g fat, 100 calories) Low-fat (2%) sweet acidophilus (5 g fat, 120 calories) Whole, fresh or evaporated cow milk, goat milk, buttermilk (8 g fat, 160 calories)
Yogurt *Per Serving: 8 g protein,* *12 g carbohydrate; fat and* *calories vary*	Nonfat, plain, or flavored with artificial sweetener, 2/3 c (5 oz) (150 mL) (0–3 g fat, 90–100 calories) Low-fat, sugar-sweetened, with fruit, 2/3 c (5 oz) (150 mL) (5 g fat, 120 calories) Plain whole milk, kefir, 3/4 c (6 oz) (175 mL) (8 g fat, 150 calories) Nonfat fruit-flavored, sweetened with sugar, 1 c (8 oz) (250 mL) (30+ g carbohydrate, 0–3 g fat, 100–150 calories) Nonfat or low-fat fruit-flavored, sweetened with sugar substitute, 1 c (8 oz) (250 mL) (0–3 g fat, 90–130 calories)
Plant Protein Sources *Per Serving: as noted*	Soy milk, regular, 1 c (250 mL) (2–3 g carbohydrate, 8 g protein, 4 g fat, 100 calories) Dried beans and peas, lentils, cooked, 1/2 c (125 mL) (15 g carbohydrate, 7 g protein, 0–1 g fat, 80 calories) Edamame (soybeans), 1/2 c (125 mL) (8 g carbohydrate, 7 g protein, 0–1 g fat, approx. 60 calories) Hummus (garbanzo bean spread), 1/3 c (75 mL) (15 g carbohydrate, 7 g protein, approx. 8 g fat, 100 calories) Refried beans, canned, 1/2 c (125 mL) (15 g carbohydrate, 7 g protein, 0–3 g fat, approx. 100 calories) Tofu, regular, 1/2 c (4 oz) (125 mL) (3 g carbohydrate, 8 g protein, 5 g fat, 75 calories)

CARBOHYDRATE FOODS

Per Serving: 15 g carbohydrate, 3 g protein, 0–1 g fat, 80 calories
Tip: Choose whole grains as often as you can.

Breads and Grains	
Breads, Rolls, Muffins, and Tortillas *Good source of fiber	Bagel, large, 1/4 Bread, white, whole grain,* rye, pumpernickel, 1 slice Buns, hot dog or hamburger, 1/2 English muffin, plain, 1/2 Pancake, 4 inches (10 cm) across, 1 Pita bread, 6 inches (15 cm) across, 1/2 Roll, regular, 1/2 Tortilla, corn or flour, 6 inches (15 cm) across, 1 Waffle, 4½ inches (11 cm) square, reduced-fat, 1
Cereals *Good source of fiber	Bran flakes, spoon-size shredded wheat,* 1/2 c (125 mL) Granola,* low-fat or regular, Grape-Nuts* 1/4 c (60 mL) Oats,* cooked, 1/2 c (125 mL) Puffed cereal, unfrosted, 1½ c (375 mL)
Grains *Good source of fiber	Bulgur wheat,* grits, cooked, tabbouleh, prepared, 1/2 c (125 mL) Pasta, barley, couscous, quinoa, cooked, 1/3 c (75 mL) Rice, white, or brown,* cooked, 1/3 c (75 mL) Wheat germ,* dry, 3 Tbsp (45 mL) Wild rice,* cooked, 1/2 c (125 mL)
Crackers and Snacks	Graham crackers, 2½ inches (6 cm) square, 3 Matzo, 3/4 oz (21 g) Melba toast, 2 x 4 inches (5 cm x 10 cm), 4 Pretzels, 3/4 oz (21 g) Rice cakes, 4 inches (5 cm) across, 2 Saltines, 6 Whole-wheat crackers, no fat added, 3–4 oz (84–112 g), 2–5

Continues ▶

CARBOHYDRATE FOODS (*continued*)

Low-Starch Vegetables

Per Serving: approx. 5 g carbohydrate, 2 g protein, no fat, 25 calories
Serving Size: 1/2 c (125 mL) cooked or vegetable juice, 1 c (250 mL) raw fresh, frozen, or canned
(frozen or canned may be high in sodium)

Amaranth
Artichoke
Asparagus
Bamboo shoots
Bean sprouts
Beets
Broccoli
Brussels sprouts
Cabbage, Chinese cabbage
Carrots
Cauliflower
Celery
Chayote (vegetable pear)
Chicory
Chilies, spicy

Cucumber
Eggplant (aubergine)
Garlic
Green beans
Green onion, scallions
Greens (collard, kale, mustard, turnip)
Jicama
Kohlrabi
Mushrooms
Nopales (cactus)
Okra
Onions
Pea pods
Radishes

Rutabaga
Salad greens
Snap peas
Spinach
Summer squash (yellow squash, zucchini)
Sweet peppers
Tomatoes (raw, canned, sauce)
Turnips
Vegetable juice (usually high in sodium)
Watercress

Starchy Vegetables

Per Serving: 15 g carbohydrate, 0–3 g protein, 0–1 g fat, 80 calories

Corn, 1/2 c (125 mL) or 1/2 large cob
Mixed vegetables with corn, peas, or pasta, 1 c (250 mL)
Parsnips, 1/2 c (125 mL)
Plantain, ripe, 1/3 c (75 mL)
Potato, baked or boiled, large, with skin, 1

Succotash (lima beans and corn), 1/2 c (125 mL)
Winter squash (acorn, butternut, pumpkin), 1 c (250 mL)
Yam, sweet potato, 1/2 c (125 mL)
Yautia, yuca (cassava), 1/2 c (125 mL)

CARBOHYDRATE FOODS (*continued*)

Fruit

Per Serving: 15 g carbohydrate, no protein, 0–1 g fat, approx. 80 calories

Fresh

Apple, small, 2 inches (5 cm), 1

Apricots, 4

Banana, extra small, 1 (4 oz) (112 g)

Berries (strawberries, blueberries, raspberries)
3/4–1 c (175–250 mL)

Cherries, 1/2 c (125 mL) (approx. 12)

Coconut, fresh (shredded), 1/2 c (125 mL)

Dates, 3

Figs, large, 2

Fruit cocktail, 1/2 c (125 mL)

Grapefruit, small, 1/2

Grapes, small, 1/2 c (125 mL)

Guava, medium, 2

Kiwifruit, large, 1

Lemon, lime, large, 1

Mango, cubed, 1/2 c (125 mL)

Melon (honeydew, cantaloupe), 1/4 (60 mL)

Orange, small, 1

Papaya, small, cubed, 1 c (250 mL)

Peach, nectarine, 1

Pear, 1/2

Persimmon, medium, 1

Pineapple, cubed, 3/4 c (175 mL)

Plum, small, 2

Tangerine, small, 2

Watermelon, cubed, 1/2 c (125 mL)

Canned

Unsweetened, 1/4–1/2 c (60–125 mL)

In sugar syrup, 1/4 c (60 mL)

Dried

Apricots, 8 halves

Figs, 2

Prunes, 3

Raisins, 1 Tbsp (15 mL)

Tamarind, 1/2 c (125 mL)

Fruit Drinks

(If the label doesn't say 100% juice, it usually contains added sugar)

Unsweetened

Apple, grapefruit, orange, pineapple, 1/2 c
(125 mL)

Apricot nectar, 1/2 c (125 mL)

Grape, prune, juice blends, 1/3 c (75 mL)

Sweetened

Carbonated juice drinks, 1/2 c (125 mL)

Cranberry cocktail, 1/3 c (75 mL)

OILS AND SOLID FATS

Per Serving: little or no carbohydrate, 5 g fat, 45 calories
Tip: Choose good fats as often as you can.

Good fats

Unsaturated fats, see page 212

Avocado, medium, 1/4

Margarine (soft), reduced-fat, 1 tsp (5 mL)

Mayonnaise, reduced-fat, 1 Tbsp (15 mL)

Mayonnaise, regular, 1 tsp (5 mL)

Olives, all types, large, 5

Salad and cooking oils (corn, olive, safflower, soybean, etc.), 1 tsp (5 mL)

Salad dressing, 1 Tbsp (15 mL)

Bad fats

Saturated fats, see pages 212–213

Bacon fat, 1 tsp (5 mL)

Butter, reduced-fat, 1 Tbsp (15 mL)

Butter, regular, 1 tsp (5 mL)

Cream, half-and-half, whipped, 2 Tbsp (30 mL)

Cream, liquid nondairy creamer, 1 Tbsp (15 mL)

Cream cheese, 1 Tbsp (15 mL)

Margarine (stick), regular, made with hydrogenated fat, 1 tsp (5 mL)

Shortening, lard, 1 tsp (5 mL)

Sour cream, regular, 1 Tbsp (15 mL)

ADDITIONAL FOODS AND DRINKS

Extras

Tip: These foods are high in fat or sugar or both; they're best saved for special occasions.

Cake with frosting, 1 small slice or 2-inch (5 cm) square

Cookies, small, 2

Danish, small, 1

Flan, with milk, 1/2 c (125 mL)

Fruit tart or pie, 1 slice

Honey, 1 Tbsp (15 mL)

Ice cream (regular), 1/2 c (125 mL)

Jam or jelly (low-sugar or light), 2 Tbsp (30 mL)

Jam or jelly (regular), 1 Tbsp (15 mL)

Juice bar (frozen, 100% juice), 1

Pudding, 1/2 c (125 mL)

Sherbet, sorbet, 1/2 c (125 mL)

Syrup (regular), 1 Tbsp (15 mL)

Syrup (sugar-free), 2 Tbsp (30 mL)

Alcoholic Beverages

Per Serving: no protein or fat; carbohydrate and calories vary

Beer, lite or nonalcoholic, 12 oz (360 mL) (approx. 5 g carbohydrate, 60–120 calories)

Beer, regular, 12 oz (360 mL) (approx. 13 g carbohydrate, about 160 calories)

Distilled spirits, 80 proof, 1½ oz (45 mL) (0 g carbohydrate, 80–110 calories)

Liqueurs, 1½ oz (45 mL) (approx. 20 g carbohydrate, 125 calories)

Mixed drinks (margarita, mojito, gin and tonic, etc.), 1 drink (approx. 12 g carbohydrate, 150–250 calories)

Wine, red, white, dry, sparkling, 4 oz (120 mL) (1–2 g carbohydrate, 80 calories)

Wine, sweet or dessert, 4 oz (120 mL) (approx. 14 g carbohydrate, 120 calories)

ADDITIONAL FOODS AND DRINKS (*continued*)

Free Foods

Per Serving: up to 5 g carbohydrate, up to 20 calories; enjoy moderate servings as often as you like

Atol (cornmeal drink), 1 c (250 mL)

Bouillon, broth, consommé

Candy, hard (sugar-free)

Chewing gum (sugar-free)

Club soda, mineral water

Coffee or tea, unsweetened or with sugar
   substitute, no milk, cream, or whitener

Gelatin (sugar-free or unflavored)

Herbs, spices

Horchata (rice drink)

Hot pepper sauces

Soft drinks (sugar-free)

Soy sauce*

Worcestershire sauce*

*Use low sodium versions to reduce salt intake.

Sugar substitutes

Approved by the U.S. Food and Drug Administration

Equal (aspartame)

Splenda (sucralose)

Sprinkle Sweet (saccharin)

Sugar Twin (saccharin)

Sweet One (acesulfame K)

Sweet-10 (saccharin)

Sweet'N Low (saccharin)

Other Resources to Explore

Academy of Nutrition and Dietetics: www.eatright.org

American Cancer Society: www.cancer.org

American Diabetes Association: www.diabetes.org

American Heart Association: www.heart.org/nutrition

Canadian Diabetes Association: www.diabetes.ca

Center for Science in the Public Interest: www.cspinet.org

Dietitians of Canada: www.dietitians.ca

Food and Nutrition Information Center: www.fnic.nal.usda.gov

Harvard School of Public Health: www.hsph.harvard.edu

Health Canada Food Guide: www.healthcanada.gc.ca/foodguide

Health Canada Licensed Natural Health Products Database:
   www.hc-sc.gc.ca/dhp-mps/prodnatur/applications/licen-prod/lnhpd-bdpsnh-eng.php

International Food Information Council Foundation: www.foodinsight.org

U.S. Department of Agriculture, Agricultural Research Service: www.ars.usda.gov

U.S. Food and Drug Administration, MyPlate: www.choosemyplate.gov

Suggested Further Reading

To learn more about the topics discussed in this chapter, we suggest that you explore the following resources:

Center for Science in the Public Interest, *Nutrition Action Healthletter* (newsletter): www.cspinet.org.

Environmental Nutrition (newsletter): www.environmentalnutrition.com.

Mayo Clinic, "Nutrition and Healthy Eating": www.mayoclinic.org/healthy-living/ nutrition-and-healthy-eating/basics/ nutrition-basics/hlv-20049477.

Tufts University, *Health & Nutrition Letter*: www.nutritionletter.tufts.edu.

U.S. Department of Health and Human Services, *Heart Healthy Home Cooking, African American Style*: www.nhlbi.nih.gov/ files/docs/public/heart/cooking.pdf.

University of California, *UC Berkeley Wellness Letter*: www.berkeleywellness.com.

Warshaw, Hope. *Eat Out, Eat Right: The Guide to Healthier Restaurant Eating*, 3rd ed. Chicago: Surrey Books, 2008.

Woodruff, Sandra, and Leah Gilbert-Henderson. *Soft Foods for Easier Eating Cookbook: Easy-to-Follow Recipes for People Who Have Chewing and Swallowing Problems*. Garden City Park, N.Y.: Square One, 2010.

CHAPTER 14

Healthy Weight Management

OUR WEIGHT AFFECTS OUR HEALTH, how we look, our ability to move, and how we feel about ourselves. Being overweight or underweight can have major effects on your pain and your life. Excess weight is associated with such painful conditions as arthritis, back pain, fibromyalgia, headache, neuropathic pain, and angina due to coronary artery disease. It increases your risk for such other chronic diseases as diabetes from high blood sugar (called type 2 diabetes) and high blood pressure. Being underweight can weaken your immune system and make you less able to fight infection. It can increase the likelihood of developing osteoporosis, which increases the risk of painful fractures. In younger women, being underweight can affect fertility and result in menstrual problems.

A healthy weight contributes to better health and a better quality of life. Managing your weight can help you manage symptoms of your pain condition, including

Special thanks to Bonnie Bruce, DrPH, RD, for her help with this chapter.

fatigue restricted movement, and pain itself. It can help prevent or hold off related health problems such as diabetes and high blood pressure. In addition, maintaining a healthy weight can help you be more active, sleep better, and do the things you want and need to do. In this chapter we spell out what defines a healthy weight, how to make changes, how to decide whether you should lose or gain weight, and how to maintain changes you make.

What Is a Healthy Weight?

Most people's weight tends to move up and down over time, even over the course of a few days. So a healthy weight is not just one specific number on the scale or some sort of "ideal" number. There is no such thing as an "ideal" weight. Your healthy weight is a range of pounds that is unique and personal to you. It is a range that will help you lower your risk of developing or further worsening health problems. Being within a healthy weight range helps you feel good in your mind and your body.

Pinpointing your healthy weight range and deciding whether you need to change your weight depend on several things. These include your age, your activity level, your health, how much and where your body fat is located, and your family history of weight-related health problems, such as high blood pressure or diabetes.

To get a sense of a healthy weight range for you, see Figure 14.1, which is a chart of height (in inches or centimeters), weight (in pounds or kilograms), and body mass index (BMI). Although not a perfect tool, the BMI is a useful, quick, and general guide for adults. Find your height and follow that line to your weight. Locate the point on the chart where your height and weight intersect. Read the number on the dashed line closest to that point. That is your BMI. You can also locate your BMI using Table 14.1 on pages 238–239. Next, refer to Table 14.2 on page 240, which tells you how your current BMI is classified.

Another way to judge your weight is to use this rough rule of thumb. Give or take 10 percent, women should weigh about 105 pounds (47 kg) for the first 5 feet (152 cm) of height and another 5 pounds (2 kg) per inch (2.5 cm) after that. Men should weigh about 106 pounds (48 kg) for the first 5 feet (152 cm) and an added 6 pounds (2.5 kg) per inch (2.5 cm). For example, for a woman who is 5 foot 5 inches (165 cm) tall a healthy weight would be 130 pounds (58 kg), and her healthy weight range would be roughly 117 to 143 pounds (53 to 64 kg). This weight range places her in the BMI "normal weight" class.

Another way to judge your weight is to measure your waist. If you are overweight and most of your body fat is around your waist (rather than on your hips and thighs), you are at higher risk for heart disease, high blood pressure, and type 2 diabetes. For nonpregnant women, this means that health risks go up with a waist size that is more than 35 inches (88 cm). For men, it is a waist circumference that is greater than 40 inches (100 cm). To measure your waist correctly, stand and place a tape measure (one that is not old and stretched out) around your bare middle, just above your hipbone. Measure your waist just after you breathe out.

Figure 14.1 **Body Mass Index (BMI) Guide**

To estimate BMI, locate the point on the chart where height and weight intersect. Read the number on the dashed line closest to this point. For example, if you weigh 154 pounds (69 kg) and are 5 feet 8 inches (68 in or 173 cm) tall, you have a BMI of approximately 23, which is in Normal Weight.

You can also calculate your BMI using this formula: $BMI = weight(kg)/height(m)^2$

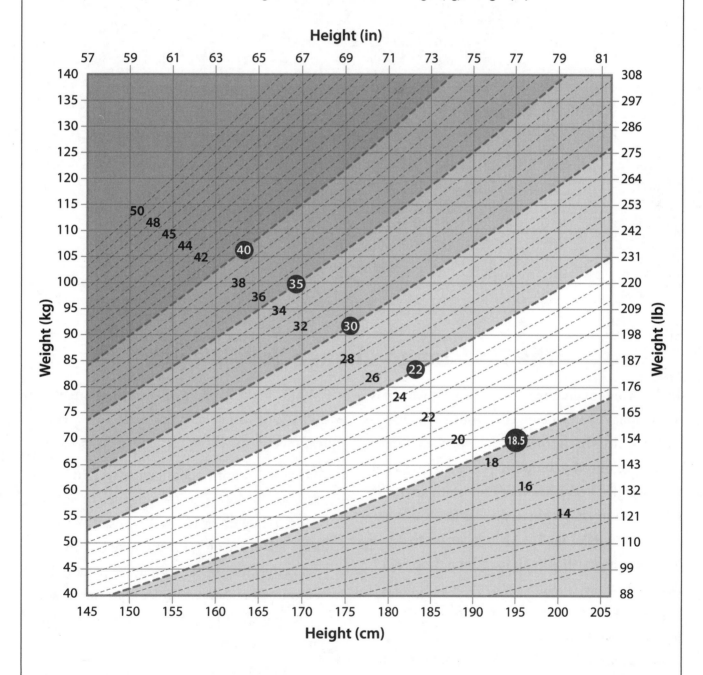

Note: For persons 65 years and older the 'normal' range may begin slightly above BMI 18.5 and extend into the 'overweight' range.

Source: Health Canada. Canadian Guidelines for Body Weight Classification in Adults. Ottawa: Minister of Public Works and Government Services Canada, 2003.

Table 14.1 **Body Mass Index**

		Normal					Overweight				
		19	**20**	**21**	**22**	**23**	**24**	**25**	**26**	**27**	**28**	**29**
Height (feet-inches)	**Weight (pounds)**											
4'10"	91	96	100	105	110	115	119	124	129	134	138
4'11"	94	99	104	109	114	119	124	128	133	138	143
5'0"	97	102	107	112	118	123	128	133	138	143	148
5'1"	100	106	111	116	122	127	132	137	143	148	153
5'2"	104	109	115	120	126	131	136	142	147	153	158
5'3"	107	112	118	124	130	135	141	146	152	158	163
5'4"	110	116	122	128	134	140	145	151	157	163	169
5'5"	114	120	126	132	138	144	150	156	162	168	174
5'6"	118	124	130	136	142	148	155	161	167	173	179
5'7"	121	127	134	140	146	153	159	166	172	178	185
5'8"	125	131	138	144	151	158	164	171	177	184	190
5'9"	128	135	142	149	155	162	169	176	182	189	196
5'10"	132	139	146	153	160	167	174	181	188	195	202
5'11"	136	143	150	157	165	172	179	186	193	200	208
6'0"	140	147	154	162	169	177	184	191	199	206	213
6'1"	144	151	159	167	174	182	189	196	204	212	219
6'2"	148	155	163	171	179	186	194	202	210	218	225
6'3"	152	160	168	176	184	192	200	208	216	224	232
6'4"	156	164	172	180	189	197	205	213	221	230	238

The Decision to Change Your Weight

To reach and maintain a healthy weight, you may need to make some changes in your eating habits and lifestyle. This is true whether you want to gain or lose weight. If you decide you need to change your weight, keep this very important advice in mind: you must decide to do this for yourself—not for friends or family. Make changes that you believe you can stick with for a long time. If you decide to make changes for someone other than yourself or plan for only short-term changes, you probably won't succeed.

To get started, review the information about action planning in Chapter 2. Consider asking your doctor to refer you to a registered dietitian for help. This is not something you need to do alone.

When making the decision to change your weight, you must ask yourself two primary questions:

- **Why do I want to change my weight?** The reasons for losing or gaining weight are personal. They differ for each of us. The most important reason for some may be physical health. For others it may be personal or emotional reasons. Think about the reasons why you want to gain or lose weight. Here are some examples:
  - To improve my symptoms (pain, fatigue, shortness of breath, restricted movement, and so on)
  - To manage my blood sugar

Table 14.1 **Body Mass Index (*continued*)**

Height (feet-inches)	Weight (pounds)	Obese										Extreme Obesity		
		30	31	32	33	34	35	36	37	38	39	40	41	42
4'10"		143	148	153	158	162	167	172	177	181	186	191	196	201
4'11"		148	153	158	163	168	173	178	183	188	193	198	203	208
5'0"		153	158	163	168	174	179	184	189	194	199	204	209	215
5'1"		158	164	169	174	180	185	190	195	201	206	211	217	222
5'2"		164	169	175	180	186	191	196	202	207	213	218	224	229
5'3"		169	174	180	186	191	197	203	208	214	220	225	231	237
5'4"		175	180	186	191	197	204	209	215	221	227	232	238	244
5'5"		180	186	192	198	204	210	216	222	228	234	240	246	252
5'6"		186	192	198	204	210	216	223	229	235	241	247	253	260
5'7"		191	198	204	211	217	223	230	236	242	249	255	261	268
5'8"		197	204	210	216	223	230	236	243	249	256	262	269	276
5'9"		203	210	216	223	230	236	243	250	257	263	270	277	284
5'10"		209	216	222	229	236	243	250	257	264	271	278	285	292
5'11"		215	222	229	236	243	250	257	265	272	279	286	293	301
6'0"		221	228	235	242	250	258	265	272	279	287	294	302	309
6'1"		227	235	242	250	257	265	275	280	288	295	302	310	318
6'2"		233	241	249	256	264	272	280	287	295	303	311	319	326
6'3"		240	248	256	264	272	279	287	295	303	311	319	327	335
6'4"		246	254	263	271	279	287	295	304	312	320	328	336	344

♦ To have more energy to do the things I want to do

♦ To feel better about myself

♦ To change the way others think of me

♦ To feel more in control of my health or my life

Jot your important reasons here:

_____

_____

_____

_____

_____

_____

■ **Am I ready to make lifelong changes?** The next step is to determine whether this is a good time to start making changes in your eating and exercise. If you are not ready, you may be setting yourself up for failure. But the truth is that there will likely never be a "perfect" time. Consider the following:

♦ Do you have a support system (someone or something) that can make it easier for you to begin and continue with your changes?

♦ Are there obstacles that will keep you from becoming more active or changing the way you eat?

♦ Will worries or concerns about family, friends, work, or other commitments affect your ability to carry out your plans successfully at this time?

Table 14.2 **Weight Classifications Based on Body Mass Index**

Body Mass Index	Weight Classification	What It Means
Less than 18.5	Underweight	Unless you have other health problems, being in this weight class may not be an issue if you are small or petite.
18.5 to 24.9	Normal weight	This is the healthy range to aim for.
25 to 29.9	Overweight	This range suggests that you are carrying extra pounds. But it may not be of much concern if you are healthy and have few or no other health problems or risk factors or are physically active and have a lot of muscle.
30 to 39.9	Obese	This range signals that it is likely you have a large amount of body fat. It puts you at increased risk for weight-related health problems.
40 and over	Extremely (morbidly) obese	This weight class pinpoints that a high proportion of your body weight is fat. It puts you at very high risk of developing or complicating serious health problems.

Table 14.3 on page 241 can help you identify some of these factors. To overcome barriers, use some of the problem-solving tools found in Chapter 2.

After you have thought about these issues, you may find that now is not the right time to start. If it is not, set a future date to revisit things. Accept that this is the right decision for you at this time, and focus your attention on other goals.

If you do decide that now is the right time, start by changing the things that are simplest, easiest, and most comfortable for you. This means working on only one or two things at a time. Do not try to do too much too quickly. Remember, slow and steady wins the race.

How to Make Changes

Two important ingredients for successfully changing your weight are to start small by taking "baby steps" and make changes that you know will work. There is no getting around it. Whether you want to lose or gain weight, you will need to change the amount and perhaps the way you eat. Making changes to something as fundamental as the way you eat can be a challenge. This may seem scary, but by starting with things that are doable, you can be successful.

Start by changing only one or two things at a time. Yes, we said this before but it is really important. For instance, instead of eating 1/2 cup of rice, eat a few tablespoons less or a few tablespoons more. To eat less, try slowing down how fast you eat. To increase calories, spread out your

Table 14.3 **Factors Affecting the Decision to Gain or Lose Weight *Now***

Things That Will Enable Me to Make My Desired Changes	Things That Will Make It Difficult for Me to Change
Example: I have the support of family and friends.	*Example:* The holidays are coming up, and there are too many gatherings to prepare for.

eating over several small meals a day. Allow yourself time to get used to these changes and then slowly change other things you are doing.

Don't attempt drastic changes. If you tell yourself you are going to walk five miles (eight km) a day every day of the week and never eat potatoes or bread again, you won't be able to stick with that for very long. You probably won't lose weight, and you will feel frustrated and discouraged. But when you make a plan to have only one piece of toast at breakfast every morning instead of two and take two 10-minute walks four times a week and stick to it, you are making good, long-term changes that will translate to success.

When you change your weight slowly over time, you have a better chance of maintaining that change. This is partly because your brain begins to recognize the changes you are slowly making as part of your regular routine or habit rather than just a passing fad. The goal-setting and action-planning skills discussed in Chapter 2 will help with this. Remember, the best weight management plan combines healthy eating and exercise and is a slow, steady path that feels right to you.

Where to Start: A Food and Activity Diary

A good starting point is to keep a diary of what you eat now and how much you exercise. Do this for a week. It will help you learn where you need to make changes. Write down:

- What and where you eat
- Why you are eating (hungry, bored, habit)
- How you feel when eating (your mood or emotions)
- Your exercise (what you are doing or not doing now)

Your diary could include a section for ideas about what you would like to do differently. Don't worry; if all your ideas don't work out right away, you can always go back to them. Our sample lifestyle tracking diary may be a useful self-management tool (see Table 14.4 on page 243).

The 200 Plan

A simple and practical plan to get you started is the 200 Plan. It involves making small daily changes in what you eat and the amount of phys-ical activity you do. The 200 Plan is straightforward: to lose weight, eat 100 fewer calories a day than you do now, and burn off an extra 100 calories a day with additional exercise. Eating 100 fewer calories and burning off another 100 calories each day can add up to a 20-pound weight change over the course of a year. If you would like to gain weight, add 100 calories to your diet while keeping your exercise level at the recommended 20 to 40 minutes most days of the week. The 200 Plan is a good way to balance eating and exercise and can help you make a long-term change in your weight. Sticking to this plan on a daily basis is essential for success.

How to change what you eat by 100 calories a day

Start by checking with the food guide, Table 13.2 on pages 226–233, which gives estimated serving sizes and calories. For example, a 1-ounce (28 g) slice of bread has close to 100 calories. By not eating one of the slices of bread on your daily lunch sandwich, right there you have cut out close to 100 calories. To consume 100 additional calories, add just two tablespoons (30 mL) of nuts to your food intake over the day.

How to burn an extra 100 calories a day

Add 20 to 30 minutes to your regular aerobic exercise routine, which could be walking, bicycling, dancing, or gardening (See Chapters 7 through 9 and the following section in this chapter for more information on exercise.) Take the stairs and park farther away from the store or work. If time is an issue, doing your exercise in three 5- to 10-minute chunks throughout the day works just as well as doing it all at once.

Table 14.4 **Lifestyle Tracking Diary**

Date	Time	What I Ate	Where I Ate	Why I Ate	My Mood or Emotions	My Exercise

Exercise and Weight Loss

Exercise can help you lose weight and keep it off. But it is very difficult to exercise enough to lose weight without also changing what you eat. It is true that the more calories you burn with exercise, the more weight you can lose. However, that is only one part of the story. The most success comes from making positive exercise and eating changes that become part of your daily habits over the long term. Many studies show that it is important to eat fewer calories and be physically active. Being active will not only help you burn calories, it will also help you build muscle (which burns more calories than fat) and give you more strength and zip. You will be able to move and breathe better, and your energy level will increase. For more information about exercise and tips for choosing activities that suit your needs and lifestyle, see Chapters 7 through 9.

Aerobic exercise (see Chapter 9) that gets your heart pumping is the best for weight loss. Walking, jogging, bicycling, swimming, and dance all do the trick. These kinds of exercises help you lose weight because they use the large muscles in the body that burn the most calories. The exercise guidelines for physical fitness in Chapter 9 are also good for weight management: 150 minutes of moderate or brisk aerobic activity a week. Exercising in 10-minute bouts works as well as longer workouts. If you can add minutes to each brief workout, that is even better.

When you add more exercise to your routine, be honest with yourself about what you can do and what is safe and enjoyable for you. If you try to exercise too hard or too long for your current condition, you are more likely to stop because of an injury, fatigue, frustration, or loss of interest. Increasing your physical activity is helpful only if you do it regularly and at a pace that is right for you. Chapter 6 has useful information on pacing activity and rest that can be helpful.

Some people become discouraged when they begin a weight management effort. The pounds may not melt off right away, or weight loss may stop. This may be true even if you are still exercising and being careful about what you eat. There are many reasons why weight loss slows. Exercise may be building muscle as well as reducing fat, and muscle weighs more than fat. You could be losing fat but the scale is not showing it. If you are seeing improvements in your body measurements or notice that your clothes fit better or are looser, this can be a signal that exercise is working even when the scale seems stuck. And remember, when you exercise regularly, even if you don't lose weight, you are doing good things for your body. Regular aerobic exercise can help give you more energy and improve your sleep. It can reduce bad cholesterol and increase good cholesterol levels, reduce your risk of heart disease, and help with depression and anxiety. And it can help your chronic pain in the long run by managing symptoms such as depression and difficult emotions.

Additional Pointers for Losing Weight

■ **Set small, gradual weight loss goals.** Break the total amount of weight you want to lose into small, reachable goals. Think in terms of, say, 1–2 pounds (0.5–1 kg) a week or 5–7 pounds (2–3 kg) a month instead of looking at the total number, especially if you have a lot of weight you would like to lose. For most people, aiming to lose just a few pounds a week is realistic and doable. When you set small goals rather than large ones, your goals are more possible and practical.

■ **Identify the exact steps you will take to lose your weight.** For example, it could be sticking to the 200 plan (page 242) or walking 20 minutes a day five days a week, not eating between meals, and eating more slowly.

■ **Keep on top of what is happening.** Keep track of your weight. Weigh yourself regularly according to a schedule that works for you.

■ **Think long-term.** Instead of "I really need to lose 10 pounds right away," tell yourself, "Losing this weight gradually will help me keep it off for good."

■ **Be "in the present" when you eat.** By focusing on what you are eating and not what you are doing (such as watching television), you will enjoy the food more, become satisfied sooner, and eat less.

■ **Eat more slowly.** If you take less than 15 or 20 minutes to eat a meal, you are probably eating too fast and not taking the time to appreciate your meal. You can enjoy food more and eat less by eating more slowly. If you find it hard to slow down, try putting your fork down on the table between bites. Pick it back up only after you have chewed and swallowed the food.

■ **Become keenly aware of your stomach.** Become aware of what it feels like when your stomach is just starting to feel full. As soon you get that signal, stop eating. Learning to recognize this feeling will take attention and practice. When you feel yourself becoming full, remove your plate immediately or get up from the table if you can.

■ **Portion out your food.** Especially when you are first starting to make changes, measure out your portions. It is amazing how easily 1/2 cup of rice can "grow" to a 1-cup serving. When you can, eat food products that are already in single-size portions.

■ **Choose smaller portions.** When eating away from home, select appetizers or first courses over entrées, or order a child's meal. This will help you eat fewer calories. Over a year, it takes only an extra 100 calories a day to put on 10 pounds. That is like eating only an extra third of a bagel a day. The food guide, Table 13.2, on pages 226–233 lists common serving sizes for a variety of foods.

■ **Clock yourself.** Make it a habit to wait about 15 minutes after eating before serving yourself another portion or starting to eat dessert or a snack. You'll often find that this is enough time for the urge to eat more food to go away.

Common Challenges of Losing Weight

"I need to lose 10 pounds in the next two weeks. I want to look good for a special event."

Sound familiar? Almost everyone who tries to lose weight wants it off fast. There are hundreds of diets promising fast and easy ways to lose weight. These promises are false. There is no "magic bullet." If it sounds too good to be true, it probably is.

During the first few days of almost any weight loss plan, your body loses mostly water, along with some muscle. This can add up to 5 or even 10 pounds. Because of this, fad diets can say they are successful. But the pounds come right back on just as soon as you return to your old ways. Also, fad diets are often badly imbalanced in the kinds and amounts of foods allowed. Because of this, you may experience light-headedness, headaches, constipation, fatigue, and poor sleep.

Rather than wasting time with fad diets, do it right. Set small, realistic goals. Do action planning, and use positive thinking and self-talk (see Chapters 2 and 5). You didn't put the weight on overnight. It won't go away overnight.

"I just can't seem to lose those last few pounds."

Almost everyone reaches a point where weight loss stops despite continued hard work. These plateaus are frustrating and can make you want to give up. Plateaus are often temporary. They can mean that your body has adapted to its lower calorie intake and higher activity level. Resist the temptation to cut calories even further. This could actually make your body burn fewer calories, making more weight loss even harder.

Ask yourself whether those last 1, 2, or even 5 pounds really make a difference. If you are feeling good and doing well with your pain management, energy level, blood sugar, and other health issues, chances are you may not need to lose more weight. If you are relatively healthy, staying active, and eating a healthy diet, it is usually not bad to carry a few extra pounds. However, if you decide that those pounds must go, try the following tactics:

- Instead of focusing on weight loss, focus on maintaining the same weight for at least a few weeks. Then go back to your weight loss plan.

- Increase your physical activity. Your body may have adjusted to your lower weight and therefore needs fewer calories, so you may need to exercise more to burn more calories. Adding more exercise could help kick-start your body into burning more calories. (You can find tips for safely increasing your exercise in Chapters 7, 8, and 9.)

- Keep thinking positive. Remind yourself of how much you have achieved. Write your achievements on sticky notes and post them where you will see them.

"I always feel so deprived of the foods I love when I try to lose weight."

You are a special person. The changes you decide to make have to meet your special likes, dislikes, and needs. Unfortunately, our brains can get channeled into unproductive thoughts instead of being supportive or encouraging, especially when it comes to losing weight. Replace unproductive thoughts with positive ones that work for you (more on positive thinking can be found in Chapter 5). Here are a couple of examples:

- Replace thoughts that include the words *never*, *always*, and *avoid*. Instead, tell yourself that you can enjoy things occasionally "but a healthier choice is better for me most of the time."

- Tell yourself that you are retraining your taste buds and that making healthier choices can help you manage your weight and feel better.

"I eat too fast or I finish eating before everyone else and find myself reaching for seconds."

If you finish meals in just a few minutes or before everyone else at the table, you are most likely eating too fast. You may be doing this for a number of reasons. You may be letting yourself get too hungry because too much time passes between meals or snacks. When you finally do get to eat, you wolf food down. You may be hurried, anxious, or stressed when you sit down to eat. Slowing down your pace can help you eat less and enjoy your food more. Here are some tips for cutting down your eating speed:

- Do not skip meals. Eat regularly to avoid becoming overly hungry.

- Make it a game not to be the first person at the table to be finished eating.

- If you find yourself saying, "I think that was good; I better have more to make sure," that

usually means you aren't paying attention to what you eat. Learn to be mindful about what you are eating and how you are enjoying it. While eating, avoid being distracted by things that take your attention away from your meal, such as friends, video games, or television.

- Take small bites, chew slowly, and swallow each bite before taking another. Chewing your food well helps you enjoy your food more and feel better after the meal. It reduces heartburn or other digestive upsets.

- Try a relaxation method about a half hour before you eat. Several methods are discussed in Chapter 5.

"I can't do it on my own."

Losing weight is challenging, and sometimes you just need some outside support and guidance. For help, contact any of the following resources:

- A registered dietitian through your health plan, local hospital, or the Academy of Nutrition and Dietetics website, (www.eatright.org). In Canada, log on to the Dietitians of Canada website (www.dietitians.ca).

- A support group such as Weight Watchers or Take Off Pounds Sensibly (TOPS), where you can meet other people who are trying to lose or maintain a healthy weight.

- A weight loss program offered by your local health department, hospital, health plan, community school, or employer.

Common Challenges of Keeping the Weight Off

"I've been on a lot of diets before and lost a lot of weight. But I've always gained it back, and then some. It's so frustrating, and I just don't understand why this happens!"

This happens to many people. It is the downside of quick-loss diets, because they typically involve drastic changes. They do not focus on lifelong changes in eating habits, exercise, and lifestyle. Typically, after you have gotten tired of the diet or have reached your goal weight, you return to your old ways, and the weight comes back on. Sometimes you even gain back more weight than you lost.

The key to maintaining a healthy weight is to develop healthy eating and exercise habits that you enjoy, that fit into your lifestyle, and that you can stick with. We have already discussed some tips earlier in this chapter. Here are a few more:

- Weigh yourself regularly and set a personal weight gain "alarm." It could be a specific number of pounds gained (perhaps 3 pounds). If you hit this mark, go back on your weight management program. The sooner you start, the faster the newly added pounds will come off.

- Monitor your activity level. Exercising three to five times a week improves your chances of keeping the weight off. Research suggests that people who successfully maintain weight loss exercise nearly an hour a day. This may seem like a lot but it includes normal activities during the day as well as planned exercise. Also remember that increasing activity does not just mean exercising longer. It can mean going faster or doing something that is harder to do, such as walking uphill or swimming with paddles.

"I eat healthy food and reasonable portions for a while. Then something happens beyond my control, and I stop caring about what I eat. Before I know it, I've slipped back into my old eating habits."

Everyone is going to slip at one time or another; no one is perfect. If it was only a little slip, don't worry about it. Just get back on your plan. If the slip is bigger, try to figure out why. Is there something taking a lot of your attention now? If so, weight management may need to take a back seat for a while. That's okay. The sooner you realize this, the better. Set a date when you will restart your weight management program. If the time is right but it is still a challenge to manage your eating, you may want to join a weight loss support group. Commit for at least 4 to 6 months and look for a group that does the following:

- Emphasizes healthy eating
- Emphasizes lifelong changes in eating habits and lifestyle patterns
- Gives support in the form of ongoing meetings and/or long-term follow-up
- Does not make miraculous claims or guarantees
- Does not rely on special meals or supplements

Common Challenges of Gaining Weight

Sometimes long-term health problems make it difficult to gain weight or keep it on. Your condition or its treatment may make it hard for you to eat because you aren't hungry. Sometimes if you are sad or depressed, your body is unable to use the food it gets, or it burns up calories faster than you can replace them.

When you aren't hungry or have trouble eating, few foods sound appealing. When this happens, it is important to keep eating. You need to eat for energy and strength. That overrides making sure that what you eat is healthy. During those times, eat whatever you can. It will probably only be temporary, and then you can return to healthy eating.

With weight gain, just like with weight loss, slow and steady wins the race. Try the 200 Plan (see page 242) and eat an extra 100 calories a day every day. This alone can result in a 10-pound weight gain over a year. Choose foods that you really enjoy, focusing on your favorites. Keep easy-to-fix or already-prepared foods handy so that you don't need to spend much time cooking.

If you experience a continual or extreme weight loss or have trouble keeping weight on, you're not alone. Let's look at some common weight management challenges and some ideas for dealing with them.

"I don't know how to add calories to my current diet."

The following are some ways to increase the calories and nutrients you eat without increasing the amount of food you eat:

- Because fat gives us many more calories than carbohydrates or protein, choose foods that are higher in fat. Remember to stick with foods that contain good fats (see page 212). For example, snack on calorie-rich foods such as avocados, nuts, seeds, or nut butter.
- Eat dried fruit or nectars instead of fresh fruit or regular juice.
- Choose sweet potatoes instead of white potatoes.
- Use whole milk instead of lower-fat dairy products. Use it instead of broth or water in soups and sauces too.
- Try a liquid supplement drink with or between meals.
- Drink high-calorie beverages such as milkshakes, malts, fruit whips, and eggnog.
- Top salads, soups, and casseroles with shredded cheese, nuts, dried fruits, or seeds.

"I just don't have much of an appetite."

Check with your doctor or a registered dietitian to see if the following tips are appropriate for you:

- Eat tiny meals or smaller meals several times a day.
- Keep some nuts or dried fruit handy, and eat a few pieces each time you walk past the bowl.
- Eat the highest-calorie foods first, saving lower-calorie foods for later (for example, eat buttered bread before cooked spinach).
- Add extra whole milk or milk powder to sauces, gravies, cereals, soups, and casseroles.
- Add melted cheese to vegetables and other dishes.

Other Resources to Explore

Dietitians of Canada: www.dietitians.ca

eaTracker: www.eatracker.ca

Health Canada: www.hc-sc.gc.ca

Healthy Weight Network: www.healthyweight.net

National Weight Control Registry: www.nwcr.ws

Shape Up America: www.shapeup.org

Weight-control Information Network (WIN): www.win.niddk.nih.gov

- Use butter, margarine, or sour cream as toppings.

- Consider keeping a snack at your bedside so that you can eat something if you wake in the middle of the night.

People come in many shapes and sizes, but if they carry too much or too little weight, it can affect their pain symptoms and overall health. There is no such thing as a perfect or "ideal" weight, but rather there is a range of pounds that is good for you. Being in a healthy weight range helps you achieve overall well-being, both for your body and your mind.

The smartest and best approach to achieving a healthy weight range involves both healthy eating and being active. Once you get to your healthy weight, it is important to keep it in a good range. Choose realistic lifelong strategies that you can stick to instead of trying quick fixes, which most often do not work. Set your sights on success by building on small changes over time.

Suggested Further Reading

To learn more about the topics discussed in this chapter, we suggest that you explore the following resources:

Ferguson, James M., and Cassandra Ferguson. *Habits, Not Diets,* 4th ed. Boulder, Colo.: Bull, 2003.

Hensrud, Donald D., ed. *Mayo Clinic Healthy Weight for Everybody.* Rochester, Minn.: Mayo Clinic Health Foundation, 2005.

Nash, Joyce D. *Maximize Your Body Potential,* 3rd ed. Boulder, Colo.: Bull, 2003.

Schoonen, Josephine Connolly. *Losing Weight Permanently with the Bull's-Eye Food Guide.* Boulder, Colo.: Bull, 2004.

Zentner, Ali. *The Weight-Loss Prescription: A Doctor's Plan for Permanent Weight Reduction and Better Health for Life.* Toronto: Penguin Canada, 2013.

CHAPTER 15

Managing Your Medicines

You MAY BE TAKING ONE OR MORE MEDICATIONS for chronic pain. You may also be taking medicines for other medical conditions. It is a very important management task to understand your medications and to use them appropriately. This chapter will provide general guidelines to help you do just that. Be sure to read this chapter first before reading Chapter 16. That chapter provides information on medicines used for chronic pain specifically.

A Few General Words About Medications

Few products are more heavily advertised than medications. If you read a magazine, listen to the radio, or watch TV, you see a constant stream of ads. These are aimed at convincing you that if you just use this pill, your symptoms will be cured. "Recommended by 90 percent of the doctors asked," they say. But be aware that they may have asked doctors who work for the company that makes the pill, or only a handful of doctors. And have you noticed that in TV ads, the benefits are presented in a slow, upbeat voice, while the side effects are recited very rapidly? It can be very confusing.

Your body is often its own healer. Given time, many common symptoms and disorders improve. The prescriptions filled by the body's own "internal pharmacy" are frequently the safest and most effective treatment. Patience, careful self-observation, and monitoring with your doctor are often excellent choices.

Medications can be an important part of managing a chronic condition—but they do not cure it. Medications generally serve one or more of the following purposes:

- **To relieve symptoms.** A nitroglycerin tablet expands the blood vessels, allowing more blood to reach the heart, thus quieting angina. Acetaminophen (Tylenol®) can relieve pain. An antidepressant medicine can lighten depression and improve mood.

- **To prevent further problems.** For example, medications that thin the blood help prevent blood clots, which cause strokes and heart and lung problems.

- **To improve or slow the progress of a disease.** Nonsteroidal anti-inflammatory drugs (NSAIDS) can help arthritis by quieting the inflammatory process. Likewise, antihypertensive medications can lower blood pressure.

- **To replace substances that the body is no longer producing adequately.** Insulin is used to manage diabetes and thyroid medication for underactive thyroid.

When you take medication to relieve symptoms such as pain, depression, or anxiety, you expect to get relief from your symptoms right away. But sometimes, medication has to build up in your body before you will experience relief. It is important to talk with your doctor or nurse practitioner about how long you need to take the medicine before deciding whether or not it is right for you.

When a medication's purpose is to lessen the consequences of disease or slow its course, you may not be aware that the medication is doing anything. This may make you think that the drug isn't working. It is important to continue taking your medications, even if you cannot see or feel how they are helping. If this concerns you, ask your health care provider.

Modern society pays a price for having such powerful pharmaceutical tools at our disposal. Besides being helpful, all medications have undesirable side effects. Some of these effects are predictable and minor, and some are unexpected and life threatening. Approximately five to ten percent of all hospital admissions are due to drug reactions. At the same time, not taking medications as prescribed is also a major cause of hospitalization.

Medication and Your Mind: Expect the Best

Medication affects your body in two ways. The first is determined by the chemical nature of the medication. The second is triggered by your beliefs and expectations. Your beliefs and confidence can change your body chemistry and your symptoms. This reaction, called the placebo effect, is an example of how closely the mind and body are connected.

Many studies have shown the power of the placebo—the power of mind over body. When people are given a placebo (pill containing no medication), some of them improve anyway. Placebos can relieve back pain, fatigue, arthritis, headache, allergies, hypertension, insomnia, asthma, irritable bowel syndrome and chronic digestive disorders, depression, anxiety, and pain after surgery. The effect will not last indefinitely but it may last for some time. The placebo effect clearly demonstrates that our positive beliefs and expectations can activate our self-healing mechanisms. You can learn to take advantage of your powerful internal pharmacy.

Every time you take a medication, you are swallowing your expectations and beliefs as well as the pill. So expect the best! Let's look at some ways to do that.

- **Examine your beliefs about the treatment.** If you tell yourself, "I'm not a pill taker" or "Medications always give me bad side effects," how do you think your body is likely to respond? If you doubt that the prescribed treatment is likely to help your symptoms or condition, this negative attitude will undermine the ability of the pill to help you. You can change these negative images into more positive ones. Review the discussion of positive thinking in Chapter 5 for guidance on how to do this.

- **Think of your medications the way you think of vitamins.** Many people associate healthful images with vitamins. Taking a vitamin makes you think you are doing something positive to prevent disease and promote health. If you regard your medications as aids to restore and promote health, like vitamins, you may obtain more powerful benefits.

- **Imagine how the medicine is helping you.** Develop a mental image of how the medication is helping your body. For example, if you are taking a pain medication, tell yourself that it is finding its way through your central nervous system and closing the pain gate. For some people, forming a vivid physical image is helpful. An antibiotic, for example, might be seen as a broom sweeping germs out of the body. Don't worry whether your image is medically correct. It's your belief in a clear, positive image that counts.

- **Keep in mind why you are taking the medication.** You are not taking your medication just because your health care provider told you to. You are taking your medication to help you live your life. Therefore it is important to understand how the medicine is helping you. Use this information to help the medicine do its job. Suppose a man with lower back pain is given an antidepressant medication to improve his pain and his mood. He has been told it will make him feel drowsy and dizzy and it will cause him to have a very dry mouth. So of course, that is what he thinks about and that is what happens. But suppose he is also told that the symptoms will likely be only temporary, and that they mean the drug is building up to a therapeutic level in his body. In a few weeks he should start to experience an improvement in his pain and mood.

These side effects indicate that the drug is starting to work. He can then take actions to counter these effects and often have an easier time tolerating them. (See Chapter 16, page 276, for tips on how to manage pain medications.)

Taking Multiple Medications

People with chronic pain often have other health problems. When this is the case, they often take many medications: analgesics for pain, medications to lower blood pressure and cholesterol, drugs to elevate mood or manage depression, antacids for heartburn, plus a handful of over-the-counter (OTC) remedies and herbs. The more medications (including vitamins and OTC remedies) you take, the greater the risk of unpleasant reactions. Also, not all drugs work together well, and when they are taken together, they sometimes cause problems. Fortunately, it is often possible to take fewer medications and lower the risks. However, you should not do this without the help of your doctor or nurse practitioner. Most people would not change the ingredients in a complicated cooking recipe or throw out a few parts when fixing something in the car. It is not that these things can't be done. It is just that if you want the best and safest results, you may need expert help.

Communicating about Medication

As a self-manager, you need to know about your medications in order to successfully manage them. How you respond to any one medication depends on your age, your metabolism, your daily activity, the waxing and waning of your symptoms, your chronic conditions, your genetics, and your frame of mind. To make sure you get the most from your medications, your doctor depends on you. Report what effect, if any, each drug you take has on your symptoms, as well as any side effects. Based on this critical information, your doctor may decide to continue, increase, discontinue, or otherwise change your medications. In a good doctor-patient partnership, there is an ongoing exchange of useful information.

Unfortunately, this vital communication is often neglected. Studies indicate that fewer than five percent of patients getting new prescriptions ask any questions about them. Doctors tend to interpret patient silence as understanding and satisfaction. Problems occur when patients do not receive enough information about medications or do not understand how to take them. In addition, all too often people do not follow instructions. Safe, effective drug use depends on your health care provider's expertise. But equally important is your understanding of when and how to take the drug. You must ask questions, and you must take the necessary precautions. (The discussion about communication in Chapter 11 can help.)

Some people are afraid to ask questions. They are afraid they will seem foolish or stupid or be perceived as challenging the doctor's authority. But asking questions is a necessary part of a healthy relationship with your health care provider.

The goal of treatment is to maximize the benefits and minimize the risks. This means taking the fewest medications, in the lowest effective doses, for the shortest period of time. Whether the medications you take are helpful or harmful often depends on how much you know about them and how well you communicate with your doctor and other health care providers.

What to Tell Your Health Care Provider

Even if your doctor or nurse practitioner doesn't ask, there is certain vital information about medications you should mention during every consultation.

Tell your health care provider if you are taking any other medications

List all the prescription and nonprescription medications you are taking, including birth control pills, vitamins, aspirin, antacids, laxatives, alcohol, and herbal remedies. An easy way to do this is to maintain an updated list of all medications along with the amount you take (dosage) and bring it with you to all medical appointments. Or bring all your medications with you. Saying that you are taking "the little green pills" isn't very helpful.

Communication about all the medications you take is especially important if you are seeing more than one health care provider. Each caregiver may not know what the others have prescribed. Knowing all your medications and supplements is essential for correct diagnosis and treatment. For example, if you have symptoms such as nausea, diarrhea, sleeplessness or drowsiness, dizziness, memory loss, impotence, or fatigue, they may be caused by a drug side effect rather than your chronic pain or other conditions. If your health care provider does not know all your medications, he or she cannot interpret your symptoms appropriately or protect you from drug interactions.

Tell your health care provider if you had allergic or unusual reactions to any medications

Describe any symptoms or unusual reactions caused by medications. Be specific: report which medication (if you know) and exactly what type of reaction. Developing a rash, fever, or wheezing after you take a medication is often a sign that you have had a true allergic reaction. If you experience any of these symptoms, call your doctor at once. Nausea, diarrhea, ringing in the ears, light-headedness, sleeplessness, and frequent urination are likely to be side effects rather than true drug allergies but you still want to mention them when you discuss medications with your provider.

Tell your health care provider what other medical conditions, besides your chronic pain, you have

Many diseases can interfere with the action of a drug or increase the risk of using certain medications. Diseases involving the kidneys or liver are especially important to mention because they can slow the metabolism of many drugs and increase toxic effects. Your provider may also avoid prescribing certain medications if you have or have had such diseases as high blood pressure, peptic ulcer disease, asthma, heart disease, diabetes, or prostate problems. Be sure to let them know if you are possibly pregnant or are breastfeeding. Many drugs cannot be safely used in those situations.

Tell your health care provider what medications were tried in the past to treat your condition(s)

It is a good idea to keep your own records of your previous prescriptions as well as your current medications. Knowing what has been tried and how you reacted will help guide the provider's recommendation for any new medications. However, the fact that a medication was not effective in the past does not necessarily mean it can't or shouldn't be tried again. Chronic pain and other diseases change, and the same medication may work the second time.

What to Ask Your Doctor, Nurse Practitioner, or Pharmacist

There is important information you need to know about your medications as a self-manager. When you discuss medications with your doctor, nurse practitioner, or pharmacist (learn more about pharmacists in the "A Special Word about Pharmacists" box in this chapter), ask the following questions:

Do I really need this medication?

Some providers prescribe medications not because it's really necessary but because they think patients want and expect drugs. Don't pressure your provider for medications. Many new medications are heavily advertised and promoted by their manufacturers. Quite a few heav-

ily marketed and prescribed medications were later found to be so hazardous that they were withdrawn. So be cautious about requesting the newest medications. Know your options. When any treatment is recommended, ask what is likely to happen if you forego or postpone treatment. Although sometimes a powerful medication is called for, other times the best medicine is none at all. If your provider doesn't prescribe a medication, consider that good news. Ask about nondrug alternatives. For chronic pain, lifestyle changes such as exercise, diet, and stress management may have better results than medications.

What is the name of this medication, and what dosage do I take?

Keep and regularly update a record of each medication you take. Note its brand name, if any; the generic (chemical) name; and the dosage prescribed (for example: Tylenol®, acetaminophen, 200 mg three times a day). Check your order when you receive it from the pharmacy. If the medication doesn't match the information in your records, ask the pharmacist to explain the difference. This is your best protection against medication mix-ups.

What is this medication supposed to do and how fast will it work?

Your health care provider should tell you why the medication is being prescribed and how it might help you. Is the medication intended to prolong your life, relieve symptoms, or improve your ability to function? For example, if you are given a medicine for high blood pressure, it is primarily to prevent later complications (such as stroke or heart disease) rather than to stop a headache. On the other hand, if you are given a pain reliever such as ibuprofen (Motrin®), the purpose is to help ease the headache. You should also know how soon you should expect results. Drugs that treat infections or inflammation may take several days to a week to show improvement. Antidepressant and some chronic pain and arthritis drugs typically take several weeks to start providing relief.

How and when do I take this medication, and for how long?

If medications are going to be effective, you must take them *when* you are told to, *in the amounts* you are told to, and *for as long as* you are told to take them. This is crucial to safe and effective use. Does "every 6 hours" mean every 6 hours while awake or every 6 hours around the clock? Should the medication be taken before meals, with meals, or between meals? What should you do if you accidentally miss a dose? Should you skip it, take a double dose next time, or take it as soon as you remember? Should you refill and continue taking the medication until you have fewer symptoms or until you finish the current medication? Some medications are prescribed on an as-needed basis. For these medications, you need to know when to begin and end treatment and how much medication to take. Work out a plan with your provider to suit your individual needs.

It is vital to take all medications properly. Yet nearly 40 percent of people report that their doctors failed to tell them how to take a medication or how much to take. If you are not sure about your prescription, contact your doctor, nurse practitioner, or pharmacist.

What foods, drinks, other medications or activities should I avoid while taking this medication?

Food may help protect the stomach from some medications, but certain foods can also make some drugs ineffective. For example, milk products or antacids block the absorption of the antibiotic tetracycline. This drug is best taken on an empty stomach. Some medications may make you more sensitive to the sun, putting you at increased risk for sunburn. Ask whether a medication will interfere with driving or operating machinery safely, or if alcohol should be avoided while taking it. Other drugs, even recreational or over-the-counter drugs, can either amplify or lessen the effects of the prescribed medication. Taking aspirin along with an anticoagulant medication, for example, can result in possible bleeding. The more medications you are taking, the greater the chance of an undesirable drug interaction. Ask about possible drug-drug and drug-food interactions.

What are the most common side effects, and what should I do if they occur?

All medications have side effects. You need to know what symptoms to look for and what to do if they develop. Should you seek immediate medical care, discontinue the medication, or call your provider? While the doctor or nurse practitioner cannot be expected to describe every possible adverse reaction, the most common and important ones should be discussed. Unfortunately, a recent survey showed that 70 percent of people starting a new medication did not recall being told about precautions and possible side effects by their physicians or pharmacists. It may be up to you to ask.

Are there any tests necessary to monitor the use of this medication?

Most medications are monitored by whether symptoms improve or worsen. However, some medications can disrupt body chemistry before any symptoms develop. Sometimes these adverse reactions can be detected by laboratory tests such as blood counts or liver function tests. In addition, the levels of some medications in the blood need to be measured on a regular basis to make sure you are getting the right amounts. Ask your provider if the medication has any of these special requirements.

If I decide I don't want to take this medication for a while or not at all, can I just stop cold turkey?

If a drug does not seem to be improving your pain or other symptoms, is not allowing you to do more, or is causing unacceptable side effects, you may be tempted to stop taking it. Some drugs, especially for chronic pain and some other conditions, cannot be stopped suddenly. They need to be "tapered" by reducing the dosage gradually. Tapering needs to be done under the supervision of your health care provider. It is important that you do not attempt this by yourself. Talk to your provider about which drugs need to be tapered and how this can be done safely.

Is there a less expensive alternative or generic medication for this medication?

Almost every drug has at least two names: a generic name and a brand name. The generic name is the drug's chemical name. It is used to refer to the medication in the scientific literature. Generic names are also used for certain drugs that are not marketed under a brand name. The brand name is the unique name given to the drug by its developer. When a drug company develops a new drug in the United States, it is granted exclusive rights to produce that drug for 17 years. If a drug is developed in Canada, the exclusive rights are for 20 years. After this period, other companies may market chemical equivalents of that drug. These generic medications are generally considered as safe and effective as the original brand-name drug but often cost much less. In some cases, your provider may have a good reason for preferring a particular brand. Even so, if cost is a concern, ask if a less expensive but equally effective medication is available.

You may also be able to save money by knowing how to use your insurance to your advantage. For example, your copayment may be less if you obtain your medications from a company designated by your insurer. Also, many pharmacies have discount programs for seniors and individuals with low income. It pays to ask and then ask again. And it is wise to shop around. Even in the same town, different stores may sell the same medication at different prices

Do you have any written information about this medication?

Your doctor or nurse practitioner may not have time to answer all your questions. You may not remember everything you heard. Fortunately, there are many other good sources of information, including pharmacists, nurses, package inserts, pamphlets, books, and websites. Several useful sources are listed at the end of this chapter.

How to Read the Prescription Label

One great source of information is the prescription label. The following illustration will help you read the labels on your prescriptions.

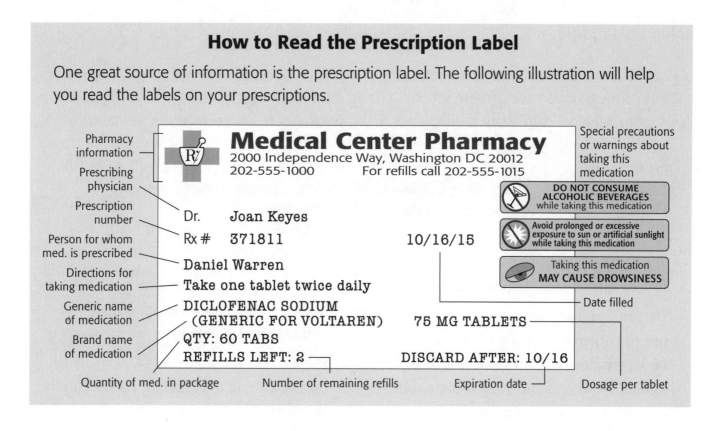

Taking Your Medicine

No matter what the medication, it won't do you any good if you don't take it. Nearly half of all medicines are not taken as prescribed. There are many reasons why people don't take their prescribed medication: forgetfulness, lack of clear instructions, complicated dosing schedules, bothersome side effects, cost, and so on. Whatever the reason, if you are having trouble taking your medications as prescribed, discuss this with your health care provider. Often simple adjustments can make it easier. For example, if you are taking many different medications, sometimes one or more can be eliminated. If you take one medication three times a day and another four times a day, your provider may be able to simplify the regimen. He or she may even prescribe

medications that you need to take only once or twice a day. Understanding more about your medications, including how they can help you, may help motivate you to take them regularly.

If you are having trouble taking your medications, ask yourself the following questions and discuss your answers with your provider or pharmacist:

- Do you tend to be forgetful?

- Are you confused about the instructions for how and when to use the medications?

- Is the schedule for taking your medications too complicated?

- Do your medications have bothersome side effects?

A Special Word About Pharmacists

Pharmacists are an underutilized resource. These professionals have gone to school for many years to learn about medications. They know how drugs act in your body and how medications interact with each other. Your pharmacist is an expert and can readily answer questions face-to-face, over the phone, or even via e-mail. In addition, many hospitals, medical schools, and schools of pharmacy have medication information services that you can call to ask questions. As a self-manager, don't forget pharmacists. They are important and helpful consultants.

- Is your medicine too expensive?

- Do you feel that your condition is not serious or bothersome enough to need regular medications? (With some diseases such as high blood pressure, high cholesterol, or early diabetes, you may not have any symptoms.)

- Do you feel that the medication is unlikely to help?

- Are you denying that you have a condition that needs medication?

- Have you had a bad experience with the prescribed medicine or another medication?

- Do you know someone who had a bad experience with the medication, and are you afraid that something similar will happen with you?

- Are you afraid of becoming addicted to the medication?

- Are you embarrassed about taking the medication, view it as a sign of weakness or failure, or fear you'll be judged negatively if people know about it?

- What are some of the benefits you might get if you take the medication as prescribed?

Self-Medication: OTC, Nonprescription, and Recreational Drugs

You may take nonprescription or over-the-counter (OTC) medications or herbs. In every two-week period, nearly 70 percent of people will take a nonprescription drug. Many OTC drugs are highly effective and may even be recommended by your health care provider. But if you self-medicate, you should know what you are taking, why you are taking it, how it works, and how to use the medication wisely.

More than 200,000 nonprescription drug products are offered for sale to the American public, representing about 500 active ingredients. In Canada, there are more than 15,000 nonprescription drug products available and 40,000 natural health products.

Nearly 75 percent of the public receives its education on OTC drugs solely from TV, radio, newspaper, and magazine advertising. The main

Remembering to Take Your Medicines

The following are some suggestions to help you remember to take your medications:

- **Make it obvious.** Place the medication or a reminder next to your toothbrush, on the breakfast table, in your lunch box, or in some other place where you're likely to "stumble over" it. (But be careful where you put the medication if children are around.) Or you might put a reminder note on the bathroom mirror, the refrigerator door, the coffee maker, the television, or some other conspicuous place. If you link taking the medication with some well-established habit such as meal times or watching the nightly news on television, you'll be more likely to remember.

- **Use a checklist or an organizer.** Make a medication chart listing each medication you are taking, the amount you take, and the time when you take it. Another option is to check off each medication on a calendar as you take it. You can purchase a medication organizer at the drugstore. This container separates pills according to the time of day you need to take them. You can fill the organizer once a week so that all your pills are ready to take at the proper time. A quick glance at the organizer lets you know if you have missed any doses and prevents double dosing. There are also websites that have printable charts to help you track your medications. PictureRx (https://mypicturerx.com) is one, but it requires a subscription. The American Chronic Pain Association (ACPA) is another (theacpa.org/communication-tools). See especially its MedCard and CARE Card.

- **Use an electronic reminder.** Get a watch or mobile phone that you can set to beep at pill-taking time. There are also high-tech pill containers that beep at a preset time to remind you to take your medication. If you have a smartphone, you can download an app that reminds you to take your medication.

- **Have others remind you.** Ask members of your household to remind you to take your medications at the appropriate times.

- **Don't run out.** Don't let yourself run out of your medicines. When you get a new prescription, determine the day when the pills will run out and mark one week before that date on your calendar. This will serve as a reminder to order your next refill. Don't wait until you take the last pill. Some mail-order pharmacies offer automatic refills, so your medications arrive when you need them.

- **Plan before you travel.** If you plan to travel, put a note on your luggage reminding you to pack your pills. Also, take along an extra prescription in your carry-on bag in case you lose your pills or your checked luggage.

message of drug advertising is that for every symptom, every ache and pain, and every problem, there is a pharmaceutical solution. While many OTC products are effective, many are simply a waste of your money. They may also keep you from using better ways to manage your condition.

If you are taking prescribed medications or using OTC medications or herbs, here are some helpful suggestions:

- **If you are pregnant or nursing, have a chronic disease, or are already taking multiple medications, consult your doctor or nurse practitioner before self-medicating.** Your provider will know if the OTC remedy will interfere or interact badly with your condition or prescription medications.

- **Always read labels and follow directions carefully.** Reading the label, including a review of the individual ingredients, may prevent you from taking medications that have caused problems for you in the past. It may also prevent double dosing on medications that you may already be taking.

A Special Word About Alcohol and Recreational Drugs

The use of alcohol and recreational drugs (both illegal drugs and prescription medications used for nonmedicinal purposes) has been increasing in recent years, particularly among people over the age of 60. These drugs, whether legal or illegal, can cause problems. They can interact with prescription medications, making them less effective or even causing harm. They can fog judgment and cause problems with balance. This can in turn cause accidents and injure both you and others. In some cases, alcohol or recreational drugs can make existing long-term conditions worse. Alcohol use is associated with increased risk of hypertension, diabetes, gastrointestinal bleeding, sleep disorders, depression, erectile dysfunction, breast and other cancers, and injury.

Ideally, you should limit alcohol use to no more than two drinks per day. "At risk" alcohol use for women is drinking more than seven drinks per week or more than three drinks per day; for men it's more than 14 drinks per week or more than four drinks in a day. This means that women of any age and anyone over age 65 should average no more than one drink per day and men under 65 should have no more than two drinks per day on average.

Consider the following two pieces of advice:

- If you are at the "at risk" level for alcohol or are regularly using recreational drugs, seriously consider cutting down or stopping their use. For more information about medical marijuana and chronic pain, see Chapter 16, page 275.

- Talk to your doctor or nurse practitioner about your use of these drugs. Health care providers are often hesitant to raise the issue because they don't want to embarrass you. It is up to you to bring up the subject. Providers will be very willing to talk about it. They have heard it all, and they will not think less of you. An honest conversation may save your life.

For example, aspirin and acetaminophen (Tylenol®) are popular medications for pain, but they are also ingredients in over-the-counter products such as cold remedies. If you don't understand the information on the label, ask a pharmacist before buying it.

- **Do not exceed the recommended dosage or length of treatment.** Only do so if you have discussed the change with your doctor or nurse practitioner.

- **Use caution if you are taking other medications.** Over-the-counter and prescription drugs can interact, either canceling or exaggerating the effects of the medications. If you have questions about drug interactions, ask your provider or pharmacist before mixing medicines.

- **Try to select medications with a single active ingredient rather than combination ("all-in-one") products.** When using a product with multiple ingredients, you are likely to be treating symptoms you don't even have. Why risk the side effects of medications you don't need? Single-ingredient products also allow you to adjust the dosage of each medication separately for optimal symptom relief with minimal side effects.

- **When choosing medications, learn the ingredient names and try to buy generic products.** Generics contain the same active ingredient as the brand-name product, usually at a lower cost.

- **Never take a drug from an unlabeled container or a container whose label you cannot read.** Keep your medications in their original labeled containers, or transfer them to a labeled medication organizer or pill dispenser. Do not mix different medications in the same container.

- **Do not take medications that were prescribed for someone else.** Even if you have similar symptoms, this is never a safe practice.

- **Drink at least a half glass of liquid with your pills.** After swallowing, remain standing or sitting upright for a short while. This can prevent the pills from getting stuck in your throat.

- **Store your medications where children or young adults cannot find them.** Poisoning from unsecured medications is a common problem among young children. Teens and young adults sometimes steal prescription drugs from relatives or the relatives of friends for recreational use. Despite its name, the bathroom medicine cabinet is not usually an appropriate place to store medications. A kitchen cabinet or toolbox with a lock is a safer option.

Medications can help or harm. What often makes the difference is the care you exercise and the partnership you develop with your doctor.

Other Resources to Explore

American Chronic Pain Association: www.theacpa.org/Communication-Tools

Health Canada—Drugs and Health Products:
www.hc-sc.gc.ca/dhp-mps/index-eng.php

Health Canada—Healthy Living: Safe Use of Natural Health Products.
www.hc-sc.gc.ca/hl-vs/iyh-vsv/med/nat-prod-eng.php

MedlinePlus—Drugs, Supplements, and Herbal Information:
www.nlm.nih.gov/medlineplus/druginformation.html

National Institutes of Health—Rethinking Drinking: Alcohol and Your Health:
www.rethinkingdrinking.niaaa.nih.gov

Natural Medicines Comprehensive Database:
www.naturaldatabaseconsumer.therapeuticresearch.com

Ontario Ministry of Health and Long Term Care—MedsCheck:
www.health.gov.on.ca/en/public/programs/drugs/medscheck

PictureRx: https://mypicturerx.com

The National Center for Complementary and Alternative Medicine (NCCAM):
www.nccam.nih.gov

WebMD—Drugs and Medications A–Z: www.webmd.com/drugs

Suggested Further Reading

To learn more about the topics discussed in this chapter, we suggest that you explore the following resources:

Castleman, Michael. *The New Healing Herbs: The Essential Guide to More Than 125 of Nature's Most Potent Herbal Remedies*, 3rd ed. New York: Rodale, 2010.

Graedon, Joe, and Teresa Graedon. *Best Choices from the People's Pharmacy*. New York: NAL, 2008.

Griffith, H. Winter, and Stephen W. Moore. *Complete Guide to Prescription and Nonprescription Drugs, 2014*. New York: Perigee Books, 2013.

Physicians' Desk Reference. *The PDR Pocket Guide to Prescription Drugs*, 10th ed. Montvale, N.J.: PDR Network, 2012.

Raman-Wilms, Lalitha. *Practical Guide to Drugs in Canada: Understanding Prescription and Over-the-Counter Drug Treatments for Everyday Ailments and Diseases*, 1st ed. Toronto: Dorling Kindersley, 2011.

Shane-McWhorter, Laura. *The American Diabetes Association Guide to Herbs and Nutritional Supplements*. Alexandria, Va.: American Diabetes Association, 2009.

Silverman, Harold M. *The Pill Book*, 15th ed. New York: Bantam Books, 2012.

CHAPTER 16

Medicines and Treatments for Chronic Pain

THERE ARE TWO STEPS TO MANAGING YOUR MEDICATIONS for chronic pain. First, you need to be informed about medicines in general and how to manage any medicine you might be taking. The second step is to be aware of the specific medications you are taking for your chronic pain condition and the intended goals of your treatment.

Please review Chapter 15 before you read this chapter. Chapter 15 contains essential information about medications in general, taking multiple medications, communicating with your doctor, nurse practitioner, or pharmacist, and self-medicating. Once you have read Chapter 15, you will be able to better understand the material in this chapter about specific medications and other treatments for chronic pain.

Special thanks to Dr. Norman Buckley, MD, FRCPC, Professor and Chair, Department of Anesthesia, Michael G. DeGroote School of Medicine, McMaster University, for his help with this chapter.

Taking Medicines for Chronic Pain

Pain medicines (which are called analgesics) and other medications can be helpful for many people with chronic pain, but they do not help everybody. Also, it is rare for medication alone to eliminate chronic pain completely. And, of course, each person may respond differently to medications. In fact, for some people, pain medicines may actually worsen pain or other symptoms over time and cause unpleasant or serious side effects. That's why it is important to balance the risks and benefits of pain medication. It is also the reason why medication is just one part of managing chronic pain along with all the other approaches discussed in this book.

Also, recall from Chapter 15 that expecting the best from your medicines is important. If you have a firm conviction that pain medicines are not for you, speak to your doctor. Your pain medicines are unlikely to work to best effect if you have negative beliefs about them. Instead focus on the many other ways to manage your pain and symptoms.

In this chapter, we talk about the medicines most commonly used to treat chronic pain and other symptoms. We do not talk about medicines that treat underlying disease conditions. (If you have angina pain, see Chapter 19.)

Treating the Disease or Treating the Pain?

Some chronic pain is the result of a known disease process. Rheumatoid arthritis is an example. The underlying cause of the pain is well understood, and there are established treatments for that cause. Medication taken to treat the disease process may also reduce the pain from the disease.

But many chronic pain conditions are not the result of a well-understood disease (see Chapter 1). The pain itself is the "disease" or the condition. With these types of pain problems, medicines are given not to treat a specific disease but to help reduce pain, increase comfort, manage other symptoms, and improve everyday functioning.

Pain from Damage to Tissues or Damage to Nerves?

When doctors or other health care providers prescribe medication for pain, they first need to decide on the most likely origin of the injury or potential injury that results in pain. The two major pain classifications that doctors use are called nociceptive pain and neuropathic pain.

Nociceptive pain is a result of damage or potential damage to tissues of the body, such as skin, muscle, joints, and bones. Nociceptive pain is also referred to as tissue-related pain. Nociceptive pain is usually due to an injury or illness that causes inflammation. Inflammation is a normal biological response: more blood is sent to the site of injury; chemicals are released that stimulate nerve endings, making the area more sensitive and painful; and fluid accumulates, causing swelling. The body's inflammatory response to injury is essential for healing, but when inflammation does not disappear over time, it can result in chronic pain. Common examples of nociceptive or tissue-related pains are back pain, whiplash, and arthritis.

Neuropathic pain is usually due to damage or potential damage to nerves or the central nervous system itself. This can involve the abnormal firing of nerves anywhere between the tips of your fingers or toes to the top of your head. Neuropathic pain is also referred to as nerve-related pain. Some examples are nerve damage after surgery or traumatic accident, post-stroke pain, shingles, diabetic neuropathy, and phantom limb pain.

Some people experience a combination of nociceptive and neuropathic pain after some surgeries or other injuries. It can also develop when pain from damaged tissues persists for a long time and leads to changes in the central nervous system and brain, which causes the body to interpret even normal sensation as painful.

Understanding the type of pain you have—whether it's due to actual or potential tissue damage, nerve damage, or both—will help you better understand why your health care provider suggests certain medications and not others for you.

Mood Disorders, Mental Health Conditions, and Pain Medication

As discussed in Chapters 4 and 5, mood disorders such as depression and anxiety can affect how a person responds to pain. So can schizophrenia, obsessive compulsive disorder, post-traumatic stress disorder, and addiction to alcohol or other drugs. These conditions can also affect how a person will respond to pain medication. While addressing a chronic pain condition, it is important to recognize and treat these other conditions with appropriate medications or counseling as well. Even if depression

or anxiety did not appear until the pain condition started, these mental health conditions may be sufficiently severe that they should be treated specifically and not just left to "get better" when the pain gets better. That is why it is essential to talk with your health care providers about how you are feeling emotionally, along with how the pain is affecting you physically.

Over-the-Counter Medicines, and Natural Products

Over-the-counter (OTC) medicines are those you can purchase without a prescription. It is important to *always* read the labels and know what the ingredients mean. Many over-the-counter medications contain ingredients that are the same as or similar to those contained in prescription medications, just in different (usually lower) doses. For example, many cold remedies also contain acetaminophen or aspirin. Some natural supplements for pain contain things like willow bark extract, which is the original source of acetylsalicylic acid (ASA or aspirin). To prevent or minimize drug interactions or the potential for overdose of some substances, your doctor and pharmacist need to know all the medications, natural products, and supplements you are taking. Review Chapters 11 and 15 for more suggestions on communicating with your health care provider about medication.

Nociceptive Pain Medications

Recall that nociceptive pain typically results from actual or potential damage to tissues due to an injury or illness. Examples of nociceptive

pain include lower back pain, whiplash, and arthritis. Various types of medications are prescribed for nociceptive pain.

Topical Pain Relievers, Acetaminophen, and Anti-inflammatory Drugs

The medical treatment for mild nociceptive (tissue-related) pain often begins with over-the-counter topical pain relievers. These are also called topical analgesics. These come in many forms—creams, liniments, gels, sprays, and patches. You apply them to your skin over a painful muscle or joint. They work by stimulating nerve endings to cause feelings of warmth, cold, or even itching to close the pain gate. There are many of these products on the market. Talk to your doctor, nurse practitioner, or pharmacist about which topical analgesic might be best for you.

Always read the label—as you should with all medications. Some topical agents contain a nonsteroidal anti-inflammatory drug (NSAID), such as diclofenac in over-the-counter Voltaren®. Other topical medicines contain aspirin-like substances called salicylates that can cause the same adverse effects as aspirin if taken in large quantities. If you are already taking aspirin or NSAID tablets—either prescription or over-the-counter—do not use topical pain relievers without telling your doctor. You may be exceeding the recommended daily dosage of these drugs if you take pills and apply a lotion or rub. *Do not* apply a topical analgesic to a wound, to broken skin, or to the face. After application, be sure to wash your hands to avoid getting these products in your eyes.

Another related group of pain relievers is over-the-counter analgesics such as acetaminophen (Tylenol®, Panadol®) or NSAIDs such as aspirin, ibuprofen (Motrin®, Advil®), and naproxen (Aleve®). As we just noted, NSAID is the brief way to refer to a nonsteroidal anti-inflammatory drug. NSAIDs are the drug of choice if your pain is due to inflammation. Even though these drugs are easy to purchase, they have potentially serious side effects, including stomach upset and bleeding, and they can affect your body's blood clotting ability. If you have a history of stomach ulcers, kidney problems, or risk factors for heart disease or are taking blood thinners, you need to be careful with these medicines. In addition, if you smoke, drink alcohol, or are over 65 years of age, you need to be careful taking aspirin or any NSAID. Talk to your doctor or pharmacist about safe dosages.

If you take acetaminophen, the amount you take is very important. Too much can cause liver problems in some people. This is a potentially serious issue for those who drink alcohol daily. Too much acetaminophen can also increase the risk of high blood pressure, heart attack, kidney problems, and bleeding ulcers. Discuss the amount you should take with your health care provider.

In some countries, such as Canada, you can buy over-the-counter acetaminophen or aspirin together with low-dose codeine (such as 222s or Tylenol® #1) in pharmacies. Codeine is an opiate (see "Opioid Medications" later in this chapter) and can cause constipation and drowsiness.

Prescription Anti-inflammatory Drugs

Some versions of over-the-counter NSAIDs are obtained by prescription. They are usually given for mild to moderate nociceptive pain due to injuries or inflammation. Examples include diclofenac (Voltaren®) and indomethacin (Indocid®, Indocin®). The same precautions for over-the-counter NSAIDs apply for these medications. If you are older or have had stomach ulcers, kidney problems, high blood pressure, or risk for heart disease, use with caution. Always take NSAIDs with food, and always report stomach upset to your doctor right away. Sometimes a doctor may give you a medication to protect your stomach when prescribing these drugs. Some NSAIDs also come in a prescription topical form to rub into painful joints or muscles. Pennsaid®, for example, contains a higher concentration of diclofenac than over-the-counter Voltaren®.

COX-2 inhibitor drugs are a newer group of NSAIDs. Celecoxib (Celebrex®) appears to have less risk of causing stomach ulcers than other NSAIDs, but it has been shown to increase the risk of cardiovascular problems such as heart attack. Your doctor will assess your risk of cardiovascular problems before prescribing this drug.

Muscle Relaxants

Muscle spasms can be a problem with such pain conditions as chronic neck or lower back pain and fibromyalgia. Spasms can also add to the discomfort for people with multiple sclerosis or spinal cord injuries. Medications such as baclofen (Lioresal®), cyclobenzaprine (Flexeril®), tizanidine (Zanaflex®), methocarbamol (Robaxin®, OTC Robaxacet®), and others can provide some relief from muscle spasm, and some have pain-reducing properties as well. For people with musculoskeletal pain such as neck and back pain, these medications may be most helpful for acute flare-ups. They are not generally recommended for chronic pain.

The main side effects of all muscle relaxants are drowsiness and dizziness. These medicines do not work directly on the muscles; rather, it is thought they work at the level of the brain

and cause sedation. Avoid driving, operating machinery, or other activities that require alertness until your response to drugs is known. These drugs should be taken with caution if you are on opioids. (We discuss opioids in more detail later in this section.)

Tramadol and Tapentadol

Tramadol (Tramacet®, Ralivia®, Zytram®, Tridural®) is similar to opioid pain relievers (see below). It is available with or without acetaminophen.

Tramadol has been available internationally for almost 30 years and is used for many types of moderate to severe pain, including lower back pain, osteoarthritis, fibromyalgia, and some neuropathic pain (see page 273). The side effects of tramadol are mainly drowsiness, nausea, and headaches, but it does not involve the same risks of stomach, liver, heart, or kidney side effects as NSAIDs or acetaminophen. Tramadol may interact with some kinds of antidepressants to increase certain side effects. These can be mild, such as shivering or diarrhea, or more serious, such as muscle rigidity or seizures. Talk to your doctor or call 911 right away if these serious side effects occur. The risk of addiction is low for tramadol.

Tapentadol (Nucynta®, Nucynta® ER) is a drug with two actions, one on opiate receptors (see below) and the other on receptors common to some anti-depressant medications. It is used to treat moderate to severe chronic pain.

Opioid Medications

Opioids are among nature's most powerful pain relievers. There is evidence that these drugs can benefit some people (but not all) who have severe

Short-Acting and Long-Acting Medications

Tramadol, tapentadol, and some opioid pain medications come in two forms: short acting and long acting. Short-acting drugs relieve pain within 15 to 30 minutes and have their best effect within one to two hours. To maintain pain relief, these drugs need to be taken every three to four hours. Doctors usually prescribe short-acting pain medicines for acute pain and for moderate to severe chronic pain to test whether the drug works before prescribing a long-acting medicine.

Long-acting (also called slow-release) pain medicines release the active drug slowly into the body. Most of these drugs provide steady pain relief for 8 to 12 hours, and some provide relief up to 24 hours or even days. Doctors usually prescribe long-acting drugs to be taken at regularly scheduled times, such as every 12 hours or once daily. Long-acting pain medications are best for people who have continuous moderate to severe chronic pain. Long-acting drugs that come in pill form should be swallowed whole and not broken, chewed, dissolved, or crushed. Tampering with the pill can lead to rapid release of the drug in your body and a potentially fatal dose.

chronic pain. Opioid medications are manufactured synthetically as well as from the sticky sap of poppy seed pods. Your body contains several types of receptors for these drugs (called opiate receptors), and different drugs have slightly different effects depending upon which receptor is most strongly affected by the drug. Examples of prescription opioids include codeine, oxycodone, morphine, hydromorphone, fentanyl, methadone, and buprenorphine. Except for methadone, these are all short-acting drugs. Some of them are available in slow-release forms as patches that release medication over several days to a week.

Opioid abuse is a growing problem. To get "high," some people crush or chew tablets for a more rapid onset and greater effect. This has led to the creation of so-called "tamper resistant" formulations such as OxyNEO (oxycodone), as well as restrictions on the availability of some drugs to reduce the rising number of overdose deaths.

Doctors administer opioids by starting with a low dose and then gradually increase the dose. They do this within certain limits until the chronic pain is relieved or unacceptable persistent side effects occur or the drug is not working. Examples of opioid side effects are nausea, dizziness, sleepiness, confusion, and constipation. Most of these side effects can be reduced or made more tolerable by carefully managing the dosage. Starting at a low dose is important because when taken in too high a dose at first, opioids can cause severe breathing problems. In extreme cases, breathing can even stop. Table 16.1 lists very important guidelines to follow when you are prescribed opioids by your doctor.

When people first start taking opioids for pain or when their dose is adjusted, they must be very careful driving or using machinery until they become accustomed to the effect of the new dose. Most people also have to take some

Table 16.1 **Opioids: Minimizing Risks**

Opioids can be part of a safe overall plan for pain management,
but when you use them, you must take care and pay attention.

Avoiding Risk to Yourself	■ Assess your known risk of addiction. (Do you have a personal or family history of alcohol or other drug abuse; history of physical, emotional, or sexual abuse in the past; or are you subject to depression?) Talk to your doctor. ■ You and your doctor should discuss and set goals for treatment. ■ Only one doctor should be prescribing your opioid. ■ Take your medication exactly as prescribed. ■ Fill all your prescriptions at the same pharmacy. ■ Urine and blood screening may be used to identify potential problems. ■ Anticipate and learn to manage common side effects such as constipation as soon as you begin the drug.
Avoiding Risk to Others	■ Do not share opioids with others—it is against the law and could seriously harm or kill them. ■ Take your prescription to a pharmacy to be filled as soon as possible. Do not leave an unfilled prescription where other people could find it and fill it for misuse. ■ Keep drugs securely stored at home in a locked box or cabinet to prevent accidental poisoning or potential misuse by others. ■ Return unused medications to the original pharmacy.
Avoiding Withdrawal Symptoms	■ Understand that symptoms will occur if you stop using your opioid. ■ Withdrawal symptoms can be uncomfortable and include nausea, diarrhea, chills, and flu-like symptoms. ■ When the time comes to stop using the opioid, know that your body has become used to the drug; your dose must be decreased slowly (tapered) under your doctor's direction.
Avoiding Overdose	■ Overdose means your ability to think clearly is impaired and your breathing could slow down or stop. This may cause brain damage, coma, and death. ■ Opioids can be safe over long periods but can be dangerous when you first start taking them or increase your dose. ■ Avoid mixing painkillers with alcohol or other drugs; this increases the risk of overdose. ■ If you or your family members notice that you show the following signs: slurred speech, crying or becoming upset easily, poor balance, or "nodding off" during conversation or activity, contact your doctor. ■ If you or your family members notice that you show signs of extreme sleepiness or they have difficulty rousing you, call 911 or other emergency services.
Travel	■ Keep your opioids in the original container from the pharmacy. ■ If you fly, keep your opioids with you in your carry-on luggage. ■ Bring a letter from your doctor documenting your need for opioids, especially if you are traveling outside your state, province, or country.

medication for constipation while taking opioids. When taken as directed, opioids do not usually cause any stomach, heart, liver, or kidney damage even over many years of use. However long-term studies in Europe show some evidence that using opioids over years may alter hormone function in both men and women. Hormonal changes may impact mood, sexual function, and fertility and increase fatigue and pain. Long-term opioid use may also accelerate osteoporosis.

Current guidelines from the United States and Canada (see Other Resources at the end of this chapter) suggest that most patients achieve adequate pain-relieving effect with a dose between 50 and 120 mgs per day of morphine or its equivalent in another drug. Higher doses increase the risk of side effects and complications, up to and including death from overdose. If higher doses of opioids are considered, it should be done only in consultation with a qualified pain specialist.

Severe chronic pain may be treated by slow-release, long-acting opioids in the form of pills or patches. These are usually taken regularly such as every 12 hours or once daily. (See page 270).

Psychological Dependence: Addiction to Opioids

One of the risks of taking opioids is the possible development of addiction. This risk may be greater in people with a history of alcohol or drug abuse (either personally or in the family), or in those who have had negative childhood experiences (physical, emotional or sexual abuse), or are subject to depression. Even when it is appropriate to treat pain with opioids, opioid prescription is complex if the patient has a history of addiction or other psychological disorders.

When we speak about addiction, we are talking about psychological dependence, or craving for the drug that is not related to the desire for pain relief. Addiction is now known to be a disease in which the drug changes the way your brain feels about pleasure and it is associated with many factors. Addiction is characterized by one or more of the following behaviors:

- **Impaired control over drug use.** Examples include repeated requests for prescriptions, using more than one doctor to obtain more drug, or using street drugs.

- **Compulsive use of the drug.** The person uses the drug all the time even when other therapies or techniques for pain management are more appropriate.

- **Continued use of the drug.** Use continues despite harm to self or others.

- **Craving for the drug.** A craving is defined as an intense desire to use the drug for the "high" feeling the drug provides.

Although it is difficult to estimate the risk of drug addiction in people with chronic pain, the consequences of addiction are very serious and sometimes fatal. It is crucial to take medications as prescribed, to monitor yourself and your behavior, and to see your doctor on a regular basis so he or she can carefully observe your response to the medication.

How to Minimize Prescription Opioids

Studies show that opioids only reduce pain by about 30%, often less. People can quickly get into the trap of thinking they just need more opioids to reduce their pain but studies show that more opioids increase health risks without better managing pain. It's important to know about the risks of opioid medication. Most people are aware that opioids carry a risk of addiction, but there are many other health risks such as disturbed sleep, sleep apnea, constipation, drug interactions, reduced fertility, hormone changes, and mood changes. These risks vary by your age, sex, and the other medications you are taking. It's important to discuss your risks with your doctor.

Often people will begin an opioid prescription and continue it for years or decades without gaining any real benefit in pain reduction. Sometimes people continue opioid medications out of fear that their pain will increase if they stop them. Studies have shown the opposite—people on high doses of opioids can have significant reductions in pain when opioids are reduced or stopped. The key is to taper wisely, and resources exist to help you with that. If you decide to take opioids, regularly take stock about how much they are helping. Ask your doctor if the benefits outweigh the risks. At the same time continue to focus on ways other than using medications to manage your pain and other symptoms. (See Chapters 4 and 5). If you use these to lower your pain a bit you will probably need less medication.

Many people want to take less opioids or stop taking them altogether. If you are interested in this, talk with your doctor. There are lots of helpful resources. One of these is an excellent book by Beth Darnall referenced at the end of this chapter.

Physical Dependence: Withdrawal from Opioids

Physical dependence is another notable effect of opioids. If you are taking opioids on a regular basis for pain, your body becomes accustomed to them. If you decrease your dosage or stop the medication, you will feel quite ill for a number of days. This is called withdrawal. Experiencing withdrawal does *not* mean that you are addicted. Withdrawal is unpleasant but usually not dangerous. However, withdrawal *may* be dangerous for people with heart disease and during pregnancy. If you are on an opioid and it is not decreasing your pain or improving your quality of life, or you wish to stop the drug or are advised to do so, you must see your doctor. Do not stop taking these drugs suddenly by yourself. Recall from Chapter 15 that some drugs need to be "tapered" by reducing the dosage gradually. Tapering needs to be done under the supervision of your doctor. Talk to your doctor about which drugs need to be tapered and how this can be done safely.

Tolerance to Opioids: Reduced Drug Effect

A third effect of opioids is called tolerance. This happens when a person needs more drug to achieve the same pain relief as a lower dose used to provide. This usually occurs when a person has been on opioids for a long time. Some people benefit from the same dose of an opioid for years, while others begin to need increasing amounts. Increasing the dose can lead to unacceptable side effects. Like physical dependence, tolerance is not addiction. If you need increasing amounts of medication to relieve your pain, talk to your doctor.

Neuropathic Pain Medications

As we discussed earlier in the chapter, neuropathic pain is usually due to damage or potential damage to nerves or the central nervous system. Neuropathic pain can involve the abnormal firing of nerves anywhere on your body. Examples of neuropathic pain include nerve damage after surgery, post-stroke pain, and shingles. Various types of medications are prescribed for neuropathic pain.

The initial treatment of neuropathic (nerve-related) pain may differ from the treatment of nociceptive (tissue-related) pain. Neuropathic pain may or may not respond to aspirin, acetaminophen, or NSAIDs. Some types of neuropathic pain can he helped with topical medications such as capsaicin (Zostrix®). Capsaicin is the chemical in chili peppers that causes burning when eaten. Lidocaine, a local anesthetic that is available in a skin patch or as a cream or gel, is also sometimes effective in treating neuropathic pain. In addition to helping with nociceptive pain, tramadol or tapentadol (see page 269) can also help some types of mild to moderate neuropathic pain.

Doctors usually begin the treatment of neuropathic pain with medications called adjuvants. These drugs were invented to treat other medical problems but turned out to have pain-relieving effects. To treat more severe kinds of nerve pain, adjuvants are often combined or used together with opioids (see page 269). Adjuvants include antidepressants and antiepileptic drugs. We discuss these drugs and others in the material that follows.

Antidepressants

Certain antidepressant medications called tricyclics (TCAs) and serotonin norepinephrine reuptake inhibitors (SNRIs) have an effect on pain that is separate from their effect on depression. If you are prescribed one of these drugs for your pain, it does not mean you are clinically depressed or that your physician believes your pain is "only in your head." To relieve pain, TCAs and SNRIs are usually prescribed at a lower dosage than when they are used to treat depression.

A third common class of antidepressants is selective serotonin reuptake inhibitors (SSRIs). SSRIs have not been found to be very effective as pain relievers, but if you have both pain and depression, they may be used to treat the depression along with other medications directed at the pain.

Examples of TCAs include amitriptyline (Elavil®), nortriptyline (Aventyl®), and desipramine (Norpramin®). Doctors prescribe TCAs for moderate pain. These drugs can be beneficial for people suffering from neuropathy, shingles, fibromyalgia, and some types of headache, facial pain, and lower back pain. TCAs are also useful for people who experience insomnia or sleeping

Why More than One Drug?

Depending on the source and mechanism of pain, there are several kinds of drugs that could be used to treat any given problem.

Sometimes combining two drugs at a low dose brings more effective relief than increasing the dose of one of them. This approach can have fewer side effects. It is very difficult to predict exactly who will respond to what drug or what combination of drugs, so it may be necessary to try a variety of drugs and combinations to find the best effect. For severe chronic pain, it often takes two or three medications used in combination to get the best balance of pain relief versus acceptable side effects. Work with your doctor and other health care providers to achieve the best result.

problems. It is important to note that moderate amounts of caffeine (more than two cups of coffee a day) may limit the pain-relieving effect of TCAs. If your doctor prescribes a TCA for you, limit your caffeine intake. (See Chapter 13, page 219, on ways to help you cut down on caffeine.)

Examples of SNRIs include venlafaxine (Effexor®), duloxetine (Cymbalta®), and bupropion (Wellbutrin®). A doctor may prescribe a SNRI if TCAs have not been effective in treating your pain.

Like opioids, the dosage for most antidepressants starts low and is increased slowly until either the dosage is effective or an intolerable side effect occurs. Side effects of antidepressants include drowsiness, dizziness, nightmares, confusion (in the elderly), dry mouth, and constipation.

Antiepileptic Drugs (AEDs)

The antiepileptic family of medications (also called anticonvulsant drugs) was initially used to treat epileptic seizures. Doctors discovered that AEDs also help some people with a variety of neuropathic pain. The two AEDs that doctors most often prescribe today are gabapentin (Neurontin®) and pregabalin (Lyrica®). The dosage for these two AEDs is increased gradually to decrease the initial side effects, such as drowsiness and dizziness. In some individuals these AEDs also cause weight gain or leg swelling. Older AEDs that are sometimes still used today are carbamazepine (Tegretol®) and valproic acid (Depakene®). Newer AEDs include topiramate (Topamax®, often prescribed for migraine prevention), lamotrigine (Lamictal®), oxcarbazepine (Trileptal®), and levetiracetam (Keppra®). Carbamazepine, valproic acid, and lamotrigine are also used as mood stabilizers for patients who suffer from bipolar mood disorders. Gabapentin and pregabalin may help to alleviate symptoms of anxiety in addition to their pain-relieving effect.

Cannabinoids (THC) Available by Prescription

Cannabinoids come from the sticky resin of the flowering tops of marijuana plants. There are research studies in the United States, Canada, and elsewhere investigating the potential role of cannabinoids for the management of chronic pain. Some studies suggest cannabinoids may be helpful for some neuropathic pain conditions, but

Personalized Medicine

Exciting new developments are happening in the field of genetics that may one day affect how we use medicine to treat pain. Based on a person's genetic makeup, it may be possible to predict who will respond to a certain type of drug and who will not. Doctors could then avoid prescribing a drug that will not work. In the future, these new developments may make it much easier to prescribe the right drug to a person in pain.

studies of effects on other types of pain have been inconclusive. Currently there are two pill forms of cannabinoids available, dronabinol (Marinol®) and nabilone (Cesamet®). There is also a liquid form for spraying in the cheek called Sativex®. The main side effect of cannabinoids is drowsiness. There are other potentially harmful physical and psychological side effects such as heart and blood pressure problems, impaired mental functioning, panic attacks, and depression. There is also a potential for addiction in people who are at risk for opioid addiction.

There are people who advocate smoking marijuana for pain. This is a controversial area of medicine, but scientific research studies are investigating the role of marijuana for chronic pain management. Some U.S. states and European countries have legalized marijuana both for medical and social use, and Canadian law currently permits use of marijuana for medical reasons with the support of a physician. But quite a bit of uncertainty about this practice remains. If marijuana is bought on the street, there is no way to know for sure how strong it is and what other chemicals may have been sprayed onto the plants as they grew. Processes are underway to better regulate the growing, dispensing, and quality and content of the drug.

Tips on Taking Medications for Pain

Most medications for chronic pain are meant to be taken on a regularly scheduled basis. Others may be prescribed on an as-needed basis. If you have medicine to take as needed when your pain is starting to escalate, don't put off taking it. It takes less medication to prevent severe pain from coming back then it does to treat pain that has gotten out of control.

All medications have side effects. Most of these effects decrease if your doctor slowly increases the dosage of the medication over time. When starting a new pain medication, try to put up with these early side effects for at least one to two weeks before giving up. Do not drive or perform other activities requiring close attention such as operating equipment if you are feeling drowsy or after a recent dose change.

A common side effect of many pain medications is dry mouth. To help with this problem, use good oral hygiene with frequent mouth rinses; keep a bottle of water with you; and try chewing sugarless gum. Another common problem caused by many medications, especially opioids, is constipation. Talk to your doctor or pharmacist about how to manage this side effect as soon as you are given a prescription for an opioid. The *Opioid Induced Constipation Conversation Guide* at www.theacpa.org/Communication-Tools can also help you with this self-management task.

Opioids are powerful drugs and need to be respected. While they can be a safe part of a pain management plan, they have also been associated with an unprecedented number of deaths due to misuse, diversion for sale on the street, and mixing with other substances. As noted earlier in this chapter, always keep all medications—especially opioids—in a secure location (not just the family medicine cupboard), and take care at the pharmacy to avoid being the target of criminal activity.

Medication for chronic pain works best when combined with exercise, psychological approaches, and other techniques and treatments described elsewhere in this book.

Other Treatments for Chronic Pain

In addition to medicines, your primary doctor, pain specialist, or other health care provider may suggest other types of interventions to treat your chronic pain. These treatments include a variety of physical, psychological and medical therapies, and self-management tools that we discuss in detail in the following material.

Acupuncture

Acupuncture is the practice of inserting thin, solid needles into one or more of 361 specific points in the skin that lie along "meridians"—lines of energy flow in the body. The area where the needles are inserted are stimulated when a practitioner twirls the needles for brief periods. The needles are so thin that virtually no pain is felt when administered by a qualified practitioner.

Acupuncture originated in China and has been used for thousands of years. Scientists are not exactly sure how it works, but they think that the needle stimulation may release endorphins and other pain-relieving substances to close the gate in the spinal cord. (See page 6). Recall from Chapter 1 that endorphins are neurochemicals that serve as the body's natural painkillers. Acupuncture may also activate the immune system and improve blood flow. Another contributing factor to the effectiveness of acupuncture may be the person's belief that it will help them. This placebo response is exactly the same as believing that medicines will work. Again, this is another example of how powerful our mind can be. (See Chapter 15, pages 252–253.)

Much research on acupuncture has been conducted in the United States, Canada, and Europe over the past 40 years. There is now solid evidence that the procedure can help some people with chronic back and neck pain, shoulder pain, osteoarthritis, and chronic headache. It is not known if acupuncture is helpful for fibromyalgia. Acupuncture is now routinely used in the United States military for pain management. As with any treatment, if you decide to have acupuncture, be sure to seek a qualified practitioner. In the United States, contact the National Certification Commission for Acupuncture and Oriental Medicine (www.nccaom.org) or the American Academy of Medical Acupuncture (www.medicalacupuncture.org). In Canada, contact the Acupuncture Foundation of Canada Institute (www.afcinstitute.com).

Exercise

Exercise is an essential component of chronic pain treatment for everyone. Various types of movement, physical activity, and exercise are discussed in Chapters 7, 8, and 9. Effective exercises include the gentle Moving Easy Program, balance exercises, aerobic activity such as walking, biking, and water aerobics, as well as resistance or weight training, yoga, and tai chi. There are many people who can help you develop a physical activity program that is right for you. Review these chapters to incorporate exercise into your overall pain treatment plan.

Injections, Nerve Blocks, and Surgery

Pain treatment options include injecting medications into painful areas of the body, injecting medications around certain nerves, surgically inserting an electrical device or medication pump into the spinal canal, or surgically cutting nerves.

Trigger point injections are injections of anesthetic into so-called trigger points, which are hard knots of muscle, ligaments, or tendons. These painful trigger points can be caused by direct pressure on a muscle, chronic muscle tension, abnormal posture, or prolonged muscle fatigue. Injecting trigger points with anesthetic

can result in temporary relief of pain. This pain relief can in turn allow the person to stretch and exercise to improve their function. Trigger points can also be managed with massage, exercise, and relaxation techniques.

A nerve block is an injection of an anesthetic or steroid medicine into an area of the body such as a sore joint, or into the space around the spinal cord. This technique has been used for more than 50 years for lower back pain, neck pain, and arthritis. Results are varied; some people experience pain relief while others do not. If there is relief, it can last from hours to days to weeks, but the effect is temporary.

For more severe pain problems, surgeons insert an electrical device called a spinal cord stimulator around the spinal canal. This reduces pain signals going to the brain. Another option is a surgically implanted small pump that delivers pain medications (such as local anesthetic and opioids) directly into the spinal fluid. Both of these techniques are very expensive and do not help everyone who undergoes the procedures. Cutting nerves surgically is usually a treatment of last resort in patients with terminal cancer who have severe pain.

Manual and Other Physical Therapies

Manual or hands-on therapy can consist of mobilization, manipulation, and massage. Mobilization involves gently moving a joint through its existing range of motion. Manipulation is a more forceful movement of a joint, sometimes beyond its range of motion. Both mobilization and manipulation can improve the range of motion of a joint, allow increased movement and activity, and reduce pain.

Massage is a form of hands-on therapy that works on the muscle and other soft tissue. It has been studied a lot and it has few risks. There are many kinds of massage therapy, including Swedish massage, sports massage, lymphatic drainage, and massage that focuses on trigger points. Massage can help relax muscles and tissues and improve blood flow to an area. It is helpful for people with chronic lower back pain, chronic neck pain, and osteoarthritis of the knee, and it may also help reduce depression. It may temporarily reduce pain, fatigue, and other symptoms for people with fibromyalgia. Studies are currently being done to assess its impact on headache.

Spinal manipulation has been studied and found to be helpful for chronic lower back pain, and it may be helpful for chronic tension-type headaches, neck-related headache, and the prevention of migraines. While it is safe for most people if performed by a qualified practitioner, there are some risks. See the National Institutes of Health fact sheet *Chiropractic: An Introduction* (www.nccam.nih.gov/health/chiropractic/introduction.htm).

Your health care provider might suggest techniques for pain management that you can do at home. One of the most common is transcutaneous electrical nerve stimulation, or TENS. With TENS, a small, battery-powered machine about the size of a pocket radio transmits electrical impulses that counteract pain. You connect two electrodes from the machine to your skin, near where you are feeling pain. When the machine is turned on, you will feel a tingling sensation or vibration that may mask pain signals. While this treatment does not help everyone, it does have some advantages. It is easy to learn, safe, inexpensive, and within your control. It can be set for different wavelength frequencies and intensities so that you can experiment with the setting that works best.

Manual therapy can be conducted by a variety of licensed health care providers, including physical therapists, chiropractors, osteopaths, and registered massage therapists. As with any treatment, be sure to seek a qualified practitioner by going to your state or provincial certification boards.

Psychological Therapies

Treatment for the body is only one part of managing chronic pain. You also need to be sure your mind and your emotions are doing okay. As discussed in Chapter 5, at times you may need help dealing with your thoughts, emotions, and feelings. This is where psychologists can be very helpful. Psychologists are highly–trained therapists who specialize in human behavior and emotional health. Talk to your health care provider about how you are feeling. He or she can ask you questions to determine if you may have an underlying depression or other disorder that can be medically treated. If you need help dealing with your emotions and stress, he or she can help you locate a qualified health psychologist in your area, or you can contact your state or provincial licensing body to find a psychologist with expertise in chronic pain.

One of the most frequently used therapies for chronic pain is cognitive-behavioral therapy, or CBT. This approach is based on the idea that what we think and feel influences how we behave, and how we behave influences our thoughts and feelings. CBT helps people think realistically about their pain by encouraging them to examine their thoughts, feelings, and behavior, including their stress responses and make positive changes. Researchers have found that CBT reduces depression and anxiety, disability, and negative or catastrophic thinking and improves everyday functioning in people who suffer from many kinds of chronic pain. This includes people who have pain conditions including lower back pain, headaches, arthritis, mouth or face pain, and fibromyalgia.

With other therapies in addition to CBT, psychologists help people learn specific ways to manage their stress responses and quiet their nervous system. Sometimes, relaxation techniques can be improved by coaching from a therapist. Coaching can be for individuals or groups. A biofeedback machine is another tool used to manage stress. In biofeedback, sensors record bodily processes such as heart rate, skin temperature, and muscle tension. Through relaxation approaches such as deep breathing and focused attention, a person can produce changes in the body and mind that improve pain and other symptoms. The biofeedback machine helps people to see how this works by recording changes that occur in the body when relaxation techniques are used.

Pain Clinics and Rehabilitation Programs

Pain clinics offer a variety of treatments and education. Some clinics are staffed only by pain physicians who offer expert advice on medications and other medical procedures, such as trigger point injections and nerve blocks. The best programs have a multidisciplinary team that may include psychologists, physical and occupational therapists, social workers, nutritionists, pharmacists, specialist nurses, exercise specialists, and others. Multidisciplinary pain programs use a combination of the treatments and techniques described in this book. Although these programs are usually for people with severe chronic pain, there are also pain assessment services and short programs for people who are less disabled by their chronic pain.

Ask your doctor or health care provider if a pain clinic is an option for you. He or she should be able to refer you to one that addresses your specific pain problem. Pain clinics are in most U.S. states and Canadian provinces. If your doctor is not able to help, try contacting your local hospital, medical school, or pain-related organizations.

Chronic pain affects everyone differently. There are a variety of medicines, treatments, and resources to help you. Finding the right combination takes patience and persistence. Work closely with all your health care providers so that you can find ways to manage your pain and do the things you want to do every day.

Other Resources to Explore

American Academy of Pain Medicine: www.painmed.org/patientcenter

American Chronic Pain Association, Resource Guide to Chronic Pain Medication & Treatment: www.theacpa.org/Consumer-Guide

American Pain Society: www.americanpainsociety.org

American Psychological Association (APA): www.apa.org

Canadian Guideline for Safe and Effective Use of Opioids for Chronic Non-Cancer Pain: www.nationalpaincentre.mcmaster.ca/documents/opioid_guideline_part_b_v5_6.pdf

Canadian Pain Society: www.canadianpainsociety.ca

Canadian Psychological Association (CPA): www.cpa.ca

Clinical Guidelines for the Use of Chronic Opioid Therapy in Chronic Noncancer Pain: www.americanpainsociety.org/uploads/pdfs/Opioid_Final_Evidence_Report.pdf

National Center for Complementary and Alternative Medicine, Acupuncture May be Helpful for Chronic Pain: www.nccam.nih.gov/research/results/spotlight/091012

National Center for Complementary and Alternative Medicine, Chronic Pain and Complementary Health Approaches: www.nccam.nih.gov/health/pain/chronic.htm

National Center for Complementary and Alternative Medicine, Massage Therapy for Health Purposes: www.nccam.nih.gov/health/massage/massageintroduction.htm

WebMD, Pain Clinic Overview: www.webmd.com/pain-management/guide/pain-clinics-overview

Suggested Further Reading

To learn more about the topics discussed in this chapter, we suggest that you explore the following resources. See also the suggested readings and other resources for Chapter 15.

Darnall, Beth. *Less Pain, Fewer Pills: Avoid the Dangers of Prescription Opioids and Gain Control over Chronic Pain*. Boulder, Colo.: Bull Publishing, 2014.

Foreman, Judy. *A Nation in Pain: Healing Our Biggest Health Problem*. New York: Oxford University Press, 2014.

CHAPTER 17

Making Treatment Decisions

YOU HEAR ABOUT NEW TREATMENTS, new drugs, nutritional supplements, and alternative treatments all the time. Hardly a week goes by without a new medical discovery of some kind showing up in the news. Drug and nutritional supplement companies run television commercials and place large ads in newspapers and magazines. E-mail inboxes are filled with promises of cures from spammers. You are bombarded with promotions for over-the-counter alternative treatments in the market and pharmacy. Your health care providers may recommend new procedures, medications, or other treatments that you don't know much about.

What can you believe? How can you decide what treatments to try?

An important part of managing your own care is being able to evaluate claims or recommendations so you can make informed decisions about your own health. It is easy to think that a special diet or new treatment may be the answer to chronic pain. We all want the "magic bullet" that will take the pain away. Unfortunately, this seldom happens with chronic pain.

In this chapter, our aim is to help you learn to ask the right questions so you can better evaluate claims and suggestions. If you are able to gather the right information, you are one step closer to making the right decisions for you and being a successful self-manager.

Questions to Ask about Treatments for Chronic Pain

There *are* treatments out there that may help you manage your pain better. But before you explore your options, you need to know how to evaluate what you hear and read. Ask yourself these important questions before making a decision about any treatment, whether it is a mainstream medical treatment or a complementary or alternative approach.

Where did I learn about this treatment?

Did your doctor or other health care provider suggest it? Was it reported in a scientific journal? Or did you read about it in a supermarket tabloid, print or TV ad, website, or flyer you picked up somewhere?

The source of the information is important. Results that are reported in a respected scientific journal are more credible than those you might see in an ad or supermarket tabloid article. Journals such as the *New England Journal of Medicine, Lancet,* and *Science* are very careful about what they approve for publication. Other scientists thoroughly review research studies before they appear in these publications. Many alternative treatments and nutritional supplements, in contrast, have not been studied scientifically. These alternative options are not as well represented in the scientific literature as medical treatments are. If you hear about something outside of a reputed mainstream media source, a scientific journal, or your doctor's office, you need to be extra careful about analyzing what you read or hear.

In reported studies, were the people who got better similar to me?

In the past, studies were often done primarily on college students, nurses, or white men. This has changed, but it is still important to find out if the people whose pain improved are like you. Are they members of the same age group, sex, and race? Did they have the same health problems as you do? Do they have similar lifestyles? If the subjects of the study aren't like you, you may not experience the same results that they did.

Could anything else have caused the positive changes attributed to the treatment?

A woman returns from a two-week stay at a spa in the tropics and reports that her chronic pain improved dramatically thanks to the special diet and supplements she received. But did the warm weather, relaxation, and pampering have even more to do with her improvement than the supplements or the diet?

If you experience positive results after starting a particular treatment, it is important to look at other things that have changed in your life.

It is common to take up a generally healthier lifestyle when starting a new treatment. Could that be playing a part in the improvement? Did you start another medication or treatment at the same time? Has the weather improved? Are you under less stress than you were before you started the treatment? Can you think of anything else that could have affected your health?

Does the treatment suggest stopping other medications or treatments?

Does a treatment that you are considering require that you stop taking another basic medication because of dangerous interactions? If the other medication is important, discuss this new treatment in detail with your health care provider before making a change.

Does the treatment suggest eating a less-than-well-balanced diet?

Some treatments may suggest that you eliminate some important nutrients or stress only a few nutrients. Maintaining a balanced diet is important for your overall health. If you change your eating habits, be sure you're not sacrificing important vitamins. Don't put excessive stress on your body by concentrating on only a few nutrients to the exclusion of others.

Can I think of any possible dangers or harm that may come from the treatment?

All treatments have side effects and possible risks. Discuss these matters thoroughly with your health care provider. Only you can decide if the potential problems are worth the possible benefit, but you must have all the information in order to make that decision.

Many people think that if something is natural, it must be good for you. This may not be true. "Natural" isn't necessarily better just because it comes from a plant or animal. The powerful heart medication digitalis comes from a plant, but the dosage must be exact or it can be dangerous. Some treatments may be safe in small doses but dangerous in larger doses.

The sale of supplements is not regulated the way the sale and distribution of medications is. Only a few countries (such as Canada and Germany) have a regulatory agency responsible for determining if what is listed on the label of a nutritional supplement is actually what's in the bottle. (See Chapter 13, page 206, for information about regulations.) Do some research about the company selling the product before you try it. Ask your doctor or pharmacist before adding any supplement to your medication regime, even if it is "natural" or herbal.

Am I willing to take on the trouble and/or expense of the treatment?

Do you have the money to give this treatment the time it needs to produce an improvement? Is your health strong enough to maintain this new regimen? Do you have the necessary support in place? Will you be able to handle it emotionally? Will this put a strain on your relationships at home or work?

If you decide to try a new treatment after asking yourself all these questions, it is very important to inform your health care provider about it. After all, you and your provider are partners, and you will need to keep your partner informed on your progress during the time you are taking the treatment.

Finding Out More about Treatment Options

The Internet is a useful resource for up-to-date information about these treatments. But be cautious. Not every piece of information on the Internet is correct or even safe. Seek out the most reliable sources by noting the author or sponsor of the site and the URL (Internet address). As we discussed in Chapter 3, addresses ending in .edu, .org, and .gov are generally more objective and reliable; they originate from universities, nonprofit organizations, and governmental agencies, respectively. Some .com sites can also be good, but because they are maintained by commercial (for-profit) organizations, their information may be biased in favor of their own products.

The National Center for Complementary and Alternative Medicine (NCCAM) is an excellent source of up-to-date reliable information about chronic pain and complementary treatments. This National Institutes of Health agency rigorously studies the usefulness and safety of complementary and alternative interventions. The webpage "Chronic Pain and Complementary Health Approaches: What You Need to Know" (nccam. nih.gov/health/pain/chronic.htm) is updated frequently because research in this area is growing quickly. Check this website every few months to keep up with the latest information on what might help chronic pain. Another source for useful information about questionable treatments is Quackwatch, a nonprofit corporation whose purpose is to combat health-related frauds, myths, fads, and fallacies (www.quackwatch.org).

Just as you should be vigilant when researching alternative treatments, you should be careful about more common treatments as well. Sometimes it is wise to refuse conventional medical treatments. For example, after reviewing the medical evidence, various medical specialty organizations have recommended that nearly 50 common treatments and procedures should *not* be done (see www.choosingwisely.org).

Making decisions about new treatments can be difficult, but a good self-manager asks the questions presented in this chapter and follows the decision-making steps in Chapter 2 to achieve the best personal results. For more information on finding reliable informational resources, see Chapter 3.

Other Resources to Explore

American Board of Internal Medicine Foundation's Choosing Wisely: www.choosingwisely.org

ConsumerLab: www.consumerlab.com

Health Canada's Licensed Natural Health Products Database:
www.hc-sc.gc.ca/dhp-mps/prodnatur/applications/licen-prod/lnhpd-bdpsnh-eng.php

National Center for Complementary and Alternative Medicine:
www.nccam.nih.gov and nccam.nih.gov/health/pain/chronic.htm

Quackwatch: www.quackwatch.org

CHAPTER 18

Managing Specific Chronic Pain Conditions

Arthritis, Back Pain, Fibromyalgia, Headache, Pelvic Pain, and Chronic Regional Pain Syndrome

*I*N THIS CHAPTER WE DISCUSS some of the more common and prevalent conditions that result in chronic pain. The more you can learn about how to recognize your particular symptoms and triggers, the better you can positively self-manage your condition and live a full and satisfying life. All of the conditions that cause chronic pain can also cause fatigue, loss of strength and endurance, and emotional distress. As we discussed in the first chapter of this book, the healthy way to live with chronic pain is to work at managing the physical, mental, and emotional concerns rooted in your particular condition. We hope the material in this chapter will help you rise to the challenge of learning how to function at your best even in the face of chronic pain and ultimately help you to achieve the things you want to do and to get pleasure from life.

Arthritis

Arthritis is a disease that causes joint and musculoskeletal pain. It consists of more than 100 different conditions that affect all ages, races, and genders. The most common form of chronic arthritis is osteoarthritis. Generally affecting older people, osteoarthritis causes sore or stiff joints, especially in the hips, knees, and lower back. It can also affect the neck and shoulders, fingers, ankles, and big toe. The cause of osteoarthritis is not precisely known, but it involves the breakdown of cartilage, the material that cushions the joint. Cartilage is like a shock absorber and when it erodes, it causes bones to rub against each other. This causes stiffness, pain, and loss of movement.

Other kinds of arthritis are due to inflammation. The most common forms are those caused by rheumatic diseases such as rheumatoid arthritis, metabolic diseases such as gout, and psoriasis. With these diseases, the lining of the joint becomes inflamed and swollen and also secretes extra fluid. As a result, the joint becomes swollen, warm, red, tender, and painful to move. If present for a time, inflammatory arthritis can also result in destruction of cartilage and bone, which can ultimately lead to deformity. The cause of the inflammation associated with many of these conditions is not precisely known, but rheumatoid arthritis and psoriatic arthritis are thought to be autoimmune diseases that cause the body's own immune system to mistakenly turn against itself.

Most arthritic diseases do not affect only the joints. Joints are crossed by tendons from nearby muscles that move the joints and by ligaments that stabilize the joints. When the joint lining is inflamed or the joint is swollen or deformed, those tendons, ligaments, and muscles can be affected. They may become inflamed, swollen, stretched, displaced, thinned out, or even broken. Also, in many places where tendons or muscles move over each other or over bones, there are lubricated surfaces to make the movement easy. These surfaces are called bursas. With arthritis, they too may become inflamed or swollen, causing a condition known as bursitis. Thus arthritis of any kind does not simply affect the joint. It can affect all of the structures in the area around the joint.

Managing Arthritis

Although arthritis can have damaging effects, you can do a lot to offset or eliminate these effects. Active self-management, the proper use of medications, and developing or maintaining supportive social relationships are key to leading a productive and satisfying life.

Important goals of arthritis self-management are to maintain the maximum possible use of affected joints and to maintain good posture. Unless the affected joints are used, they will slowly lose mobility, and the surrounding muscles and tendons will weaken. Good posture is important to reduce strain placed on other parts of the body. For example, if arthritis affects the joints of one leg, that leg may be favored during walking. This can cause extra burdens on other body areas that result in even more pain.

The key to attaining joint mobility and good posture is exercise, an essential part of any chronic pain management plan. Exercise will not make arthritis worse. In fact, failing to exercise can increase arthritis symptoms because of loss of joint mobility, muscle strength, and overall physical conditioning. To maintain joint mobility and healthy cartilage, you will need to move the affected joints through their full range of motion several times a day. Consult with a health care provider such as a physical therapist to learn the best way to move your joints safely. She or he can also examine your posture and provide ideas on improving your posture when doing different activities.

Gentle flexibility exercises such as the Moving Easy Program (MEP) and balance exercises are good ways to start increasing your activity. The MEP can also help with stiffness that can occur after periods of rest such as sleeping and prolonged sitting. Appropriate exercise programs for people with arthritis are described in Chapters 7, 8, and 9. Review this material to get started on a more active lifestyle.

As with all chronic pain conditions, other symptoms are frequently part of living with arthritis (see page 13). If you suffer from fatigue, review the sections on fatigue and sleep problems in Chapter 4. Pacing is an especially important fatigue and pain self-management skill. Review the ten pacing tips in Chapter 6 so that you can better balance your activity with rest periods. Of course, having a regular fitness program is a key strategy in managing fatigue and many other related symptoms.

Arthritis can cause stress, anxiety, emotional difficulties, and sometimes depression. If you suffer from any of these symptoms, Chapters 4 and 5 are especially important for you to read. You will learn many ways to manage these symptoms and how to recognize when you need to seek help and support. Remember that you do not have to do this alone. Effective ways to communicate with your family, friends, and members of your health care team are discussed in Chapters 10 and 11. The pain and discomfort of arthritis can also impact intimate relationships. See Chapter 12 for more information on how to approach this sensitive subject with your partner.

Because the pain of arthritis is often located in one area of the body, self-management approaches such as the use of heat or cold can be helpful for joint pain and stiffness. Read pages 44–48 in Chapter 4 on tools for managing localized pain. Another important area of arthritis self-management is nutrition and maintaining a healthy weight. Read Chapters 13 and 14 to help you plan healthier meals and achieve a healthy weight. If you are overweight, losing even a few pounds can reduce the strain on joints such as hips, knees, and feet.

Sometimes when joint function remains limited, assistive devices can be of benefit. Many types of devices are available, including braces, canes, special shoes, grippers, and reachers. If you need help making decisions about devices that could be most useful to you, consult an occupational therapist. They have specialized knowledge in this area and can help make daily living easier for you.

Because arthritis consists of many different conditions, your medical treatment will be specific to the type of arthritic condition you have. Your doctor will prescribe medications to prevent or control inflammation, swelling, and pain and to improve your physical function. The most commonly prescribed medications

Resources for Arthritis

To learn more, type in the specific type of arthritis you have into the search engines on any of the following sites:

Arthritis Foundation: www.arthritis.org

Arthritis Society: www.arthritis.ca

Canadian Arthritis Network: www.arthritisnetwork.ca

Canadian Orthopaedic Foundation: www.canorth.org

National Institutes of Health: www.niams.nih.gov and www.nccam.nih.gov/health/arthritis

For more in-depth information about living with arthritis and osteoporosis, see: Lorig, Kate, Halsted Holman, David Sobel, Diana Laurent, Virginia González, and Marian Minor. *Living a Healthy Life with Chronic Conditions*. Boulder, Colo: Bull Publishing, 2012.

---

for the pain of osteoarthritis and some rheumatic diseases are acetaminophen and mild or strong anti-inflammatory drugs (NSAIDS). (See Chapter 16 for information on these and other medications you may be prescribed, including antidepressants.) Other strong medications such as "disease-modifying" drugs, corticosteroids, and new biological agents may also be prescribed for the treatment of some inflammatory arthritis conditions. These stronger medications are powerful and need to be well managed. Take the time to develop a good relationship with your pharmacist and health care team so that you have all the information you need to manage your medications safely. Read Chapter 15 to review your role in managing all the medications you take.

Sometimes, despite self-management and drug treatments, joints are damaged to the point where they no longer work effectively. Fortunately, modern surgical techniques allow for replacement of many types of joints, and replacement joints often function almost as well as natural joints. This is especially true for hips and knees. Modern surgery is efficient, and recovery is usually rapid.

Chronic Back Pain

If you suffer from chronic back pain, you are not alone. Back pain is one of the most common medical conditions in Western countries. There are 30 bones or vertebrae that make up the spinal column. These bones are divided into four regions: the neck area, the middle or thoracic area, the lumbar or lower back area, and the sacrum or coccyx, which is a group of bones fused together at the base of the spine. Muscles that attach to the spinal bones support the bones of the back.

The strong muscles in our abdomen also support the spine. Spinal bones or vertebrae are separated from each other by jelly-like cushions (called intervertebral discs) that act as shock absorbers as the body moves. A critical structure is the spinal cord, which contains the many nerves that travel to our brain. The bones of the back surround and protect the spinal cord. A healthy back is straight, strong, flexible, and pain-free.

Back pain can develop anywhere along the spine. The two most common areas for pain to occur are the neck and the lower back. Pain can be localized in one area or can spread to a wider area. Neck pain can spread to the shoulders and upper back; lower back pain can spread to the buttocks and down one or both legs.

Nearly everyone experiences back pain sometime in his or her life. It can be caused by many things, including poor posture, weak back muscles or weak abdominal muscles, lifting heavy objects incorrectly, twisting, excess body weight, and repetitive activities that require lifting or bending. Sometimes neck or other back pain is the result of a poorly designed workstation—for example a computer that is too high or low, or a chair that does not provide back support. Back pain can also result from motor vehicle or other accidents. An example is whiplash, a common neck injury that results from rear-end automobile accidents.

Most back pain gets better within one month. But for a small number of people, back pain becomes chronic. About 10 percent of chronic back pain is caused by arthritis or other diseases. See your health care provider to rule out disease-related causes for your back pain. Most people with chronic back pain have "nonspecific" back pain that is related to the muscles and ligaments that surround and support the spine, and not the spine itself. As with most chronic pain, changes occur in the central nervous system and the brain that perpetuate the pain. But you can take action to calm your nervous system to reduce your pain and improve your life.

Red Flags: Chronic Back Pain

Rarely, symptoms of chronic neck and back pain are warning signs of a more serious problem. Seek immediate medical help if any of the following accompany your back pain:

- Numbness or tingling in the buttocks, groin, and inner thighs (the parts of the body that would contact a saddle if you were riding a horse) and/or sudden loss of control of urination or bowel movements. This may mean that important nerves are being compressed. This is an emergency.

- Numbness, tingling, or weakness in arms and hands (if you have neck pain) or legs and feet (if you have lower back pain)

- Severe worsening of pain, especially at night or when lying down

- Unexplained weight loss or fever

- Difficulty breathing or swallowing along with neck pain

Managing Chronic Back Pain

The experience of chronic back pain is different for everyone. The location and intensity may be different. The impact it has on everyday functioning and family life also varies. If back pain starts when you are in your 30s or 40s, it may affect job and financial security. Job change and job loss are difficult to cope with. Review Chapter 4 (pages 70–73) for more about coping with job loss.

Even though your back may cause serious pain, there are many ways you can learn to manage the pain and live a full, satisfying life. The most effective approach is to combine self-management techniques, such as the ones in this book, and care from your health care providers. Research has shown that staying physically active and developing a regular exercise program improves pain and function in people with chronic back pain. Sometimes, exercising can hurt a bit; remember that as long as you are exercising in a safe manner, "hurt" does not equal "harm." The muscles and ligaments of your back have already healed, so being involved in regular physical activity will not harm them further unless you overdo it. So go slow. Always consult with your health care provider about the type of exercise to avoid before beginning an exercise program. Chapters 7, 8, and 9 can help you get started with exercising. There are specific suggestions about exercise and chronic neck and back pain in these chapters.

Emotional distress and depression can make chronic back pain harder to deal with. That's why it is very important to learn and use the coping skills and relaxation techniques in Chapters 4 and 5. Communicating with your family and maintaining intimacy with your partner can be challenging with back pain. Read Chapters 10 and 12 as you address these challenges. Another key self-management technique for chronic back pain is pacing. Look at Chapter 6 to begin implementing these strategies and get more accomplished with less pain.

Healthy eating and weight management are other key self-management goals. Carrying excess weight can really impact your back pain by causing increased stress on muscles in your back and abdomen and on your joints. See Chapters 13 and 14 for information on these topics. Research findings are consistent about smoking being a risk factor for many types of chronic musculoskeletal pain problems such

Resources for Chronic Back Pain

To learn more about chronic back pain, type the term "back pain" into the search engines on any of the following sites:

American Chronic Pain Association: www.theacpa.org

Arthritis Society: www.arthritis.ca

National Institutes of Health: www.ninds.nih.gov/disorders/backpain

Toward Optimized Practice (TOP), Low Back Pain: www.topalbertadoctors.org/cpgs/885801

WebMD: www.webmd.com/back-pain

as back pain. This is true especially if you are under the age of 50. If you smoke, talk to your health care provider about ways to stop.

Heat and cold applications, acupuncture, and massage, especially when combined with physical activity and self-management education, have been shown to help people with chronic lower back pain. More studies are being done on chiropractic spinal manipulation treatment.

Some studies have shown a positive impact from spinal manipulation, while others have not. In addition to these types of treatments, your health care provider may prescribe medications such as acetaminophen, mild anti-inflammatory medicines, low-dose antidepressants, muscle relaxants, and other more powerful medications if pain is severe. Please see Chapter 16 for more specific information about pain medications.

Fibromyalgia

The term fibromyalgia is made up of three root words: "fibro" means fibrous or connective tissue, "myo" means muscle, and "algia" means pain. Fibromyalgia literally means pain in muscle and connective tissue. Connective tissues are the tendons and ligaments that connect muscles to bones and bones to bones in your body. The pain and tenderness of fibromyalgia last longer than three months, are widespread, move from one area of the body to another, and change over time. Up until 2010, a health care provider would diagnose fibromyalgia only if a person had 11 to 18 trigger points as well as widespread pain. (Trigger points are sensitive areas over muscle and are painful when touched.) Since 2010, new guidelines for the diagnosis of fibromyalgia have been developed based on the latest research evidence. While people with fibromyalgia may have a number of trigger points, trigger points are not required for a diagnosis of fibromyalgia.

Fibromyalgia also displays other common symptoms, including fatigue, sleep disturbance, problems with thinking and memory (called "fibro fog"), depression, and anxiety. You might also experience headache, irritable bowel or bladder, painful menstrual cycles, or other painful problems. Sometimes fibromyalgia occurs with other chronic painful diseases such as osteoarthritis or rheumatoid arthritis.

Fibromyalgia is two times more common in women than in men. It can develop at any age, including childhood. The cause of fibromyalgia is not known but is likely due to multiple factors. New research suggests that certain genes may make you more likely to develop fibromyalgia. Also, it may be associated with early negative childhood experiences, including abuse. What scientists know for sure is that if you have fibromyalgia, there are abnormalities in the processing of pain in your central nervous system and your other body systems such as the stress/response system and systems that regulate sleep and mood.

Managing Fibromyalgia

Like other chronic pain conditions, fibromyalgia can be managed. And, like all chronic pain conditions, the goals of fibromyalgia treatment are to manage symptoms, be as healthy as possible, and maintain or improve physical and social functioning. The latest guidelines state that regular

Fibromyalgia Resources

To learn more about fibromyalgia, visit the following sites (type the term "fibromyalgia pain" into the search engines on any of the more general health sites listed below):

American Chronic Pain Association: www.theacpa.org

Chronic Pain & Fatigue Research Center, University of Michigan:
 www.fibroguide.med.umich.edu

Fibromyalgia Network: www.fmnetnews.com

FM-CFS Canada: www.fm-cfs.ca

Medline Plus: www.nlm.nih.gov/medlineplus/fibromyalgia.html

National Institute of Arthritis and Musculoskeletal and Skin Diseases: www.niams.nih.gov

Women's Health Matters: www.womenshealthmatters.ca

physical activity is the cornerstone of fibromyalgia treatment. No one specific type of exercise is recommended; you can engage in a combination of aerobic, strengthening, flexibility, and balance exercises. Your exercise options can be very gentle like slow walking, the Moving Easy Program (see Chapter 8), gentle yoga, or tai chi, and also include more vigorous exercise once you build up your stamina. Exercise can be done in water or on dry land, either at home or in a group. The best exercise is the one that you will do. Review Chapters 7, 8, and 9 for more ideas about exercise.

Fibro fog is the term used to describe the problems with thinking and memory that can accompany fibromyalgia. You can best manage fibro fog by pacing your activities (Chapter 6) and taking some of the specific actions described in Chapter 4 on pages 69–70. You can learn how to manage other fibromyalgia-related symptoms you experience by reviewing the appropriate sections of Chapters 4 and 5. Of course, eating well and maintaining a healthy weight are part of optimizing your overall health. Explore Chapters 13 and 14 for guidelines for healthy eating and weight management.

Your health care provider will likely prescribe medications to help manage some of your symptoms. Most of the medications used for the treatment of fibromyalgia are discussed in Chapter 16. Be sure to also review Chapter 15 for more general information about medications and how to manage them.

Headache

Headache is one of the most common pain conditions. The World Health Organization recently reported that 47 percent of adults worldwide experienced headache in the past year. For many people, headaches occur infrequently, are not severe, and last only a short time. But, there is another group of headache sufferers who deal with headache pain on a regular basis—daily, weekly, or monthly. Persistent or chronic headache can wear you down, make you depressed and anxious, and negatively impact your quality and enjoyment of life.

What is a headache? Headache is pain that occurs in any region of your head. It can be on one or both sides of your head, on the top or the back of your head, or both. It can also be pinpointed in a specific spot. If pain is located in your face, mouth, or jaw, it may be termed orofacial pain. Headache pain can be sharp and jabbing, throbbing and pounding, or dull and achy. It can be mild or it can be so severe that it is disabling. It can come on gradually or suddenly and can be gone in an hour or last for many days at a time. Depending on the type of headache, a person may also have other symptoms such as nausea or extreme sensitivity to light and noise. In short, headache is often quite different for different people.

Physicians classify headaches into two types: primary or secondary headache. Primary headaches are caused directly by activity in your blood vessels, muscles, and nerves in your head and neck, as well as any chemical activity taking place in your brain. Common examples of primary headache are tension headaches, migraine, and cluster headaches. Secondary headache is a symptom of another health condition that stimulates the pain-sensitive nerves in your head. Many conditions can cause secondary headache. Dehydration, fever, and infection such as colds or flus can result in secondary headaches. More serious problems can also bring on headache, including high blood pressure, stroke, blood clots, head injury, arthritis in your neck, or other pain conditions in your face or jaw. A common but not well understood cause of secondary headache is the overuse of pain medicines, sometimes called rebound headache. Ask your health care provider to take a careful medical history from you and perform tests to rule out any disease-related causes for your headaches.

Managing Headache

If you are a person who gets headaches often, you may not be able to get rid of them entirely. But self-management strategies, such as the ones in this book, can help reduce the number and severity of your headaches.

One of the first things you can do is identify triggers that might bring on your headaches or make them worse. Become a "headache detective" and keep a diary for at least two weeks or, even better, for a month. When you get a headache, stop and take a few minutes to write down the events or actions that led up to the onset of the pain. Consider what might have triggered it or made it worse. Many things can affect headache. You may have sensitivities to certain foods, alcohol or other beverages, or strong odors. Chapter 13 (page 219) lists some common food triggers. You may be under excess stress or be upset or emotional about something going on in your life. Have you skipped meals or changed your activity pattern? Are there any changes to your posture—resulting from a change in the chair or desk you use, for example—that might cause neck or shoulder strain? Are you fatigued or sleeping poorly? Are you going through hormonal changes? Does the weather seem to be a factor? In addition to identifying triggers, it is important to note what you do when you get a headache. Keep a record of the self-management strategies you try, including medications, and

Red Flags: Headache

Occasionally headache symptoms signal a new serious health problem. Seek immediate emergency care if you experience the worst headache of your life, a sudden severe headache different from your usual headache, or headache with one or more of the accompanying symptoms:

- confusion or trouble understanding speech
- trouble speaking
- changes in vision
- trouble walking
- numbness, weakness, or paralysis on one side of the body

- dizziness or fainting
- high fever, greater than 102°F to 104°F (39°C to 40°C)
- stiff neck
- nausea or vomiting not related to the flu or overconsumption of alcohol

whether they help. The lifestyle diary in Chapter 14 on page 242 can help you get started on your detective work or serve as the basis for making your own chart.

After you have kept your diary for a few weeks, begin to look for patterns. Remember, sometimes a combination of things can trigger pain. If you identify some possible triggers, divide them into triggers you can avoid (certain foods or drink), triggers you can't avoid but can learn to manage (stress, emotional reactions, fatigue, poor posture), triggers you can minimize (missed meals, late nights), and triggers that are not in your control (hormonal or weather changes). Being aware of the triggers that can be controlled, even partially, is the first step to managing your headaches.

Once you have a sense of your headache patterns and triggers, you can start planning how you will avoid, manage, or minimize these triggers. Chapters 4 and 5 discuss methods to self-manage stress, strong emotions, fatigue, poor sleep, and other factors that might impact your headache. The information in Chapter 6 on pacing can help you plan to balance your activity and

rest and stay below your headache "threshold." Your headache threshold is the point at which you start to feel a headache coming on. You may find that if you take action as soon as you have signs that you will have a headache (like taking a short walk, doing a relaxation or breathing exercise, taking medication, etc.), you can prevent or reduce the intensity of the headache.

Living an overall healthy lifestyle is also important for headache self-management. Regular moderate exercise can give you an overall sense of well-being, reduce stress and anxiety, lift your mood, and reduce the frequency of headache attacks. Chapters 7, 8, and 9 discuss ways to increase your physical activity and exercise. If you suffer from migraine headaches, you may need to be careful when you exercise. Work out at a moderate pace, not too fast or too hard. Stay hydrated and don't exercise if you have not eaten. Eliminating food triggers and eating a healthy diet with regular meals is also important. Read Chapters 13 and 14 for more information on nutrition. Also, be sure to communicate with your family, friends, and coworkers about how they can support you when you do get a

Headache Resources

To learn more about headache, visit the following sites (type the term "headache pain" into the search engines on any of the more general health sites listed below):

American Academy of Orofacial Pain: www.aaop.org

American Headache Society Committee for Headache Education: www.achenet.org

American Headache Society: www.americanheadachesociety.org

Help for Headaches (Canada): www.headache-help.org

National Headache Foundation: www.headaches.org

National Institute of Neurological Disorders and Stroke: www.ninds.nih.gov

Toward Optimized Practice (TOP), Headache: www.topalbertadoctors.org/cpgs/10065

headache. Chapter 10 can help you learn how to communicate in a positive way.

Medications can be effective in managing headache, but they need to be taken with care. Review Chapters 15 and 16 about the management of medications. Over-the-counter medicines such as aspirin, acetaminophen (Tylenol®, Panadol®), and anti-inflammatory medicines such as Advil® and Motrin® can be used. But they should not be taken for more than 14 days in a month. This is because the overuse of pain medications can be the cause of daily or frequent headaches in some people. This is not addiction, but a side effect of taking too much of any given drug. If you are taking multiple medications or high doses for headache and have frequent or daily headache, talk to your health care provider about the possibility of medication overuse and how you can reduce the amount you take. If you suffer from severe migraine or cluster headaches, your health care provider may prescribe other types of headache medicine.

Chronic Pelvic Pain

Pelvic pain refers to pain in the lower part of your abdomen and the structures related to the pelvis. This pain affects the area directly below your belly button down to your hips. The pelvis includes organs involved in reproduction and sexuality such as the womb or uterus, the vagina, and the vulva in women and the penis, testicles, and prostate gland in men. The pelvis also includes the bladder, bowel, and many muscles, nerves, bones, and soft tissue. Chronic pelvic pain can occur in any of these structures as well as in the lower back, buttocks, or thighs.

Most women experience pelvic pain at times because of menstruation. But there are many other possible reasons for pelvic pain. In women and men, reasons for pelvic pain include infection, abnormal tissue growth, and diseases of the urinary tract or bowel. Pelvic pain can also be caused by damage to nerves, tissues, or bones, or injury that causes tender, tight, or weakened muscles in the lower abdomen, lower part of the pelvis (called the pelvic floor muscles), or the buttocks. In men, chronic pelvic pain can be caused by prostatitis, or inflammation of the prostrate gland. If your pelvic pain is due to a known cause, treatment is specific to that cause. Treatments can include various medications to cure the infection or disease or to manage troublesome symptoms; surgery to remove a growth, cyst, or tumor; and physical therapy and exercise to stretch tight muscles and trigger points.

Sometimes the cause of pelvic pain is complex and treatments do not work. The pain persists and becomes chronic. Like other kinds of chronic pain, chronic pelvic pain is a condition in its own right because of abnormal nerve activity patterns in the pelvic region, the central nervous system, and the brain.

Chronic pelvic pain is different for everyone. It can be mild to severe. It can feel dull, sharp, burning, or cramping. It might be there all the time or you might only notice it at certain times such as when having a bowel movement, passing urine, during sexual activity, or after you sit for long periods of time. It may not be very bothersome most days, or it may frequently interfere with sleep, work, and enjoyment of life.

There are two additional challenges that people with chronic pelvic pain face. First, it is often difficult to talk about pelvic pain to other people, even your health care professionals. The relationship of pelvic pain to sexual, urinary, or bowel functions can stifle conversation and make you want to hide it from others. Researchers refer to this as a "culture of secrecy." This can be problematic because just like anyone who experiences any kind of chronic pain, people with chronic pelvic pain need supportive relationships and need to be

taken seriously. Secrecy means that you may not talk openly to friends, family, or even your doctor about your pain problem. This can leave you feeling isolated and alone. This can be compounded by the second special consequence of chronic pelvic pain, which is that some symptoms can be potentially embarrassing. Symptoms such as unpredictable urinary or bowel incontinence or gynecological discharge can lead to fear of embarrassment or damage your self-confidence. These issues can contribute to your solitude if you decide to avoid social occasions.

Managing Chronic Pelvic Pain

While chronic pelvic pain is complex and challenging, there are many things you can do to improve your quality of life. Your role in the management of pelvic pain begins with open communication. Open communication will help you build a trusting relationship with members of your health care team so that you feel comfortable talking with them. You will likely be referred to medical and other specialists. Prepare for these visits by reading Chapter 11, pages 181–185. It is important to be aware that you may be asked about any past or current sexual or physical abuse, because abuse is associated with pelvic pain for some people. If you are a victim of abuse, it may be hard to talk about these things, but it is very important that you do in order to get the help you need.

Chronic pelvic pain has been described as an emotional roller coaster of anger, depression, guilt, anxiety, frustration, and fear. Sometimes, the cause of pelvic pain results in infertility and related feelings of loss and grief. The management of these difficult emotions can be aided by the self-management tools described in Chapter

4, pages 57–69, and Chapter 5 on how to use your mind to manage symptoms. Sometimes, self-management is not enough and you may require additional help to deal with your emotions. A support group or professional counseling may be the answer. Talk to your health care provider about your feelings, and seek emotional support from family and friends.

Your health care provider may recommend analgesics and other medicines to manage your symptoms. Review Chapters 15 and 16 so that you understand the pain medications and other medicines you are advised to take and your key role in medication self-management. Your provider may also suggest other forms of treatment or products. When deciding on what treatments to try, refer to Chapter 17 on evaluating treatments and Chapter 2, pages 22–23, on decision making. This information can help you if you feel unsure of what path to pursue in seeking treatment.

As with all chronic pain conditions, when you experience chronic pelvic pain you need to pay attention to your overall health, including issues relating to nutrition, weight, and exercise.

Eating well, maintaining a healthy weight, and getting enough physical activity will improve your overall sense of well-being, increase your energy, and improve many other symptoms. Read Chapters 13 and 14 on nutrition and Chapters 7, 8, and 9 on physical activity. In addition to a flexibility and aerobic exercise program, you may be referred to a physical therapist for assessment and treatment of pain in the muscles and tissues of the lower abdomen and pelvic floor. Ask if there are specific exercises you should not do or exercise machines you should not use. For example, to reduce nerve irritation, you may be advised not to do abdominal "crunches," not to use an elliptical machine, and to avoid bicycling or to use a well-padded seat or padded clothing if you do bicycle. You may also be given special pelvic floor and abdominal exercises that will help relax and strengthen muscles in this area.

Sexual concerns are common with pelvic pain. Read Chapter 10 on communication and Chapter 12 on sex and intimacy for more information about concerns relating to this area of your life.

Chronic Pelvic Pain Resources

To learn more about chronic pelvic pain, visit the following sites (type the term "pelvic pain" and/or "prostatitis" into the search engines on any of the more general health sites listed below):

BC Women's Centre for Pelvic Pain and Endometriosis: www.womenspelvicpainendo.com

International Pelvic Pain Society: www.pelvicpain.org

Interstitial Cystitis Association: www.ichelp.org

Interstitial Cystitis Network: www.ic-network.com

Mayo Clinic: www.mayoclinic.org

Medscape: www.emedicine.medscape.com

Prostatitis Foundation: www.prostatitis.org

WebMD: www.webmd.com

Complex Regional Pain Syndrome (CRPS)

Complex regional pain syndrome (CRPS) is a difficult chronic pain condition. It is also known as causalgia or reflex sympathetic dystrophy (RSD). CRPS most often affects a limb—an arm, hand, finger, leg, foot, or toe—but it can occur in other parts of the body as well. If you have CRPS, you may have continuous burning or "pins and needles" type pain in the affected limb, have increased sensitivity to even light touch, and experience changes in the skin around the painful area. The skin can change color and look pale, blotchy, blue, or very red. It can feel cold or very warm compared to the unaffected limb. The skin might look swollen, shiny, and thin. There can be changes to fingernails and toenails and even changes in hair growth in the area. You might also have abnormal sweating near the painful area. Muscles and joints in the affected area can be become stiff and go into spasm. In some people, CRPS moves up the limb and spreads to the opposite limb.

The exact cause of CRPS is not known but is likely due to multiple causes. There is often a triggering event that starts the pain in the first place. The most common initial causes are crushing injuries, sprains (even mild ones such as a twisted ankle or wrist), bone fractures, or surgery. It is also attributed to other causes such as heart attack, stroke, or infection. A key indicator for the presence of CRPS is that the pain is much more severe than expected from the original injury or illness. CRPS results from damage to nerves that travel from the limbs to the central nervous system in the spinal cord and brain. The nerves in your limbs are part of the sympathetic

nervous system. Among other things, the sympathetic nervous system controls the flow of blood to limbs, skin temperature, and our response to stress. The skin changes in CRPS can be caused by damage to nerves in the sympathetic nervous system. This damage is also why being cold makes the pain of CRPS feel worse.

CRPS is not easy to diagnose, especially in the early stages. Other conditions have similar symptoms, so your doctor will conduct a careful examination to eliminate other treatable conditions such as arthritis syndromes, muscle diseases, a blood clot in a vein, or diabetes. CRPS is most common in women who are in their 40s and older. For most people, CRPS symptoms go away after a year, especially in younger children and teenagers or in adults if they are treated early. But for others, CRPS can linger for many years and lead to disability.

Managing Complex Regional Pain Syndrome

Managing CRPS is a learning process for both you and your health care team. You may need to undergo multiple tests, procedures, and treatments before finding ones that provide some pain relief. Review Chapters 15 and 16 that discuss your role in managing medications and other treatments for chronic pain. Because CRPS is difficult to manage, it is very important for you to work closely with all members of your health care team and keep them informed about what is working and what is not improving your quality of life. Along with symptoms that accompany all chronic pain conditions such as those discussed in Chapter 4, CRPS can pose some especially difficult problems and concerns. These include the impact of heightened emotions, negative thinking, and fear and avoidance of movement. In the following material, we talk about these one at a time.

High levels of emotion and stress can make the pain of CRPS much worse. The sympathetic nervous system that controls our response to stress is directly involved in CRPS. This is not the case for many other chronic pain conditions. That is why managing your emotions and monitoring your stress levels is so important when you have CRPS. Read more about depression, anger, and stress in Chapter 4, pages 57–69. If you are dealing with the stress of unemployment, also read pages 70–73. Learning and practicing self-management techniques to reduce stress and quiet the mind and the nervous system can really help with the stress that is part of CRPS. Examples of techniques that employ the mind to address stress are found in Chapter 5. Another useful strategy is pacing. The suggestions in Chapter 6 can help reduce your stress while still allowing you to achieve the things you want and need to do.

Another challenge you might have is excessive negative thinking, sometimes called catastrophic thinking. This happens when you can't stop thinking about pain and how bad it is. Read the sections in Chapter 5 on the use of distraction, positive realistic thinking, and relaxation. If these techniques do not work for you, talk to your health care provider and seek professional help.

The third major challenge for people with CRPS is fear and avoidance of movement. Because

the affected limb is often very painful, you may want to protect it by moving as little as possible. But not moving the affected limb will cause many problems, including muscle wasting, weakness of muscles and bones, joint stiffness, and contractures (shortening and hardening of muscles that can lead to deformed and rigid joints). It will also decrease your daily functioning. A physical therapist needs to be part of your health care team as soon as you are diagnosed with CRPS. She or he will start you on a program of exercise to maintain the function of your affected limb as well as help you develop an exercise program for your overall health. Read Chapters 7, 8, and 9 to learn more about starting and maintaining an effective exercise program.

A recent research study in the journal *Chronic Illness* asked men and women with CRPS what advice they would offer another person recently diagnosed with the condition. The people in the study said they would tell newly diagnosed people that they must play an active role in self-management. Patients who have had CRPS for some time cautioned that effective self-management can only happen if a person feels in sufficient control of the condition and his or her life. They identified three important things that help a person with CRPS feel more in control. The following is their advice:

■ **First, accept the condition.** Once a diagnosis is established, you need to stop looking for a cure and accept that you have this condition. Part of acceptance is setting realistic goals and being kind to yourself. Another important point: acceptance is hard and it takes time to get there. Review pages 92–96 in Chapter 5 to learn more about coming to terms with your condition.

- **Second, gain the right support.** Getting support from members of your health care team and from family and friends is critical. You need people to talk to—people who understand. Sometimes this means building a new support network. Read Chapter 10 on ways to improve communication and Chapter 3 on resources to learn as much as you can about finding the support you need.

- **Third, become informed about the condition and learn what works best for you.** Being informed and learning more about CRPS from reputable information sources such as the ones in this book (including those listed in the "Complex Regional Pain Syndrome Resources" list below) can provide reassurance and help you accept and live a good life with this condition. Your CRPS symptoms are also experienced by others. You are not alone.

Complex Regional Pain Syndrome Resources

To learn more about Complex Regional Pain Syndrome, visit the following sites (type the term "Complex Regional Pain Syndrome" into the search engines on any of the more general health sites listed below):

Mayo Clinic: www.mayoclinic.org

National Health Service, United Kingdom: www.nhs.uk

National Institute of Neurological Disorders and Stroke: www.ninds.nih.gov/disorders/reflex_sympathetic_dystrophy

PainHEALTH, University of Western Australia: www.painhealth.csse.uwa.edu.au

RSDSA: www.rsds.org/index2.html

Reflex Sympathic Dystrophy Canada: www.rsdcanada.org

WebMD: www.webmd.com

CHAPTER 19

Managing Angina Pain, Coronary Artery Disease, and Related Conditions

A NGINA IS A COMMON, AND OFTEN CHRONIC, painful symptom of coronary artery disease. Angina occurs when an area of the heart does not receive enough oxygen-rich blood due to poor circulation. The pain from angina may be on the left side of the chest over the heart, but it can also radiate to the back, shoulders, arms, neck, and jaw. For some, it may be just a vague sense of discomfort or weakness. In addition to angina and coronary artery disease, in this chapter we also discuss two other problems of the circulatory system common among people with angina: high blood pressure and peripheral vascular disease.

Special thanks to the following individuals for their help with this chapter: Dr. Michael McGillion, RN, PhD, Assistant Professor and Heart and Stroke Foundation Michael G. DeGroote Endowed Chair of Cardiovascular Nursing Research, McMaster University; Shelley Gershman, RN, Research Coordinator, McMaster University; Dr. Sheila O'Keefe-McCarthy, RN, PhD, Adjunct Scientist, Ross Memorial Hospital; and Noorin Jamal, RN(EC), MN-NP, University Health Network, Toronto, Canada

Coronary Artery Disease

Coronary artery disease is the most common form of heart disease. It causes most heart attacks and heart failure. Coronary arteries are blood vessel "pipelines" that wrap around the heart (see Figure 19.1). They deliver the oxygen and nutrients the heart needs to perform its job. Healthy arteries are elastic, flexible, and strong. The inside lining of a healthy artery is smooth, so blood flows easily. Unhealthy arteries narrow when they become clogged with cholesterol and other substances. This thickening or hardening process is called atherosclerosis.

Atherosclerosis is a gradual process that occurs over many years. The first step is damage to the wall of the artery. This can be caused by high cholesterol, high triglycerides, diabetes, smoking, or high blood pressure. This damage allows LDL cholesterol (the "bad" cholesterol) to enter the artery wall and cause inflammation. Some people experience this problem as early as their teens.

Over time, more cholesterol is deposited in the damaged arteries and the fatty areas grow larger and larger. These fatty areas are plaques. Plaque is a sticky, yellow material made up of cholesterol, calcium, and waste products from cells in your body. Plaques can completely block off blood flow in an artery, causing reduced blood circulation and oxygen supply to the heart muscle. Plaques can also crack open, causing a blood clot to form at the injured site. In both cases, blood flow to the heart is blocked, and the person may experience angina (temporary chest pain) or a heart attack. If not treated immediately, a heart attack can cause permanent damage to the heart muscle. When a part of the heart muscle has been damaged, that part can no longer help the heart pump blood.

There are a number of risk factors for coronary artery disease. You can control some of these factors, but not all of them. The risk

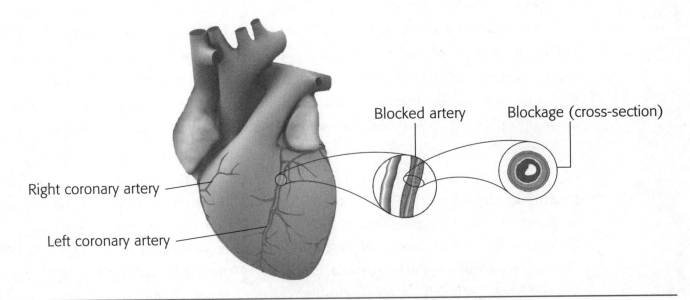

Figure 19.1 **The Arteries of the Heart**

factors for coronary artery disease that you can't control include:

- Age—The older you get, the more at risk you are for coronary artery disease.

- Sex—Men over the age of 55 and women who are postmenopausal are at higher risk for coronary artery disease.

- Family history—You are at higher risk for coronary artery disease if a close family member such as a parent or sibling developed it before age 55 or before menopause.

- Ethnicity—First Nations of Canada, Native Americans, African, or South Asian individuals are more likely to have high blood pressure and are at greater risk of coronary artery disease and stroke than the general population.

The risk factors for coronary artery disease that you can control include:

- High blood pressure— High blood pressure is consistently higher than 140/90 when measured in a clinic or 135/85 when measured using a blood pressure cuff at home. (We discuss blood pressure figures in more detail on pages 236–240.)

- Diabetes—This includes type 1 diabetes, type 2 diabetes, and gestational diabetes.

- High cholesterol—LDL (bad) and HDL (good) cholesterol must be evaluated in relation to each other.

- Being overweight—A person with a body mass index (BMI) over 25 is considered to be overweight. (For more on BMI, see Chapter 14, pages 236–239)

- Smoking—This includes exposure to secondhand smoke.

- Lack of exercise—Those who are physically inactive are twice as likely to be at risk for coronary artery disease than those who are physically active.

- Stress—People who experience prolonged periods of stress are more susceptible to atherosclerosis, high blood pressure, and high cholesterol.

- Excessive alcohol consumption—Excess is defined as more than 10 drinks per week for women and more than 15 drinks per week for men.

More About Cholesterol

Cholesterol is a waxy fat that is found in all cells of the body and can be measured in your blood. You need cholesterol in order to make hormones, vitamin D, and substances that allow food to be digested. The body makes enough cholesterol for your body to function properly, but it is not good to have too much cholesterol in your blood. High blood cholesterol level is a major risk factor for heart disease. High cholesterol can lead to a buildup of plaque in the artery walls, narrowing your arteries and not leaving enough space for the blood to flow freely. This narrowing of the space in your arteries can lead to angina pain because the heart is not able to receive enough blood and oxygen to work properly.

There are "good" and "bad" forms of cholesterol. Low-density lipoprotein (LDL) is known as the bad cholesterol because high levels of it in your blood causes the buildup of plaque in your arteries. One way to remember is to think of LDL as "lousy" (L) cholesterol. High-density lipoprotein (HDL) is good cholesterol because it helps protect your body from developing heart disease by carrying away the LDL from your

When Should I Test My Cholesterol?

Some general rules for testing your cholesterol are if:

- You are male and over 40.
- You are female and over 50 or postmenopausal.
- You have heart disease, stroke, diabetes, or high blood pressure.
- You have a family history of heart disease or stroke.
- Your waist measures more than 40 inches (102 centimeters) for men or 35 inches (88 centimeters) for women. For persons of Chinese or South Asian descent, if your waist measures more than 35 inches (90 centimeters) for men or 32 inches (80 centimeters) for women.

Table 19.1 Guidelines for Cholesterol Values

Total cholesterol (U.S. and some other countries)	Total cholesterol (Canada and most of Europe)	
Below 200 mg/dL	Below 5.2 mmol/L	Desirable
200–239 mg/dL	5.2–6.2 mmol/L	Borderline high
240 mg/dL and above	Above 6.2 mmol/L	High
LDL (bad) cholesterol (U.S. and some other countries)	**LDL cholesterol (Canada and most of Europe)**	
Below 70 mg/dL	Below 1.8 mmol/L	Ideal for people at very high risk of heart disease
Below 100 mg/dL	Below 2.6 mmol/L	Ideal for people at risk of heart disease
100–129 mg/dL	2.6–3.3 mmol/L	Near ideal
130–159 mg/dL	3.4–4.1 mmol/L	Borderline high
160–189 mg/dL	4.1–4.9 mmol/L	High
190 mg/dL and above	Above 4.9 mmol/L	Very high
HDL (good) cholesterol (U.S. and some other countries)	**HDL cholesterol (Canada and most of Europe)**	
Below 40 mg/dL (men) Below 50 mg/dL (women)	Below 1 mmol/L (men) Below 1.3 mmol/L (women)	Poor
40–49 mg/dL (men) 50–59 mg/dL (women)	1–1.3 mmol/L (men) 1.3–1.5 mmol/L (women)	Better
60 mg/dL and above	1.6 mmol/L and above	Best
Triglycerides (U.S. and some other countries)	**Triglycerides (Canada and most of Europe)**	
Below 150 mg/dL	Below 1.7 mmol/L	Desirable
150–199 mg/dL	1.7–2.2 mmol/L	Borderline high
200–499 mg/dL	2.3–5.6 mmol/L	High
500 mg/dL and above	Above 5.6 mmol/L and above	Very high

Source: www.mayoclinic.org/diseases-conditions/high-blood-cholesterol/in-depth/cholesterol-levels/art-20048245 arteries. To remember its meaning, think of the H as a sign for "healthy" cholesterol.

Tryglycerides are another form of fat in your body. When you eat a meal, your body stores any calories it doesn't immediately need into triglycerides. These triglycerides are stored in your fat cells. Triglycerides are released by hormones in your body for energy between meals. Over time, consuming more calories than you burn can lead to having high triglycerides (hypertriglyceridemia).

High levels of cholesterol in your body are often linked to uncontrolled diabetes, being overweight, or a high alcohol intake. You can control your cholesterol levels by losing weight, eating a heart-healthy diet, exercising regularly, quitting smoking, and drinking alcohol in moderation. If these lifestyle changes are not enough, medications will be added to lower cholesterol levels. Recommended blood levels of cholesterol (total, LDL, and HDL) and triglycerides tend to range by country, as shown in Table 19.1. These recommended levels are guidelines only and may change. So, talk to your health care provider about getting your levels checked and what your results mean for your health.

Angina

As previously mentioned, angina is a common symptom of coronary artery disease. It is often brought on by emotional stress or physical exertion and is usually relieved with medication or rest.

Symptoms of Angina

Sometimes angina will not be experienced as chest pain; it can also be experienced as pressure, tightness, squeezing, or a vague sense of discomfort. Some people (especially women) may only experience some of the following symptoms:

- Persistent indigestion with or without nausea
- Breathlessness
- Cold sweats
- Cramping or burning pain
- Numbness in arms, shoulders, or wrists
- Weakness
- Unusual tiredness
- Sleep disturbances

Angina episodes are *not* heart attacks, and angina pain does *not* mean that the heart is permanently damaged. Angina is, however, a warning sign of increased risk of a heart attack or heart failure. A heart attack occurs when the heart is damaged because the blood supply to an area of the heart has been cut off. The pain of a heart attack generally lasts longer, is more severe than angina pain, and it is not alleviated by resting or taking prescription medicine.

It is important to note that angina symptoms usually last only for a few minutes. Changes in the nature of your usual angina pain are cause for concern. If episodes become more frequent, occur at rest, or last longer than they have previously, seek medical help immediately. It is also important to note that for some, angina may be "atypical." When angina is atypical, the common symptoms are not experienced. Instead, the individual with atypical angina may feel vague forms of chest discomfort along with additional

Seek Emergency Care Immediately

If you are having symptoms that might mean a heart attack, *you must seek medical care immediately.* New treatments are available that can dissolve blood clots, restore blood flow, and prevent heart or brain damage. However, these treatments *must be given within hours of the heart attack*—the sooner, the better. In the United States and Canada, call 911 or emergency services if you have any of the following symptoms:

- Severe, crushing, or squeezing chest pain

- Pain or discomfort in one or both arms, the back, neck, jaw, or stomach

- Chest pain lasting longer than five minutes when there is no apparent cause and it is not relieved by rest or heart medications

- Chest pain occurring with any of the following: rapid or irregular heartbeat, sweating, nausea or vomiting, shortness of breath, light-headedness or passing out, or unusual weakness

- For women, chest pain may not be present. Instead, symptoms such as chest discomfort, rapid or irregular heartbeat, sweating, persistent indigestion with or without nausea or vomiting, shortness of breath, light-headedness or passing out, or unusual weakness may indicate a heart attack.

If you think you are having a heart attack:

1. Stop what you are doing.

2. Sit down.

3. Call 911. (Do not try to drive yourself to the hospital.)

4. If you are not allergic to aspirin, take one adult (325 mg) or four baby (81 mg) aspirin tablets.

Minutes matter! Fast action can save lives—maybe your own. Don't wait more than five minutes to call 911 or your local emergency response number.

---

symptoms listed above. There is some evidence to suggest that women are more prone to atypical angina, particularly prior to menopause. This may be because women tend to have blockages not only in their main arteries but also in the smaller arteries that supply blood to the heart.

Types of Angina

The major types of angina include stable angina, refractory angina, unstable angina, variant or Prinzmetal's angina, and microvascular angina.

Each of these is described in detail in the following material.

- **Stable angina.** Stable angina is the most common form of angina. It usually follows a predictable pattern. Stable angina can vary with respect to how often it occurs, how severe it is, and factors that trigger it. The pain typically comes at about the same point during exertion or exercise or while under emotional stress. It is relieved with rest, medication, or both. Other triggers of stable angina include extreme cold or heat, eating heavy meals, consuming alcohol, and smoking cigarettes.

■ **Refractory angina.** Refractory angina is a severe form of stable angina that cannot be controlled by typical treatments for coronary artery disease such as medication, angioplasty, or coronary artery bypass surgery. (Common coronary artery disease treatments are discussed later in this chapter on pages 316–319). Refractory angina requires specialized treatments. For information on these treatments, talk with your health care provider.

■ **Unstable angina.** Unstable angina is more severe than stable angina. It does not follow a predictable pattern and may occur with or without physical exertion. It may not be relieved by rest or medication. Unstable angina is a dangerous condition requiring emergency medical attention.

■ **Variant angina.** Variant angina, also known as Prinzmetal's angina, is a rare form of angina that usually happens when a person is at rest during the night. It is caused by coronary artery spasm and is characterized by severe chest pain. Almost 70% of people who experience variant angina have severe atherosclerosis in at least one coronary artery (see page 304). The pain from variant angina can be relieved with medication.

■ **Microvascular angina.** Microvascular angina is a severe form of chest pain that typically lasts longer than other types of angina. People who experience it do not have any disease of the coronary arteries that can be detected with currently available technology. In other words, there is no visible blockage of a coronary artery. Medication may or may not be helpful in relieving microvascular angina. This condition is sometimes referred to as cardiac syndrome X.

High Blood Pressure

High blood pressure (hypertension) increases the risk of coronary artery disease. Blood pressure is a measurement of the amount of pressure in an artery, expressed as two numbers. The higher first number is the pressure in the artery when the heart contracts and pushes out a wave of blood. The lower second number is the pressure when the heart relaxes between contractions. Both numbers are important because a high reading for either can compromise the ability for your heart to function normally, especially over time.

High blood pressure is often called the silent disease because most people who have it have no symptoms. Because they feel perfectly well, they find it hard to believe that anything is wrong and so they may not seek treatment. However, the silent disease may not stay silent. Over years, untreated high blood pressure can damage blood vessels throughout the body. In some people this damage can cause strokes, heart attacks, heart failure, or damage to the eyes or kidneys. To prevent these serious complications, it is extremely important to get your blood pressure checked regularly even if you feel perfectly well.

What is normal blood pressure? A healthy blood pressure is below 120/80 (described as "120 over 80"). A condition called prehypertension is indicated by a reading that is above 120/80 but below 140/90. Hypertension is 140/90 or higher. For most people, lower blood pressure is accompanied by less risk of complications. It's important to note that if you have diabetes, your acceptable blood pressure range may be even lower. Consider having a discussion with your primary care provider about the blood pressure range that would be the right target for you.

Hypertension is diagnosed when blood pressure measurements are high at two or more separate times. Except in severe cases, the diagnosis is never based on a single measurement because everyone's blood pressure varies from minute to minute. That's one reason it is important to have repeated measurements of your blood pressure.

Some people's blood pressure tends to go up only in the health care provider's office. This is a stress reaction called "white-coat hypertension." That is another reason why it is helpful to have additional measurements for both diagnosing hypertension and monitoring blood pressure treatment.

There are many ways to get your blood pressure checked. Ask at the pharmacy, fire station, or senior center. You can even get a machine and take your blood pressure at home. Collect three or four blood pressure readings and see how they vary, depending on what you are doing. Take the results with you to your health care professional.

People can often lower their blood pressure by eating a low-sodium diet, exercising, maintaining a healthy weight, limiting alcohol, and using prescribed medications. Don't be reluctant to take these medications due to fear of side effects. Many people with high blood pressure actually feel better (less fatigue, fewer headaches, and so on) when they are on the medications.

Peripheral Vascular Disease

Peripheral vascular disease (PVD) occurs when the arteries in the legs harden, form plaque deposits, and narrow (atherosclerosis). Atherosclerosis in the legs is usually the result of the same disease process that happens with atherosclerosis in coronary artery disease (see page 304).

The main symptom of peripheral vascular disease is leg pain when walking. Some people may also experience leg sores that don't heal or heal slowly. Treatments are similar to those for coronary artery disease (which we discuss in detail later in this chapter). They include stopping smoking, exercise, medications, and sometimes surgery to help restore blood flow to the legs.

Diagnosing Coronary Artery Disease

Sometimes the symptoms of coronary artery disease are clear and "classic," such as angina pain in the chest during physical activity. But others have atypical angina and experience only vague symptoms. Fortunately, there are now many tests available to determine the presence and severity of coronary artery disease. The following are the most common tests for coronary artery disease:

■ **Blood tests.** Blood tests to measure cholesterol and triglycerides estimate your risk of coronary artery disease. They are also used to monitor the effects of cholesterol-lowering medications. If you are having chest pains, your physician may order tests to confirm the diagnosis of a heart attack.

■ **Electrocardiogram.** An electrocardiogram (EKG or ECG) measures patterns of electrical currents produced by your heartbeat. This test requires you lie still for only a few minutes. Ten thin wires are attached to your chest, arms, and legs. The electrical patterns of your heartbeat are recorded by the wires and plotted on a paper graph for your health care provider to read. The EKG is a "snapshot" of your heart's activity. It can show a lack of oxygen to the heart, a heart attack, heart enlargement, and irregular heart rhythm. The test may need to be repeated to see if a heart attack is occurring. Sometimes a portable monitor is worn for several hours or days to detect abnormal heart rhythms that come and go. An EKG cannot predict the risk for a future heart attack.

■ **Echocardiogram.** This test uses sound waves (ultrasound) to generate a moving picture of the heart. A computer converts echoes and displays them on a monitor to show the shape, texture, and movement of heart valves as well as the size and function of the heart chambers. It provides a more detailed picture of the heart than can be seen in an X-ray. This test does not involve radiation exposure, does not require any special preparation, and does not cause any pain or discomfort. To prepare, a gel is spread on the chest to help transmit the sound waves, and a device called a transducer is moved over the chest wall. An echocardiogram is very helpful in determining if there is any type of dysfunction of the chambers or valves of the heart. It may also be done while you exercise (stress testing) to see how your heart responds to stress.

■ **Stress test.** Sometimes problems appear only when the heart is under increased stress. (In this case stress refers to something that makes the heart work harder, not emotional stress.) A stress test is done while a person is exercising on a treadmill or stationary bicycle or after a doctor injects a chemical to stimulate the heart without exercising. If the test is performed while you are exercising, you begin to walk on the treadmill or pedal the bike, and the intensity of the exercise increases every 2 to 3 minutes. Your blood pressure, heart rate, EKG tracing, and any angina pain or discomfort are monitored throughout the test and for a few minutes afterward. The test is stopped if you experience angina or become short of breath. While a positive test result may suggest the presence of coronary artery disease, sometimes stress tests can give false results, especially in women. Sometimes, people with coronary artery disease will have a negative test, and people with no coronary artery disease have a positive test. It is a safe test, and is often done in conjunction with another test to confirm the results.

- **Nuclear scan.** During this test, a weak radioactive substance is injected into a vein. Then a scanner or special camera takes two sets of pictures—with and without stress (induced by exercise or medication). By comparing the pictures, your doctor evaluates blood distribution to the heart muscle and how well your heart is pumping.

- **Cardiac catheterization and coronary angiography.** For this procedure, a long plastic tube called a catheter is inserted through a major blood vessel (usually in the groin) and gently guided into the heart. A dye is then injected into the catheter. This allows your coronary arteries to show up on X-rays. This test helps your physician decide the best treatment if the arteries are clogged. It can also give information about the function of the heart muscle and the valves.

Prevention and Treatment of Coronary Artery Disease

There are three general approaches to help prevent and treat coronary artery disease and angina: lifestyle changes, medications, and procedures and surgery. Most people will benefit from one or more of these. In this chapter we first address the lifestyle changes and nondrug treatments and then we discuss medications, and procedures and surgery.

Lifestyle Changes and Nondrug Treatments

Heart attacks and high blood pressure can often be prevented or controlled by adopting the following lifestyle changes and/or nondrug treatments:

- **Not smoking.** Smoking damages the inner lining of the blood vessels and raises blood pressure. Quitting is the best thing you can do for your health. Fortunately, there are now a variety of support programs (from telephone counseling to online and group programs) and medications (from nicotine gum and patches to calming medications) that can help you quit and stay quit.

- **Exercising.** Exercise strengthens your heart. It can also lower your cholesterol and blood pressure and help you control your weight. Inactive people double their risk for coronary artery disease. Even small amounts of daily physical activity can lower your risk of coronary artery disease and help you feel better and have more energy (see Chapters 7, 8, and 9).

- **Eating well.** The higher your cholesterol level, the greater your risk for coronary artery disease. Lowering the amount of cholesterol in your diet can reduce the risk of heart attacks and strokes (see Chapter 13). Unfortunately, not all cholesterol can be controlled by what you eat or drink. The body also makes cholesterol, and medications may be necessary. (See pages 305–307 for more on cholesterol.)

■ **Maintaining a healthy weight.** Being overweight makes your heart work harder, raises your cholesterol and blood pressure, and increases your chances of developing diabetes. Carrying excess weight around the midsection is a particular risk factor for coronary artery disease. Regular exercise and healthy eating are the most important steps to lose weight and maintain a healthy weight. (See Chapter 14.)

■ **Managing emotional stress.** Stress increases your blood pressure and heart rate, which can damage the lining of the blood vessels. This can lead to coronary artery disease. (See Chapters 4 and 5 for ways to manage stress.)

■ **Limiting alcohol.** Drinking a little (one drink per day for women, two drinks per day for men) may *reduce* the risk of coronary artery disease, but drinking more or binge drinking (more than five drinks at one time) can *increase* the risk of both coronary artery disease and high blood pressure. If you do use alcohol, limit your consumption.

■ **Controlling diabetes.** If you have diabetes, your risk for coronary artery disease more than doubles because high blood sugar damages blood vessels. By controlling your blood sugar and taking certain heart-protective

medications, you can greatly lower the risk of heart attack and stroke.

Exercising with Coronary Artery Disease

Exercise can be both safe and beneficial for many people with coronary artery disease and angina. To make the most of your exercise, work closely with your health providers to find the best exercise program for your needs. Remember that regular, well-chosen exercise is an important part of treatment and rehabilitation. It can lower your risk for future problems, reduce the need for hospitalization, and improve your quality of life.

When not to exercise if you have coronary artery disease or angina

Coronary artery disease and angina can limit the kinds and amount of exercise you do. Follow your health care provider's advice about exercise and exertion if you have poor circulation to the heart. If your condition is severe, your health care provider may want to change your treatment before giving you clearance to exercise. For example, if you have poor circulation to the heart muscle, your doctor may recommend medications, bypass surgery, or "balloon" angioplasty to improve blood flow to the heart before clearing you for exercise activities. (See the material later in the chapter on page 317 for more on heart procedures and surgeries.)

Tips for safe exercise with coronary artery disease or angina

If you do not have any restricting conditions or a health care provider's advisory, it is safe for you to begin the exercises in this book (see Chapters 7, 8, and 9). The following are special considerations for people with coronary artery disease:

- Strengthening activities such as isometrics, weightlifting, or rowing can increase blood pressure and stress your heart needlessly. This can be dangerous if you have high blood pressure or your heart has poor circulation. If strengthening exercises are part of your fitness program, pay special attention and make sure you do not hold your breath while you exercise. Remember to breathe out as you exert. One way to be sure to breathe is to count out loud or breathe out through pursed lips.

- If you have not exercised since your coronary artery disease began, supervision by experienced professionals is a good way to start. Most communities have cardiac rehabilitation programs or professionally staffed gyms at a local hospital or community center.

- When exercising, keep the intensity well below the level that causes symptoms such as angina or severe shortness of breath. For example, if you get angina during an exercise treadmill test when your heart is beating at 130 beats per minute, you should not let your heart get above 115 beats per minute when you exercise. If you cannot easily judge your intensity to stay below your "symptom zone," wear a pulse rate monitor (available at medical supply and sporting good stores) and check your heart rate at any time. Other ways to monitor the intensity of your exercise are the talk test or a perceived exertion scale (see Chapter 9, page 151, and the Borg Scale of Perceived Exertion that follows.

- If your heart has poor circulation, avoid activities that cause you to strain. Try safer and more helpful conditioning activities such as light calisthenics, walking, swimming, and stationary bicycling.

- Always remember that if you develop new or different angina symptoms, while at rest or while exercising, you should stop what you are doing and contact your health care provider.

The Borg Scale of Perceived Exertion

Some people with coronary artery disease and angina find it helpful to use a scale to monitor their physical exertion. The Borg Scale is one method of monitoring your level of effort on a scale from 6 to 20, with 6 being "no exertion at all" and 20 being "maximal exertion"—the most strenuous ever experienced (see page 315). More information on how to use the scale can be found online at the Center for Disease Control and Prevention website at:

www.cdc.gov/physicalactivity/everyone/measuring/exertion.html

Exercising with Peripheral Vascular Disease

People with peripheral vascular disease can experience pain in the legs during exercise. The good news is that conditioning exercises can help improve endurance and reduce leg pain for most people. Start with short walks or bicycling (see Chapter 9), and continue to the point when you start to have leg pain. Slow down or stop and rest until the discomfort eases and then start again. Repeat this cycle for 5 to 10 minutes. Many people find they can gradually increase the length of time they can walk comfortably or exercise with this method. A good goal is to be able to keep going for 30 to 60 minutes, which is long enough to get noticeable fitness ben-

Borg Scale of Perceived Exertion

6	No exertion at all	
7	Extremely light	
8		
9	Very light	9 corresponds to "very light" exercise. For a healthy person, it is like walking slowly at his or her own pace for some minutes.
10		
11	Light	
12		
13	Somewhat hard	13 on the scale is "somewhat hard" exercise, but it still feels OK to continue.
14		
15	Hard (heavy)	
16		
17	Very hard	17 "very hard" is very strenuous. A healthy person can still go on, but he or she really has to push him- or herself. It feels very heavy, and the person is very tired.
18		
19	Extremely hard	19 on the scale is an extremely strenuous exercise level. For most people this is the most strenuous exercise they have ever experienced.
20	Maximal exertion	

Source: The Borg RPE Scale®. Scales with instructions can be obtained from Borg Perception: www.borgperception.se.

efits too. If leg pain continues to prevent you from being physically active, talk to your health care provider about your options. Remember, arm exercises won't usually cause leg pain, so be sure to include them as an important part of your overall conditioning program.

Healthy Eating and Tracking your Weight

Maintaining a healthy weight is a key way to managing coronary heart disease and angina. Healthy eating is an important step to lose weight and maintain a healthy weight.

Eat Healthy, Low-Sodium Foods and Avoid Trans Fat

People with coronary artery disease and angina need to eat healthy to prevent their arteries from hardening or getting clogged. Review the section on oils and fats in Chapter 13 on page 212. Most of the fat you eat should come from the good (unsaturated) fats and very little from the bad (saturated) fats. You should eat little to no trans fat. If you have coronary artery disease and angina, increase the amount of fiber you eat. Fiber is plentiful in oats, barley, dried beans and peas, lentils, apples, citrus fruits, carrots, and psyllium seed. Fiber consumption can help you manage high blood cholesterol, a major risk factor for coronary artery disease.

To learn more about healthy eating, including how to make healthy choices, and increase fiber in your eating plan, see Chapter 13.

Track Your Weight

It is important to weigh yourself properly and frequently if you want to catch trends that may indicate health problems. Here's how to do it:

- Weigh yourself daily at about the same time every day. We suggest weighing every morning, just after waking up (after urinating and before eating).

- Weigh yourself with the same amount of clothing on or without clothing.

- Use the same scale. Check to be sure it is set to zero and resting on a hard surface before weighing yourself.

- Write your weight in a daily log (a journal or calendar works well).

- Weigh yourself again if you have doubts about the scale or your weight.

- Bring your daily weight log to all your medical appointments.

- Call your health care professional if you gain two or more pounds in a day or five or more pounds in five days, or if you experience shortness of breath or increased swelling of feet or ankles.

To learn more about maintaining a healthy weight, see Chapter 14.

Medications for a Healthy Heart

A variety of medications are available to treat coronary artery disease and angina, high blood pressure, and peripheral vascular disease. In the past, medications were prescribed only if lifestyle changes such as healthy eating and exercise failed. Newer research suggests that combining certain medications with lifestyle changes provides the greatest benefit.

Nitrates for Angina

Nitrates are medications that alleviate chest pain by expanding blood vessels to increase the flow of oxygen-rich blood to the heart and decrease cardiac workload. Examples include nitroglycerin (Nitrostat®, Nitro-Bid®, and Nitro-Dur®) and isosorbide dinitrate (Isordil®). Nitrates are categorized as immediate release (act quickly) or extended release (act over time) formulations. Immediate release formulations are used to prevent or manage an angina attack. These include spray or tablets, both of which are applied under the tongue. Extended release formulations are used as maintenance therapy to keep coronary vessels open. These include patches, which deliver nitrates through the skin, and pills, which are swallowed.

Nitroglycerine is often taken under the tongue (as a pill or a spray) at the first sign of angina. You must speak to your health care provider for specific guidance on using nitroglycerine, depending on your situation. You can also take nitroglycerine before activity to prevent an angina attack rather than just using it when you are having an attack. To learn more about this, speak to your health care provider. Always carry your nitroglycerine with you and be sure your supply is fresh. Arrange with your pharmacist to have your prescription refilled regularly. Nitroglycerine is sensitive to light, so be sure to keep it in the container the pharmacy provided.

Other Common Heart Medications

Table 19.2 on pages 318–319 lists other common medications for managing coronary artery disease and high blood pressure. If you have these conditions, consult your health care provider to find out if some or all of these heart-protective medications are right for you. If one medication is not working for you or is causing side effects, discuss this with your provider. Usually an alternative medication can be found that will work. These medications are not addictive and usually can be used safely over many years to reduce the risk of coronary artery disease and high blood pressure. Do not start or stop these medications without discussing it with your health care provider. Read Chapter 15 for information on how to be better able to manage the medications you take.

Because research on medications changes rapidly, consult your health care provider, a pharmacist, or a recent drug reference book for the latest information.

Heart Procedures and Surgery

When using medications alone is not sufficient to manage coronary artery disease and angina, several types of heart procedures and surgery may be helpful.

- **Coronary or "balloon" angioplasty.** Coronary angioplasty relieves the symptoms of coronary artery disease by opening the blockages and improving blood flow to the heart. In this procedure, a catheter with a balloon at the tip is inserted into the artery to widen a narrow passage in the vessel. Your physician may choose to insert a tiny mesh tube called a stent to help keep the narrowed vessel open. Many stents contain medications that may help prevent the artery from clogging up again.

- **Coronary artery bypass surgery.** Bypass surgery creates a new route for blood flow to your heart. During a bypass, a surgeon uses a blood vessel from your leg or chest wall to create a detour around the blockage in the coronary artery. One or more blocked arteries may be bypassed. The surgery usually requires several days in the hospital, and the recovery time can be weeks to months.

The medical community can do a lot to prevent coronary artery disease and manage angina. People with these conditions can live long, full lives. The combination of healthy lifestyle and selective use of medications and cardiac procedures has dramatically lowered the risk of heart attack and early death. You also have an important job to do. It is up to you to eat well and exercise, manage stress, and take your medications as prescribed. If you do not do your part, your health care team will be much less effective.

However, even with good care, people with coronary artery disease and angina need to plan for the future. Specifically, they need to make their wishes known regarding end-of-life issues and medical care. The next chapter has more on this vital self-management task.

Table 19.2 **Medications for Managing Coronary Artery Disease and High Blood Pressure***

Medication	How It Can Help You	Comments
Blood thinners or anticoagulants, e.g., coated baby aspirin (81 mg), warfarin (Coumadin®), clopidogrel (Plavix®)	Blood thinners lower the risk of a blood clot. This decreases the risk of a heart attack and stroke, especially if you have already had a heart attack or stroke or have diabetes.	Aspirin can cause stomach irritation and may even cause small ulcers and bleeding. Usually, taking the low-dose (81 mg) aspirin with a special coating or with food can prevent stomach problems. Although aspirin can reduce the overall risk of strokes caused by blood clots, it can slightly increase the risk of having a certain type of stroke from bleeding.
Cholesterol-lowering statins, e.g., lovastatin (Mevacor®), simvastatin (Zocor®), atorvastatin (Lipitor®), pravastatin (Pravachol®) Resins, e.g., cholestyramine (Questran®), colestipol (Colestid®)	Statins and resins lower your LDL (bad) cholesterol by blocking the production of cholesterol in the liver. They also increase your HDL (good) cholesterol and may help prevent blood clots and inflammation inside your arteries. The latest evidence suggests that even if your cholesterol levels are normal, if you have coronary artery disease or diabetes, taking a statin medication can lower your risk of future coronary artery disease or stroke.	People who take statins daily are much less likely to have a heart attack or to die from a heart attack or stroke. If you have severe muscle pain, severe weakness, or brown urine while taking one of these drugs, contact your health care professional immediately. Statins may be combined with other drugs to lower cholesterol and reduce triglycerides.
Calcium channel blockers, e.g., amlodipine (Norvasc®), felodipine (Plendil®), nifedipine (Adalat®, Procardia®), verapamil (Calan®, Isoptin SR®), diltiazem (Cardizem®, Dilacor®)	These medications relax the muscles around the arteries, lowering blood pressure. This makes it easier for your heart to pump blood.	Some calcium channel blockers may cause heart failure to become more severe.
Angiotensin-converting enzyme (ACE) inhibitors, e.g., lisinipril (Prinivil®, Zestril®), captopril (Capoten®), enalopril (Vasotec®) Angiotensin receptor blockers (ARBs), e.g., losartan (Cozaar®)	ACE inhibitors and ARBs relax blood vessels so that blood flows more easily to the heart. This allows oxygen-rich blood to reach the heart. They lower blood pressure and can help reduce symptoms and improve survival in heart failure. They are also used to treat and prevent kidney problems, especially in people who also have diabetes.	Some people taking ACE inhibitors develop a mild cough or tickle in the back of the throat. If the cough is not very bothersome, it is not necessary to stop the medication. If the cough is annoying, an ARB can sometimes be substituted or alternatively, another type of ACE inhibitor can be tried.

Table 19.2 **Medications for Managing Coronary Artery Disease and High Blood Pressure (*continued*)***

Medication	How It Can Help You	Comments
Beta-blockers, e.g., atenolol (Tenormin®), metoprolol (Lopressor®, Toprol XL®), propranolol (Inderal®), acetabutol (Sectral®), nadolol (Corgard®), carvedilol (Coreg®)	Beta-blockers reduce the workload of the heart by relaxing the heart muscle and slowing the heart rate. This allows your heart to pump blood more easily. Beta-blockers are used to treat high blood pressure, heart failure, irregular heartbeats, blocked arteries, and angina. This medication reduces the chance of sudden death (without symptoms or warning) from heart attack in people with coronary artery disease. If you monitor the intensity of your exercise by heart rate, be aware that because beta-blockers slow your heart rate, they may change your target heart rate range and maximal heart rate. Ask your health care provider about this.	Early side effects usually go away over time. You may need to take a beta-blocker for two to three months before you feel better. But throughout this time, it can protect your heart from getting weaker. People with poorly controlled asthma and diabetes need to discuss whether they can use beta-blockers with their health care provider.
Antiarrhythmics, e.g., amiodarone (Cordarone®), flecainide (Tambocor®), various beta-blockers and calcium channel blockers	These drugs help the heart beat more slowly or more steadily.	Various medications may be used in combination to slow your heart rate. You may be prescribed more than one antiarrhythmic agent to get a good response from your body.
Diuretics, e.g., hydrochlorothiazide (HCTZ®, Esidrix®), furosemide (Lasix®), chlorthalidone (Hygroton®), bumetanide (Bumex®), triamterene + hydrochlorothiazide (Dyazide®, Maxzide®)	Diuretics ("water pills") reduce the amount of fluid in the body. Your body gets rid of this excess fluid when you urinate. A decrease in the amount of excess fluid decreases the amount of work your heart needs to do and can help reduce blood pressure, swelling, and the buildup of fluids in the lungs. Certain diuretics have been shown to reduce the risk of heart attack and stroke.	If you take your last dose of diuretic medication no later than 6:00 P.M., you may not need to get up as often at night to urinate. Depending on the medication, you may need to take extra potassium.

*Because research on medications is changing rapidly, we suggest you consult your physician, pharmacist or a recent drug reference book for the latest information.

Other Resources to Explore

American Heart Association (AHA): www.heart.org

American Stroke Association: www.strokeassociation.org

Canadian Cardiovascular Society (CCS): www.ccs.ca

DASH Diet: www.nhlbi.nih.gov/health/health-topics/topics/dash

Heart and Stroke Foundation of Canada (HSF):
   https://ehealth.heartandstroke.ca/HeartStroke/BPAP.Net/Tracker.aspx

Heart and Stroke Foundation of Canada (HSF): www.heartandstroke.com

HeartHub: www.hearthub.org

Mayo Clinic, Diseases and Conditions—High Cholesterol:
   www.mayoclinic.org/diseases-conditions/high-blood-cholesterol/in-depth/cholesterol-levels
   /art-20048245

National Heart, Lung, and Blood Institute (NHLBI): www.nhlbi.nih.gov

National Institute of Neurological Disorders and Stroke: www.ninds.nih.gov

National Institutes of Health: health.nih.gov

National Stroke Association: www.stroke.org

Office on Women's Health: www.womenshealth.gov

Persistent Cardiac Pain Resource Centre: www.cardiacpain.net

WomenHeart—The National Coalition for Women with Heart Disease: www.womenheart.org

Suggested Further Reading

To learn more about the topics discussed in this chapter, we suggest that you explore
the following resources:

American Heart Association. *To Your Health: A Guide to Heart-Smart Living.* New York: Clarkson Potter, 2010.

American Medical Association. *Guide to Preventing and Treating Coronary Artery Disease: Essential Information You and Your Family Need to Know about Having a Healthy Heart.* Hoboken, N.J.: Wiley, 2008.

Casey, Aggie, Herbert Benson, and Ann MacDonald. *Mind Your Heart: A Mind/Body Approach to Stress Management, Exercise, and Nutrition for Heart Health.* New York: Free Press, 2004.

Casey, Aggie, Herbert Benson, and Brian O'Neill. *Harvard Medical School Guide to Lowering Your Blood Pressure.* New York: McGraw-Hill, 2005.

Granato, Jerome. *Living with Coronary Artery Disease: A Guide for Patients and Families.* Baltimore: Johns Hopkins University Press, 2008.

Heart and Stroke Foundation. *Recovery Road: An Information Guide for Heart Patients and their Families.* www.heartandstroke.com/site/c.ikIQLcMWJtE/b.3751099/k.C320/Heart_disease__Recovery_Road.htm

Heller, Marla. *The DASH Diet Action Plan: Proven to Lower Blood Pressure and Cholesterol Without Medication.* New York: Grand Central Life & Style, 2011.

Ornish, Dean. *Eat More, Weigh Less: Dr. Dean Ornish's Life Choice Program for Losing Weight Safely While Eating Abundantly.* New York: Quill, 2001.

Ornish, Dean. *The Spectrum: A Scientifically Proven Program to Feel Better, Live Longer, Lose Weight, and Gain Health.* New York: Ballantine, 2008.

Rippe, James M. *Heart Disease for Dummies.* Hoboken, N.J.: Wiley, 2004.

Taylor, Jill Bolte. *My Stroke of Insight: A Brain Scientist's Personal Journey.* New York: Viking, 2009.

CHAPTER 20

Planning for the Future: Fears and Reality

CHRONIC PAIN IS RARELY A LIFE-LIMITING CONDITION, but it can accompany diseases that become progressively worse. Also, people with chronic pain can develop additional conditions as they age. They often worry about what will happen to them if their condition becomes truly disabling. They fear that at some time in the future they may have problems managing their condition and their lives.

One way people can deal with fears of the future is to take control and plan for it. You may never need to put your plans into effect, but you will be reassured knowing that you will be in control if the events you fear come to pass. In this chapter, we examine the most common concerns and offer some suggestions that may be useful.

What If I Can't Take Care of Myself Anymore?

Regardless of our state of health, most of us fear becoming helpless and dependent. But this fear is even greater among people with potentially disabling health problems. And it usually has financial, social, and emotional components as well as physical concerns.

Physical Concerns of Day-to-Day Living

As your health condition changes, you may need to consider changing your living situation. This may involve hiring someone to help you in your home or moving to a place where more help is provided. How you make this decision depends on your needs and how they can best be met. Your physical, financial, social, and emotional needs all must be considered.

Start by evaluating what you can do for yourself and what activities of daily living require some kind of help. Activities of daily living are the everyday things such as getting out of bed, bathing, dressing, preparing and eating meals, cleaning house, shopping, and paying bills. Most people can do all of these things, even though they may have to do them slowly, with some modification, or with help from gadgets.

Some people, though, may eventually find one or more of these tasks no longer possible without help from somebody else. For example, you may still be able to fix meals but no longer can do the shopping. Or if you have problems with fainting or sudden bouts of unconsciousness, you might need to have somebody around at all times. You may also find that some things that you enjoyed in the past, such as gardening, are no longer pleasurable. Using the problem-solving steps discussed in Chapter 2, analyze the situation and make a list of the potential problems. Once you have this list, solve the problems one at a time.

First, write down every possible solution you can think of for each problem. For example:

Can't go shopping

- Get daughter to shop for me
- Find a volunteer shopping service
- Shop at a store that delivers
- Ask a neighbor to shop for me
- Shop for groceries on line and have them delivered
- Get home-delivered meals

Can't be by myself

- Hire an around-the-clock attendant
- Move in with a relative
- Get a Lifeline Emergency Response system
- Move to a board-and-care home
- Move to a retirement community

Select the solution that seems the most workable (step 3 of problem solving). It will depend on such things as your finances and the availability of family or other resources. Sometimes one solution will be the answer for several problems. For instance, if you can't shop and can't be alone, and household chores are becoming difficult, you might consider a retirement community that offers meals, regular house cleaning, and transportation for errands and medical appointments.

A good self-manager often makes use of other resources (step 6 in the problem-solving steps in Chapter 2). Your local hospital, senior center, or center for people with disabilities can provide information about resources in your community. They can also give you ideas about how to deal with your care needs. For our retirement community example, look up the independent living center or agency that assists people with disabilities in your area. It should be able to direct you to an out-of-home care facility appropriate for you.

It may help to discuss your wishes, abilities, and limitations with a trusted friend, relative, or a professional such as a social worker or occupational therapist. Sometimes another person can spot things you may overlook or would like to ignore. Several kinds of professionals can be of great help. Social workers are good for helping you decide how to solve financial and living arrangement problems and for locating appropriate community resources. Some social workers are trained in counseling and can assist you with emotional and relationship problems that may be associated with your health condition or advancing age.

An occupational therapist can assess your daily living needs and suggest assistive devices or rearrangements in and around your home to make life easier. They can be especially helpful for people with chronic pain who have limited movement. Occupational therapists can also help you figure out how to keep engaging in pleasurable activities.

If for any reason you are admitted to the hospital, you will see a discharge planner before you go home. This person (usually a nurse) will check to make sure you know how to care for yourself and you have the help you need. It is very important that you be honest with this person. If you have concerns about your ability to care for yourself, say so. Solutions are almost always available, and the discharge planner is a real expert. However, the planner can help only if you share your concerns.

To get your financial affairs in order, consult a lawyer. He or she can help you preserve your assets, prepare a proper will, and perhaps execute a durable power of attorney for both health care and financial management (see page 335). If finances are a concern, contact a local agency such as a senior center for the names of attorneys who offer free or low-cost services. Your local bar association chapter can also refer you to a list of attorneys who are competent in this area. These attorneys are often specialists in elder law, but they generally are familiar with the laws applying to younger persons with disabilities as well.

Make changes in your life slowly, one step at a time. You don't need to change your whole life to solve one problem. Remember that you can always change your mind, so leave your options open. If you think that moving out of your own place to another living arrangement (relatives, care home, or elsewhere) is the right thing to do, don't give up your present home until you are settled in your new home and are sure you want to stay there.

If you think you need help at home, hiring someone is less drastic than moving. If you can't be alone and you live with a family member who is away from home during the day, going to an adult or senior day care center may be enough to keep you safe and comfortable while your family is away. In fact, adult day care centers are ideal places to find new friends and activities geared to your abilities.

Finding In-Home Help

If you find that you cannot manage alone, the first option usually is to hire somebody to help. Most people just need a person called a home aide or something similar. These are people who provide no medically related services that require special licensing but do help with bathing, dressing, meal preparation, and household chores.

There are a number of ways to find somebody. The easiest, but most expensive, is to hire someone through a home care agency. You can find these companies online or listed under "home care" or "home nursing" in the Yellow Pages. These are usually (but not always) private, for-profit businesses that supply caregiver staff to individuals at home. The fees are usually about double what you would expect to pay for someone you hire directly. The advantage is that the agency assumes all personnel and payroll responsibilities. It guarantees the skill and integrity of the attendant and can replace an ill or no-show attendant right away. It also pays the staff directly, so you do not have to pay the attendant.

Most of these agencies also can provide licensed staff who are certified to handle more medically involved tasks. Unless you are bedridden or require some procedure that must be done by someone with a certain category of license (such as a registered nurse), a home aide will most likely be the most appropriate and least expensive choice for your needs.

Other types of agencies act as referral services. They maintain lists of prescreened attendants or caregivers, and you select the one you wish to hire. The agency may charge a placement fee, usually equal to one month's pay of the person hired. It will assume no liability for the skill or honesty of these people, so you'll need to check references and interview carefully. Look online or in the Yellow Pages under the listing for "home nursing agencies" or "home nursing registries." Some agencies provide both their own staff and registries of staff for you to select from.

Senior centers and centers serving the disabled are also resources for finding a home aide. They often have listings of people who have contacted them about their home attendant services or who have posted a notice on a bulletin board there. These job seekers are not screened. You must interview carefully and check references before they start working for you.

Many experienced home care attendants advertise in the classified "employment wanted" section of the newspaper or on websites such as Craigslist. You can find a competent helper this way, but the advice again is to interview and check references carefully.

Probably the best source of help is word of mouth—a recommendation from someone who has employed a person or knows of a person who has worked for a friend or relative. Putting the word out through your family and social network may lead you to a jewel.

Home sharing may be a solution for the person who can offer living space to someone in exchange for help. This works best if you primarily need help with household and garden chores. Some people may also be willing to provide personal care, such as help with dressing, bathing, and meal preparation. Look for community agencies or government bureaus that match home sharers and home seekers. Voluntary organizations, church or religious organizations, and even universities may offer this service.

In the United States, every county has an Area Agency on Aging. You can find your local agency in the phone book or online. These are excellent places to call when you are looking for resources. In Canada, most provinces have government senior services organizations and community services councils that are valuable resources.

Finding Out-of-Home Care

If you are considering a move out of your home, you have several options to find the lifestyle and level of care you need. When you are looking, consider the levels of care that are offered. These usually include independent living, where you have your own apartment or small house; assisted living, where you get some help with dressing, taking medications, and other tasks; and skilled nursing, which includes help with all common daily activities and some medical care.

Retirement communities

If you require very little personal care but recognize the need to live in a more protected setting (security, emergency response services, and so on), consider a retirement community. These can consist of owned units, rental units, or so-called life care facilities in the United States. Government-subsidized facilities are also available for low-income applicants. Even if you are

not of retirement age, many facilities accept younger people. For example, some take residents at age 50 or younger if one member of the household is the minimum age.

There are almost always waiting lists for retirement communities, even before they are built and ready for occupancy. If you think such a place would be right for you, get on the waiting list right away, even if it will be a couple years before you think you want to move. You can always change your mind or decline if you are not ready when a space is available. If you have friends living in local retirement communities, ask to be invited for a visit and a meal. In this way you can get an inside view. Some communities have guest accommodations where you can arrange to stay for a night or two before you commit to a lease or contract.

Residential care homes

Residential care homes are also known as board-and-care homes in the United States or assisted living in Canada. These homes are licensed to provide nonmedical care and supervision for individuals who cannot live alone. The living arrangements can be family-like or more of a boardinghouse, hotel-type setting.

In either type of facility, the services to the residents are the same: all meals, assistance with bathing and dressing as needed, laundry, housekeeping, transportation to medical appointments, assistance with taking medications, and general supervision. The larger facilities usually have professional activities directors. When considering a residential care home, it is important to evaluate the setting and the residents already living there to make sure you will fit in. For example, some of these facilities may cater to individuals who are mentally confused. If you are mentally clear, you would not find much companionship there.

Although all homes are required by law to provide wholesome meals, make sure the cuisine is to your liking and can meet your dietary needs. If you need a salt-free or diabetic diet, for instance, be sure the operator is willing to prepare your special diet.

The monthly fees for residential care homes vary, depending on whether the facilities and services are basic or luxurious. Compare costs, review your budget and needs, and take your time making a decision.

Skilled nursing facilities

Also called a nursing home, extended care facility, or convalescent hospital, the skilled nursing facility provides the most comprehensive care for severely ill or disabled people. Sometimes, a person who has had a stroke or a hip replacement is transferred from the hospital to a skilled nursing facility for a period of rehabilitation before going home. Recent studies have shown that almost half of all people over 65 will spend some time in a nursing home, many of them only for a short time.

Skilled nursing facilities provide medically related care for people who can no longer function without such care. This means that professional nursing staff may administer medications by injection or intravenously and manage feeding tubes, respirators, and other high-tech equipment. Nursing home patients are usually physically limited, so staff also help them get in and out of bed, eat, bathe, and use the bathroom. For people who are partially or temporarily disabled, the facility might provide physical, occupational, and speech therapy, wound care, and other services.

Not all nursing homes provide all types of care. Some specialize in rehabilitation and therapies, and others specialize in long-term custodial care. Some provide high-tech nursing services, and others do not.

Nothing seems to inspire more fear than the prospect of having to go to a nursing home. Horror stories in the news help foster anxiety about the awful fate that will befall anyone who has the misfortune to have to go there. But it must be remembered that nursing homes serve a critical role in our communities. When one really needs a nursing home, usually no other care situation will meet this need.

Public scrutiny is valuable to ensure proper standards of care. If you are not satisfied with the level of care you receive, contact your local elected representative or advocacy group. In the United States, each nursing home is required by law to post in a prominent place the name and phone number of the "ombudsman," a person assigned by the state licensing agency to assist patients and their families with problems related to their nursing home care. Or look online or in the Yellow Pages under "social service organizations" for agencies that can help you with this. In Canada, provincial ministries of health monitor all care facilities.

Most nursing homes provide humane and competent care. If you need to move to a nursing home, there may be several options in your area. Have family or friends visit several facilities and make recommendations. If you don't know where to start, seek out the help of a hospital discharge planner, social worker, or similar professional.

Will I Have Enough Money to Pay for My Care?

In addition to fearing physical dependence, many people fear not having enough money to pay for their needs. Being sick often requires expensive care and treatment. If you are too ill or disabled to work, the loss of income, and especially the loss of your health insurance coverage, may present an overwhelming financial problem. You can, however, avoid some of the risks by planning ahead and knowing your resources.

Make it your business to find out which health benefits are covered and which are not by your personal and employer health insurance plans and your state, provincial, and federal health and disability plans. Some plans may cover home care and nursing home care. Some may provide benefits to you and your dependent children if you are too sick or disabled to work. Given how complex this can be, we suggest you contact your local senior center, disability center, Area Agency on Aging in the United States, and other appropriate government departments to find trustworthy sources of information.

I Need Help but Don't Want Help. Now What?

Every human being emerges from childhood reaching for and cherishing every possible sign of independence—your driver's license, your first job, your first credit card, the first time you go out and don't have to tell anybody where you are going or when you will be back, and so on. In these and many other ways, you have demonstrated to yourself as well as to others that you are "grown up"—in charge of your life and able to take care of yourself without help.

If a time comes when you must face the realization that you can no longer manage completely on your own, it may seem like a return to childhood and allowing somebody else to be in charge of your life. This can be very painful and embarrassing.

Some people in this situation become extremely depressed and can no longer find any joy in life. Others resist recognizing their need for help, thus placing themselves in possible danger and making life difficult and frustrating for those who would like to be helpful. Still others give up completely and expect others to take total responsibility for their lives, demanding attention and services from their children or other family members. If you are having one or more of these reactions, you can help yourself feel better by developing a more positive response.

To be able to stay in charge of your life, it is important to understand the concept of "changing the things I can change, accepting the things I cannot change, and being able to know the difference." You must be able to evaluate your situation accurately. You need to identify the activities that require the help of somebody else (going shopping and cleaning house, for instance) and those that you can still do on your own (getting dressed, paying bills, writing letters or e-mails). Another way to approach this is to get help from others for the things you least like to do, giving you the time and energy to do the things you want to do.

This means making decisions, and as long as you are making the decisions, you are in charge. It is important to make a decision and take action while you are still able to do so, before circumstances intervene and the decision gets made for you. That means being realistic and honest with yourself. Decision-making tools can be found in Chapter 2.

Some people find that talking with a sympathetic listener is comforting and helpful. This can be either a professional counselor or a sensible close friend or family member. An objective listener can often point out alternatives and options you may have overlooked or were not aware of. The person can provide information or contribute another point of view that you would not have come upon yourself. Talking things over with someone else can be an important part of the self-management process.

Be very careful, however, when evaluating advice from somebody who has something to sell you. There are many people whose solution to your problem just happens to be whatever it is they are selling. This may include health or burial insurance policies, annuities, special and expensive furniture, "sunshine cruises," special magazines, or health foods with magical curative properties.

When talking with family members or friends, be as open and reasonable as you can. At the same time, make them understand that you will reserve for yourself the right to decide how much and what kind of help you will accept. They will probably be more cooperative and understanding if you say, "Yes, I do need

some help with _____ but I still want to do _____ myself." More tips on asking for help can be found in Chapter 10.

Lay the ground rules with your helpers early on. Insist on being consulted about the things that affect you. Ask to be presented with choices so that you can decide what is best for you as you see it. If you objectively weigh all suggestions and not dismiss every option out of hand, people will consider you able to make reasonable decisions and will continue to give you the opportunity to do so.

Be appreciative. Recognize the goodwill and efforts of people who want to help. Even though you may be embarrassed, you will maintain your dignity by accepting with grace the help that is offered. If you are truly convinced you are being offered help you don't need, decline it with tact and appreciation. For example, you can say, "I appreciate your offer to have Thanksgiving at your house, but I'd like to continue having it here. I could really use some help, though— maybe with the cleanup after dinner."

If you are unable to come to terms with your increasing dependence on others, consult a professional counselor. This should be someone who has experience with the emotional and social issues of people with disabling health problems. Your local agency that provides services to the disabled can refer you to the right kind of counselor. The national organization dedicated to serving people with your specific health condition (Chronic Pain Association, Arthritis Foundation or Society, Canadian Pain Coalition, etc.) can also direct you to support groups and classes to help you deal with your condition. Look under "social service organizations" in the Yellow Pages, or find what you need online.

Similar to the fear of becoming physically dependent is the fear of being abandoned by family members who you expect to provide help and companionship. Tales of being "dumped" in a nursing home by children who never come to visit haunt many people. They worry that this may happen to them.

When you recognize that you can't go on alone, you need to reach out to family and friends for help. Expecting rejection, some people fail to do this. They try to hide their need, fearing it will cause loved ones to withdraw. Yet families often complain "If we'd only known . . . " when it is revealed that a loved one had needs for help that were unmet.

If you really cannot turn to close family or friends because they are unable or unwilling to become involved in your care, there are agencies dedicated to providing for such situations. Contact the "adult protective services" program of your local social services department or such nonprofit organizations as the Family Service Association. They should be able to connect you to a "case manager" who can organize the resources in your community to provide the help you need. The social services department at your local hospital can also put you in touch with the right agency.

Grieving: A Normal Reaction to Bad News

When we experience any kind of a loss, we go through an emotional process of grieving and coming to terms with the situation. The loss can be small, such as losing one's car keys, or big, such as facing life with chronic pain or losing a life partner.

A person with a health problem such as chronic pain experiences a variety of losses. These may include loss of confidence, loss of self-esteem, loss of independence, loss of the lifestyle we knew and cherished, loss of employment, and perhaps loss of a positive self-image if our condition has an effect on appearance (such as rheumatoid arthritis).

Psychiatrist Elisabeth Kübler-Ross has written extensively about loss. Here is how she describes the stages of grief:

- **Shock**, when one feels both a mental and physical reaction to the initial recognition of the loss

- **Denial**, when the person thinks, "No, it can't be true," and proceeds to act as if it were not true

- **Anger**, when we fume "Why me?" and search for someone or something to blame (the doctor for not diagnosing it earlier, the job for causing too much stress, etc.)

- **Bargaining**, when we promise to behave better from now on ("I'll never smoke again," "I'll follow my treatment regimen absolutely to the letter," or "I'll go to church every Sunday, if only I can get over this")

- **Depression**, when awareness sets in, we confront the truth about the situation, and experience deep feelings of sadness and hopelessness

- **Acceptance,** when we recognize that we must deal with what has happened and make up our minds to do what we have to do

People do not pass through these stages in a linear fashion. We are more apt to flip-flop between them. Don't be discouraged if you find yourself angry or depressed again when you thought you had reached acceptance.

Facing Death

Fear of death is something most of us begin to experience only when something brings us face-to-face with the possibility of our own death. Losing someone close, having an accident that might have been fatal, or learning you have a health condition that may shorten your life usually causes you to consider the inevitability of your own eventual passing. Even then, many people try to avoid facing the future because they are afraid to think about it.

Your attitudes about death are shaped by your central attitudes about life. This is the product of your culture, your family's influences, perhaps your religion, and certainly your life experiences.

If you are ready to think about your own future—about the near or distant prospect that your life will most certainly end at some time—then the ideas that follow will be useful to you. If you are not ready to think about it just yet, put this chapter aside and come back to it later.

Practical Preparations

The most useful way to come to terms with your eventual death is to take positive steps to prepare for it. This means attending to all the necessary details, large and small. If you continue to avoid dealing with these details, you will create problems for yourself and those around you.

There are several components to this process:

- **Decide and then convey to others your wishes for your last days and hours.** Do you want to be in a hospital or at home? When do you want procedures to prolong your life stopped? At what point do you want to let nature take its course when it is determined that death is inevitable? Who should be with you—only the few people who are nearest and dearest, or all the people you care about and want to see one last time?

- **Make a will.** Even if your estate is a small one, you may have definite preferences about who should inherit what. If you have a large estate, the tax implications of a proper will may be significant. A will also ensures that your belongings go where you would like them to go. Without a will, some distant or "long lost" relative may end up with your estate.

- **Plan your funeral.** Write down your wishes, or actually make arrangements for your funeral and burial. Your grieving family will be very relieved not to have to decide what you would want and how much to spend. Prepaid funeral plans are available, and you can purchase the type of burial space you'd like and in the location you prefer.

■ **Draw up a durable power of attorney covering your medical and financial affairs.** This is called a representation agreement in Canada. You want one for health care and one for your financial affairs. You should also discuss your wishes with your personal physician, even if he or she doesn't seem interested. (Your physician may also have trouble facing the prospect of losing you.) Have some kind of document or notation such as an advance directive included in your medical records that indicates your wishes in case you can't communicate them when the time comes. (See pages 335–340 for more on this important topic.)

The person you want to handle things after your death needs to know about your wishes, your plans and arrangements, and the location of necessary documents. You will need to talk to her or him, or at least prepare a detailed letter of instructions and give it to someone who can be counted on to deliver it to the proper person at the appropriate time. This person should be close enough to you to know when that time is at hand. You may not want your spouse to have to take on these responsibilities, for example, but he or she may be the best person to keep your letter and know when to give it to your designated agent.

You can purchase a kit at any well-stocked stationery store in which you place a copy of your will, your durable powers of attorney, information about your financial and personal affairs, and other important papers. Another useful source to help organize this information is "My Life in a Box" (see the Resources section at the end of this chapter). This kit contains forms that you fill out with bank and charge account details, insurance policies, the location of important documents, your safe deposit box and its key, and so on. This is a handy, concise way to get everything together that anyone might need to know about. If you choose to keep these documents on your computer, be sure others have access to your passwords and accounts.

Emotional Preparations

After the practical matters are attended to, turn to your emotional needs. Finish your dealings with the world around you. Mend your relationships. Pay your debts, both financial and personal. Say what needs to be said to those who need to hear it. Do what needs to be done. Forgive yourself. Forgive others.

Talk about your feelings about your death. Most family and close friends are reluctant to initiate such a conversation but will appreciate it if you bring it up. Initiate "courageous conversations," as author Jane Blaufus describes in her book written about her husband's sudden death. You may find there is much to say to and to hear from your loved ones. If you find that they are unwilling to listen to you talk about your death and the feelings you are experiencing, find someone who is comfortable and empathetic doing so. Your family and friends may be able to listen to you later on. Remember, those who love you will also go through the stages of grieving when they have to think about the prospect of losing you.

A large component in facing death is fear of the unknown. You may wonder: "What will it be like?" "Will it be painful?" "What will happen to me after I die?" Most people with a terminal disease are ready to die when the time comes. Many just "slip away," with the transition between the state of living and no longer living hardly identifiable. People who have been brought back to life after being in a state of clinical death report experiencing a sense of peacefulness and clarity and were not frightened.

A dying person may sometimes feel lonely and abandoned. Regrettably, many people cannot deal with their own emotions when they are around a person they know to be dying. They may deliberately avoid his or her company, or engage in superficial chitchat broken by long, awkward silences. This is often puzzling and hurtful to those who are dying. They need companionship and solace from the people they love and count on.

You can sometimes help by telling your family and friends what you want and need from them—attention, entertainment, comfort, practical help, and so on. A person who has something positive to do is more able to cope with difficult emotions. If you can engage your family and loved ones in specific activities, they can feel needed and can relate to you around the activity. This will give you something to talk about and occupy time, or at least it will provide a definition of the situation for them and for you.

Palliative Care and Hospice Care

In everyone's life there comes a point when regular medical care is no longer helpful and it is time to prepare for death. At this stage of life, medical and other care is aimed at making the person as comfortable as possible and providing a good quality of life. In most parts of the United States and Canada, as well as in many other parts of the world, both palliative care and hospice care are available to serve this function. Palliative care is available for those expected to live more than six months. Most hospices accept people who are expected to die within six months, although this does not mean you will not receive care if you live longer than six months.

Thanks to modern medicine, we often have several weeks or months, and sometimes years, to make final preparations. This is when hospice care is so useful. It provides the terminally ill person with the highest quality of life possible. At the same time, hospice professionals help both the person and the family prepare for death with dignity. Today most hospice care programs are in-home—the person stays in his or her own home and the services come to them. There are also residential hospices where people can go for their last days.

Often people wait until the last few days before death to ask for hospice care. They somehow see asking for it as "giving up." By delaying hospice care, they often put an unnecessary burden on themselves, as well as family and friends. Consider as well that, at least for some diseases, studies show that people who receive hospice care actually live longer than those who receive more aggressive treatment.

The same is true of families that say they can cope without help. This may be true, but the person's final days may be much better if hospice tends to all the medical issues so that family and friends are free to give love and support.

If you, a family member, or a friend is in the end stage of illness, you should find and make use of your local hospice. It is a wonderful final gift.

Making Your Wishes Official: Advance Directives for Health Care

Although none of us have absolute control over our own deaths, our deaths are, like the rest of our lives, something we can help manage. You can have input, make decisions, and probably add a great deal to the quality of your death. Proper management can lessen the negative impact of your death on your family and friends. That is the role of an advance directive—to help you manage medical and legal issues as well as help you plan for both expected and unexpected end-of-life situations.

What Are Advance Directives?

Advance directives are written instructions about what kind of care you would like to receive if and when you are not able to make medical decisions for yourself—for example, if you are unconscious, in a coma, or mentally incompetent. Usually an advance directive describes both the types of treatments you want and those you do not want. There are different types of advance directives.

Living Wills

A living will is a document that states the kind of medical or life-sustaining treatments you want if you become seriously or terminally ill. A living will, however, does not let you appoint someone to make those decisions for you. (Note that in Canada, living wills have limited legal force, as the term does not appear in Canadian legislation.)

Durable power of attorney for health care

A durable power of attorney (DPA) for health care does two things: it allows you to name someone to serve as your agent or substitute decision maker, and it gives guidelines to your agent about your health care wishes. (In Canada, the equivalent term to DPA is powers of attorney for person, representation agreements, or medical proxies, depending on the jurisdiction. We will refer to DPA for the rest of this section, but the discussion applies equally to Canada.) You can let your agent make the decisions, but many people prefer to give instructions according to their own wishes. This guidance can cover a broad range of care, from aggressive life-sustaining measures to the withholding of these measures.

A DPA for health care allows you to appoint someone else to act as your agent only in matters relating to health care. It does not give this person the right to act on your behalf in other ways, such as handling your financial matters. In general, a DPA is more useful than a living will because it allows you to appoint someone to make decisions for you, and it can be activated at any time when you are unable to make decisions due to any illness, accident, or injury. A living will is valid only in the case of a terminal illness. The only time a DPA may not be the best choice is if there is no one you trust to act on your behalf. We include detailed information on preparing a durable power of attorney for health care in the pages that follow.

Do Not Resuscitate orders

A do not resuscitate (DNR) order is a request not to be given cardiopulmonary resuscitation (CPR) if your heart stops or if you stop breathing. A DNR can be included as part of a living will or durable power of attorney for health care; however, you do not need to have either of those in order to have a DNR order. Your doctor can put a DNR in your medical chart so it can guide the actions of the hospital and any health care provider. You can also post a DNR on your refrigerator so that emergency personnel will know your wishes. Without a DNR order, hospital or emergency personnel will make every effort to resuscitate you. DNR orders are accepted in all states and throughout Canada.

Advance directives and mental health

Although advance directives for health care are generally used for end-of-life situations, they may also be prepared to direct the type of mental health treatment you wish to receive in the event you become incapacitated due to mental illness. Under U.S. federal law, in most states you may combine advance directives for health care and mental health care in one document and appoint an agent to act on your behalf for both issues. Some states, however, require separate documents. This allows you to choose different agents for health care and mental health

care. For more information on mental health advance directives and the specific practices in your state, check the website of the National Resource Center on Psychiatric Advance Directives (www.nrc-pad.org). In Canada, practices on mental health care directives differ by province. For more information, check with your local health care authority or hospital, or contact your local branch of the Canadian Mental Health Association (www.cmha.ca).

Power of attorney

In both the United States and Canada, a power of attorney (POA) is a document that gives someone you appoint the power to make your financial or business decisions. If you are no longer able to make these decisions and you need to pay for care but you have not granted POA to someone, your family or friends (or even sometimes the state) will have to go to court to address your financial obligations. This can be very expensive. You may want to talk to your lawyer about the advantages and disadvantages of a POA.

Preparing a Durable Power of Attorney for Health Care

Adults should prepare a durable power of attorney for health care. Unexpected events can happen to anyone at any age. This is a different document from a regular power of attorney. The DPA for health care applies only to health care decisions. You do not need to see a lawyer to draw up a durable power of attorney. You can do this by yourself with no legal assistance.

To prepare a durable power of attorney for health care first choose your agent or substitute decision maker. It can be a friend or family member. It cannot be the physician who is providing your care. Your agent should probably live in your area. If the agent is not available on short notice to make decisions for you, he or she is not much help. You can also name a backup or secondary agent who can act for you if your primary agent is not available.

Be sure that your agent thinks like you or at least would be willing to carry out your wishes. You must be able to trust that this person has your interests at heart and truly understands and will respect your wishes. He or she should be mature, composed, and comfortable with your wishes. Sometimes a spouse or child is not the best agent because they are too close to you emotionally. For example, if you do not want to be resuscitated in the case of a severe heart attack, your agent has to be able to tell the doctor not to resuscitate. This could be very difficult or impossible for a family member. Be sure your agent is up to this task. You may want your agent to be someone who will find this job less of an emotional burden than a partner or child would.

In summary, look for the following characteristics in an agent:

- Someone who will be available should they need to act for you

- Someone who understands your wishes and is willing to carry them out

- Someone who is emotionally prepared and able to carry out your wishes, and will not feel burdened by doing so

Finding the right agent is a very important task. It may mean talking to several people. These may be the most important interviews you will ever conduct. We talk more about discussing your wishes with family, friends, and your doctor later in this chapter.

After you have identified an agent, determine what you want. This process will be guided by your beliefs and values. Some DPA forms provide several general statements concerning medical treatment. These can help convey your directions to your agent. Here are some examples:

- *I do not want my life to be prolonged and I do not want life-sustaining treatment to be provided or continued (1) if I am in an irreversible coma or persistent vegetative state or (2) if I am terminally ill and the application of life-sustaining procedures would serve only to artificially delay the moment of my death or (3) under any other circumstances where the burdens of the treatment outweigh the expected benefits. I want my agent to consider the relief of suffering and the quality as well as the extent of the possible extension of my life in making decisions concerning life-sustaining treatment.*

- *I want my life to be prolonged, and I want life-sustaining treatment to be provided unless I am in a coma or vegetative state that my doctor reasonably believes to be irreversible. Once my doctor has reasonably concluded that I will remain unconscious for the rest of my life, I do not want life-sustaining treatment to be provided or continued.*

- *I want my life to be prolonged to the greatest extent possible without regard to my condition, the chances I have for recovery, or the cost of the procedures.*

If you use a form containing such suggested general statements, all you need to do is initial the statement that applies to you.

Other forms allow you to make a "general statement of granted authority," in which you give your agent the power to make decisions. In this case, you do not write out the details of what these decisions should be. Instead you are trusting that your agent will follow your wishes. Since these wishes are not explicitly written, it is very important to discuss them in detail with your agent.

All forms also have a space in which you can write out any specific wishes. You are not required to give specific details, but you may want to do so.

Knowing what specifics to address is a little complicated. None of us can predict the future or know the exact circumstances in which the agent will have to act. You can get some idea by asking your doctor what he or she thinks are the most likely developments for someone with your condition. You can then use this information to direct your agent on how to act. Your directions can discuss outcomes, specific circumstances, or both. If you discuss outcomes, the statement should focus on which outcomes would be acceptable and which would not (for example, "resuscitate if I can continue to fully function mentally").

There are several decisions you need to make when directing your agent or substitute decision maker on how to act in your behalf:

- Generally, how much treatment do you want? This can range from the very aggressive to the very conservative—that is, either doing many things to sustain life or doing almost nothing to sustain life, except to keep you clean and comfortable.

- Given the types of life-threatening events that are likely to happen to people with your condition, what sorts of treatment do you want and under what conditions?

- If you become mentally incapacitated, what sorts of treatment do you want for other illnesses, such as pneumonia?

Although each state and Canadian province has different regulations and forms for advance directives, the information presented here should be useful wherever you live. Check out some of the websites at the end of this chapter for forms you can download. You can also find them at your local health department, Area Agency on Aging, hospitals, or even the offices of your health care providers. For information about advance directives in other countries, visit the Growth House website (www.growthhouse.org). If you move to another state or province or if you travel a lot, it is best to check with a lawyer in your destination jurisdiction to see if your document is legally binding there.

One final very important note: Do not put your durable power of attorney in your safe deposit box. No one will be able to get it when it is needed.

Sharing Your Wishes with Others

Writing down your wishes and having a durable power of attorney is not the end of the job. If you really want your wishes carried out, it is important that you share them fully with your agent, your family, and your doctor. This is often not an easy task.

Before you can have this conversation though, everyone involved needs to have copies of your DPA for health care. Once you have completed the documents, have them witnessed and signed. In some places you can have your

DPA notarized instead of having it witnessed. Make several copies; your agents, family members, and doctors will all need to have one. It is also a good idea to give one to your lawyer.

When you are ready to talk about your wishes, remember that people don't like to discuss the death of a loved one. Don't be surprised that when you bring up this subject, if the response is, "Oh, don't think about that," "That's a long time off," or "Don't be so morbid; you're not that sick." Unfortunately, this is usually enough to end the conversation. Your job as a good self-manager is to keep the conversation progressing. There are several ways to do this.

After you have given copies of your DPA to the appropriate family members or friends, ask them to read it. Then set a specific time to discuss it. If they give you one of the avoidance responses, explain that you understand this is a difficult topic, but it is important. This is a good time to practice the "I" messages discussed in Chapter 10—for example, "I understand that death is a difficult thing to talk about. However, it is very important to me that we have this discussion."

Another strategy is to get blank copies of the DPA form for all your family members and suggest that you fill them out together. This could even be part of a family get-together. Present this as an important aspect of being a mature adult and responsible family member. Making this a family project involving everyone may make it easier to discuss. Besides, it will help clarify everyone's values about death and dying.

If these two suggestions seem too difficult or impossible to carry out, consider writing a letter or e-mail or preparing a video or CD that can then be sent to family members. Talk about why you feel your death is an important topic to discuss and that you want them to know your wishes. Then state your wishes, providing reasons for your choices. At the same time, send them a copy of your DPA for health care. Ask that they respond in some way, or set aside some time to talk in person or on the phone.

As mentioned, when deciding on your agent, it is important to choose someone with whom you can talk freely and exchange ideas. If your agent is not willing or unable to talk to you about your wishes, you have probably chosen the wrong person. Remember, just because someone is very close to you does not mean that he or she really understands your wishes or is able to carry them out. This topic should not be left to an unspoken understanding unless you don't mind if your agent decides differently from what you wish. For this reason, it is essential to choose someone who is not as close to you emotionally and then talk things out with that person. This is especially true if you have not written out the details of your wishes.

Talking with Your Doctor

From our research, we have learned that people often have a more difficult time talking to their doctors about their wishes surrounding death than to their families. In fact, only a very small percentage of people who have written DPAs for health care or other advance directives ever share these with their physician.

Even though it is difficult, it is important to talk with your doctor about your preferences. First, you need to be sure that your doctor's values are similar to yours. If they are not, it may be difficult for him or her to carry out your wishes. Second, your doctor needs to know what you want. This allows him or her to take appropriate actions such as writing orders to resuscitate or not to use mechanical resuscitation. Third, your doctor needs to know who your agent or substitute decision maker is and how to contact this person. If an important decision has to be made and your wishes are to be followed, the doctor must talk with your agent.

As surprising as it may seem, many physicians find it hard to talk to their patients about their end-of-life wishes. After all, doctors are in the business of keeping people alive and they don't like to think about their patients dying. On the other hand, most doctors want their patients to have durable powers of attorney for health care. These documents relieve both you and your doctor from pressure and worry. Therefore, be sure to give your doctor a copy of your DPA for health care so that it can become a permanent part of your medical record.

Plan a time with your doctor when you can discuss your wishes. This should not be a side conversation at the end of a regular appointment. Rather, start a visit by saying, "I want a few minutes to discuss my wishes in the event of a serious problem or impending death." When put this way, most doctors will make time to talk with you. If the doctor says there is not enough time to discuss these matters, ask when you can make another appointment to do so. This is a situation where you may need to be a little assertive. Sometimes a doctor, like your family members or friends, might say, "Oh, you don't have to worry about that; let me do it," or "We'll worry about that when the time comes." Again, take the initiative, using an "I" message to communicate that this is

important to you and that you do not want to put off the discussion.

Sometimes doctors do not want to worry you. They think they are doing you a favor by not describing all the unpleasant things that might happen to you in case of serious problems. You can help your doctor by telling him or her that having control and making decisions about your future will ease your mind. Not knowing or not being clear on what will happen is more worrisome than being faced with the facts, unpleasant as they may be, and dealing with them.

If you still feel it could be hard to talk with your doctor, bring your agent with you when you have this discussion. The agent can facilitate the discussion and at the same time make your doctor's acquaintance. It opens the lines of communication so that if your agent and physician have to act to carry out your wishes, they can do so with few problems. This also gives everyone a chance to clarify any misunderstandings.

If you aren't able to talk with your doctor, it is still important that he or she receive a copy of your DPA for health care for your medical record. When you go the hospital, be sure the hospital has a copy of your DPA as well. If you cannot bring it, be sure your agent knows to do so. This is important, as your doctor may not be in charge of your care in the hospital.

Now that you have done all the important things, the hard work is over. However, remember that you can change your mind at any time. Your agent may no longer be available, or your wishes might change. Be sure to keep your DPA for health care updated. Like any legal document, it can be revoked or changed at any time. The decisions you make today are not forever.

Other Resources to Explore

Benefits Check Up: www.benefitscheckup.org

Canadian Bar Association: www.cba.org

Canadian Hospice Palliative Care Association: www.chpca.net

Canadian Mental Health Association: www.cmha.ca

Caring Connections, National Hospice and Palliative Care Organization: www.caringinfo.org

Five Wishes (Aging with Dignity): www.agingwithdignity.org

Growth House, Improving Care for Dying: www.growthhouse.org

Leading Age: www.leadingage.org

My Life in A Box—A Life Organizer: www.mylifeinabox.com

National Council on Aging: www.ncoa.org

National Resource Center on Psychiatric Advance Directives: www.nrc-pad.org

PLAN Institute: www.institute.plan.ca

Making your wishes known about how you want to be treated in case of serious or life-threatening illness is one of the most important tasks of self-management. The best way to do this is to prepare a durable power of attorney for health care and share it with your family, close friends, and physician.

Suggested Further Reading

To learn more about the topics discussed in this chapter, we suggest that you explore the following resources:

Atkinson, Jacqueline M. *Advance Directives in Mental Health: Theory, Practice and Ethics.* London: Jessica Kingsley Publishers, 2007.

Blaufus, Jane. *With the Stroke of a Pen: Claim Your Life.* Ancaster, Ont.: Blaufus Group, 2011.

Callahan, Maggie, and Patricia Kelley. *Final Gifts: Understanding the Special Awareness, Needs, and Communications of the Dying.* New York: Simon & Schuster, 2012.

Doukas, David John, and William Reichel. *Planning for Uncertainty: Living Wills and Other Advance Directives for You and Your Family,* 2nd ed. Baltimore: John Hopkins University Press, 2007.

Godkin, M. Dianne. *Living Will, Living Well: Reflections on Preparing an Advance Directive.* Edmonton: University of Alberta Press, 2008.

Kübler-Ross, Elisabeth. *On Death and Dying.* New York: Scribner, 2014.

Kuhl, David. *Facing Death, Embracing Life: Understanding What Dying People Want.* Toronto: Doubleday Canada, 2006.

Kurz, Gary. *Cold Noses at the Pearly Gates: A Book of Hope for Those Who Have Lost a Pet.* New York: Citadel Press, 2008.

Long, Laurie Ecklund. *My Life in a Box: A Life Organizer,* 4th ed. Fresno, Calif.: AGL, 2010.

Olick, Robert S. *Taking Advance Directives Seriously: Prospective Autonomy and Decisions Near the End of Life.* Washington, D.C.: Georgetown University Press, 2001.

Pettus, Mark C. *The Savvy Patient: The Ultimate Advocate for Quality Health Care.* Sterling, Va.: Capital Books, 2004.

Sitarz, Daniel. *Advance Health Care Directives Simplified.* Carbondale, Ill.: Nova, 2007.

Stolp, Hans. *When a Loved One Dies: How to Go On After Saying Goodbye.* Hampshire, England: O Books, 2005.

Wilkinson, James A. *A Family Caregiver's Guide to Planning and Decision Making for the Elderly.* Minneapolis, Minn.: Fairview, 1999

Helpful Hints for Everyday Living

THE FOLLOWING HELPFUL HINTS are alternative ways to approach daily activities that may be difficult or impossible for you to do. We'll start with the first thing you do in the morning: getting out of bed. Many people with chronic pain experience stiffness after lying in bed all night and find it difficult to get moving without experiencing even more pain. We'll look at helpful ways to approach this morning routine, and then we'll move on to other common activities throughout the day. Many of these hints may help you solve some of your everyday problems with chronic pain.

Getting Out of Bed

1. Before getting out of bed in the morning, try doing a few simple stretches. This will begin to loosen up stiff muscles as well as get your blood circulating.

   - While lying flat on your back, point your toes down away from your body. Hold for 10 seconds and then bring your feet back toward your shoulders, toes extended upward.

   - Do the same thing with your hands. Point your fingers down, away from your body and then bring your hands back toward your shoulders, fingers extended upward.

   - Remain lying on your back and take in a deep breath. Hold for 10 seconds and then slowly release the air from your lungs. Repeat this three times.

   - Lying on your side, body outstretched, slowly bring your knees up toward your chest. Hold this position for 10 seconds and then slowly return your body to a straight position.

2. Getting out of bed can be a problem in itself. Try these tips:

   - Slowly bring yourself to a sitting position on the edge of the bed. Sit there for a few moments before you stand up.

   - If you have difficulty sitting up, swing your legs over the edge of the bed, allowing them to dangle. Then slide to the edge of the bed until your feet hit the floor. Slowly roll your body out of bed, allowing your feet to support your weight.

   - Place a chair beside your bed when you retire for the night. Upon awakening, use the chair for support by putting your weight on it as you slowly get out of bed.

3. Instead of making the bed immediately, allow yourself time in the morning to relax over a cup of coffee or tea without trying to accomplish anything but waking up in a leisurely way. Then, make your bed just before taking your shower.

Making Breakfast

1. Prepare as much as you can the night before. For example, set up the coffeemaker so that all you have to do is hit the "on" switch. Set the table so it's ready for breakfast when you wake up. Ask a family member to help.

2. If you find it difficult to prepare a large breakfast for your family, try ready-made healthy products: prepared fiber cereal, yogurt, fruit, nuts, whole-grain breads, etc.

3. Give yourself enough time in the morning to eat breakfast. Good nutrition is important, and feeding your body in the morning is especially important.

Getting Dressed

1. Sit on the edge of the bed to put on socks and pants.

2. If you have to stand to get certain clothes on, rest your body against a wall to maintain balance and distribute your weight.

3. Have a convenient place where you can sit down to put on your makeup or shave.

4. When brushing your teeth, stand upright. Bending over the sink puts a lot of pressure on your back.

Making the Bed

1. Instead of making a proper bed, just pull the covers up.

2. Instead of cover sheets, blankets, and bedspread, consider buying a duvet (also called a comforter). It is lightweight, warm in winter and cool in summer, and takes only a second to straighten up so your bed is made in a flash.

3. Conserve your time and energy by following these tips:

   ■ As you get out of bed, toss the covers back up over the bed so they will be in position when you come back later to tidy up.

   ■ Make one side of the bed, placing the pillow in position and the bedspread or duvet over the pillow before going to the other side of the bed. This will save many steps walking from one side of the bed to the other.

   ■ When you do have to bend over to make the bed, don't bend at the waist. Bend at the hips and knees. This will take considerable strain off your back muscles.

   ■ Ask someone to help you make the bed. One of your basic rights is to ask for assistance when needed.

4. Remember, you don't have to make the bed. Just shut the door to the bedroom. An unmade bed does not mean you are lazy but rather that you have placed your attention on other things that are more important to accomplish during the day. Consider making it only when you'll have visitors or before going away for any length of time, such as a weekend visit to a relative's house.

At Work

1. If you must sit all day, make sure your chair is the proper height from the floor. Your knees should be bent at slightly more than a 90 degree angle and your feet should rest comfortably flat on the floor. A small, tilted footrest may be useful to take strain off your knees and back.

2. Do not sit hunched over your desk. Relax your shoulders and neck. It is important to keep your neck in alignment with your spine.

3. If you work at a computer, it is crucial to have a chair with appropriate armrests and back and neck support. Talk to your employer about evaluating your workstation for comfort and efficiency.

4. It is okay to cross your legs while sitting. When you feel tired, simply cross one leg over the other for several minutes, then switch sides.

5. If you sit at a desk all day, take a few minutes each hour to stand up and walk around. Get some water, go make photocopies, or just walk around your work area—anything to get moving for a little while.

6. If you must lift objects at work, make sure you bend from the hips and knees. Bending this way puts most of the strain on the large muscles of your legs rather than the small muscles of your back.

7. If you stand over a worktable all day, find a stool to sit on that will permit you to work at the same level as standing. You can also stand on a cushioned mat, which will ease the strain on feet and knees.

8. Make sure your worktable is at a level that will permit your arms to fall naturally on the top. If the work surface is too high or too low, it will cause increased strain.

9. To help take strain off your back, stand with one leg raised slightly off the ground, resting on a ledge. Alternate legs when you tire of one position.

Cleaning the House

1. The entire house does not need to be cleaned in one day. Break up the chores so you can do the work over several days.

2. Gently wheel your vacuum from the storage area, don't lift it.

3. Bend at the knees when you need to reach something on the floor. If you have knee problems, talk with your health care provider or health supply store about purchasing a "reacher" so you don't have to bend over.

4. When ironing, place one foot on a small stool several inches off the ground. After a while, alternate feet.

5. Sit when you feel you need to. You can do such chores as loading the dishwasher from a sitting position.

6. Store frequently used items at waist-high level.

7. Organize your work to avoid multiple trips up and down the stairs. For example, clean the downstairs bathroom on one day and the upstairs bathroom on another.

8. Try not to rush while working. Take your time to do the work, and take rest breaks.

9. Place the laundry basket on a table next to the washing machine so you do not have to bend over to sort the clothes.

10. Put an extension on your broom or duster so you do not have to strain to reach hard-to-get places.

11. Make housekeeping a family project and share responsibility.

Working in the Kitchen

1. Look into devices that can make your job quicker and easier, such as special utensils to help open jars, peel potatoes, etc. There are also kitchen implements with large grips that can reduce discomfort.

2. While standing in the kitchen, open the cupboard door below you and place a foot on the ledge to take the strain off your back. Alternate feet when you feel the need.

3. Sit down to do tasks if that is more comfortable—but remember to get up and walk around.

4. When you bring ice cream home from the store, place individual scoops into small plastic bags and refreeze it. Ice cream is usually softer and easier to scoop when it's fresh from the store and hasn't been in the freezer for a while.

5. When making cookies, make two batches of dough—one for now and one to freeze for another time.

6. On days when you are feeling good, prepare double recipes for dinner and freeze half for the days when you don't feel up to cooking.

7. Roll out pie crust on the kitchen counter, which is higher than your table.

8. Be sure to set time aside to relax between jobs in the kitchen.

Grocery Shopping

1. Have a list of needed items in the order they appear in your local stores to avoid taking extra steps for forgotten items.

2. At the checkout, distribute your purchased items evenly between two bags so that no bag is too heavy.

3. Carry bags close to your body.

4. Avoid plastic shopping bags if you can. They put more strain on your arms, shoulders, and back than brown bags that you carry in your arms, close to your chest.

5. Make extra trips to the car with several lighter packages rather than carry fewer heavy packages.

6. Avoid placing grocery bags in the back seat of your car. It is too difficult to lift them out from that position. Instead, put grocery bags in the trunk.

7. Don't hesitate to ask store employees for assistance bringing your bags to the car.

Driving

1. Make sure your seat and headrest are in the proper position. Adjust your seat so you can reach the pedals comfortably. You don't want to be leaning too far back or forward; rather, your neck should be gently balanced on the top of your spine.

2. Place a small pillow in the small of your back to give added support to your back.

3. If you are going to be driving for a long period of time, allow enough time for frequent stops to stretch.

Recreation Time

1. If you plan a vacation, make sure you allow enough time to rest if it is a long trip.

2. If you get tired when travelling by car, have someone else do the driving while you relax in the passenger or back seat.

3. When dining out, wear comfortable clothes and don't be shy to take a back support with you if you need one. The same goes for going out to movies.

4. Entertaining at home should be planned well enough in advance so you do not do all your chores in one day. Spread your chores over several days, and make food that is easy to prepare and serve.

5. When doing activities like shopping or sightseeing, take time to sit down and relax for a few minutes every so often. It will actually increase the time you feel you are able to be on your feet.

6. Work at building up your tolerance over a long period of time so you can pursue hobbies you enjoy—woodworking, sewing, gardening, sports, whatever.

Sleeping

1. If you have back trouble, lie on your back and place a small pillow under your knees to take the pressure off your back. But be careful. Over time, this may give you trouble with your knees, so alternate this position with other positions, such as lying on your side.

2. When lying on your side, have both knees slightly bent. Try putting a pillow between your knees for extra comfort.

3. If you have neck problems, consider trying a special neck pillow. This pillow is higher under your neck than your head. It will keep your neck in the proper position with the rest of your spine while you are sleeping.

4. Try to avoid sleeping on your stomach; it puts strain on your spine.

By recognizing the challenges you face due to chronic pain, trying different ways to work around them, and maintaining a positive attitude, you will find that anything is possible. You can live a healthy life with chronic pain!

Index